Rotator Cuff Injuries

Patrick J. McMahon

Editor

Rotator Cuff Injuries

A Clinical Casebook

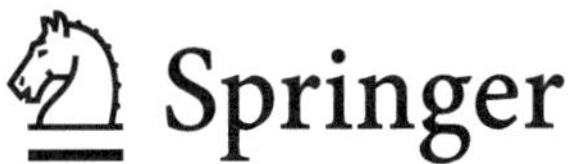 Springer

Editor
Patrick J. McMahon
McMahon Orthopedics and Rehabilitation
Department of Bioengineering
University of Pittsburgh
Pittsburgh, PA
USA

ISBN 978-3-319-63666-5   ISBN   978-3-319-63668-9   (eBook)
DOI 10.1007/978-3-319-63668-9

Library of Congress Control Number: 2017954942

This Springer imprint is published by Springer Nature
The registered company is Springer International Publishing AG
The registered company address is: Gewerbestrasse 11, 6330 Cham, Switzerland

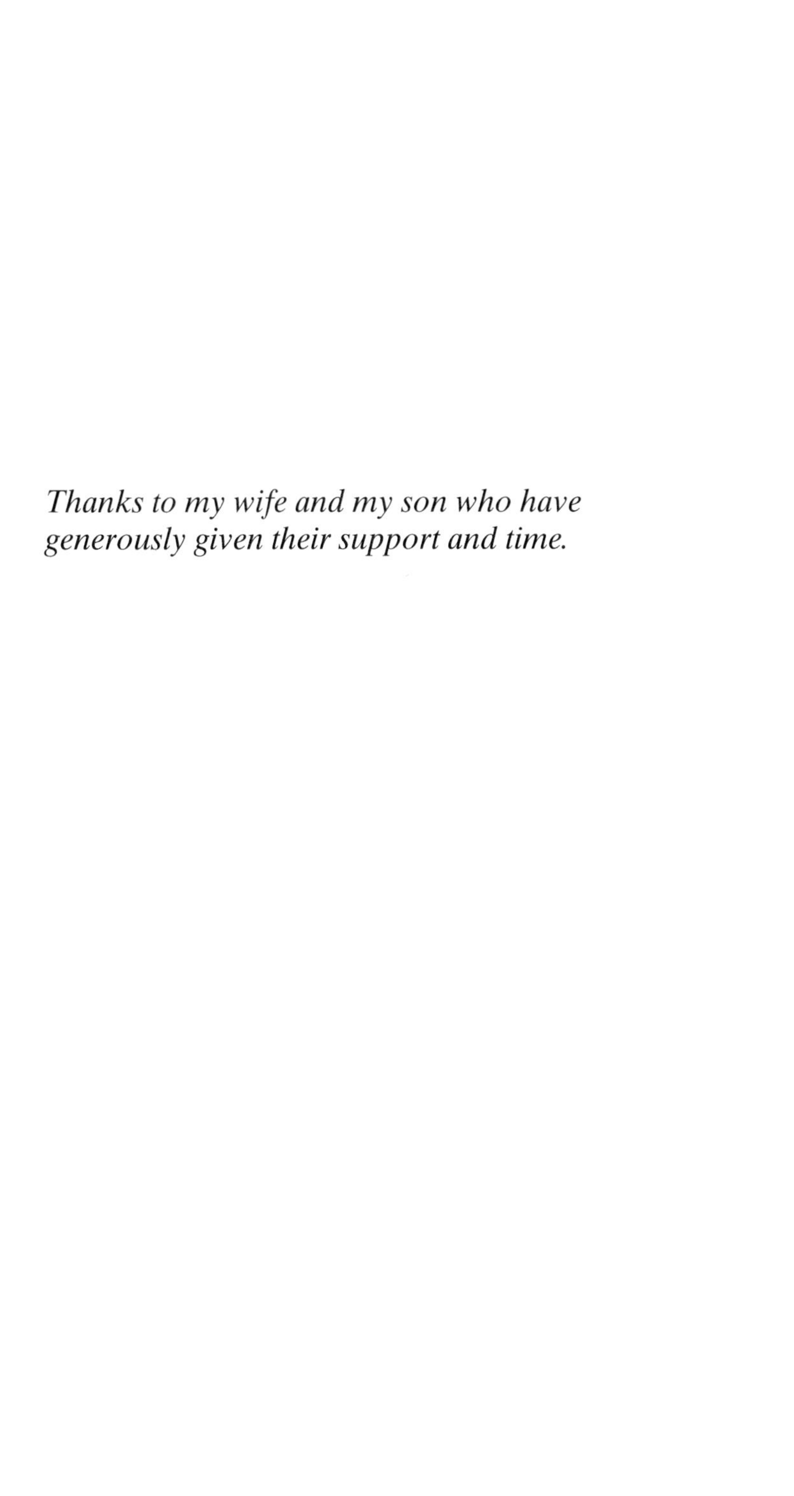

Thanks to my wife and my son who have generously given their support and time.

Preface

Over the last several years, the diagnosis and treatment of rotator cuff injuries have improved. But despite this, care is sometimes uncertain. For example, when a patient first presents to a clinician's office, there are no good criteria for deciding whether treatment should be nonoperative. This is partly because rotator cuff injuries are common and often without symptoms, especially in the elderly. And in those that have symptoms, some are able to cope with them. It is also partly because some rotator cuff tears have the potential to worsen. Most experienced surgeons have had the unpleasant experience with an individual returning to their office several years after diagnosis of a small tear that has now become massive. A surgeon who chooses to repair all the torn rotator cuff tears must face the reality that about 25% fail to heal. These retears occur more often in severe rotator cuff tears, but other factors impair the healing as well.

This book provides detailed instructions in an easy-to-read, case-based format for treatments of patients with rotator cuff injuries. This includes tools for diagnosis, clinical decision-making for both nonoperative and operative management, surgical planning and techniques, postoperative rehabilitation and outcomes. Nonoperative, arthroscopic, and open surgical techniques in the treatment of rotator cuff injuries are detailed by experts in the field. From common rotator cuff tendonitis to complex revision surgery, biological augmentation, tendon transfer, and shoulder arthroplasty, the chapters are in a standard format, including clinical pearls and pitfalls to avoid. Reverse total shoulder arthroplasty, an effective treatment for some who have little other hope for diminishing their pain and improving their function, is also included. In recent years, there has been more interest in the biology of healing the torn rotator cuff, specifically in injectables that may aid healing.

This casebook will be an excellent resource for orthopedic surgeons, residents, and fellows alike, as well as sports medicine specialists and all professionals who treat injuries to the shoulder.

Pittsburgh, PA, USA   Patrick J. McMahon, M.D.

Contents

Contributors

Joseph Abboud, M.D. Department of Shoulder and Elbow Surgery, Rothman Institute — Thomas Jefferson University, Philadelphia, PA, USA

Jesse W. Allert, M.D. Shoulder and Elbow Service, Florida Orthopaedic Institute, Tampa, FL, USA

Alexander Bitzer, M.D. Division of Surgery, Department of Orthopaedic Surgery, The Johns Hopkins University, Baltimore, MD, USA

Richard Blalock, M.D. Vanderbilt University Medical Center, Nashville, TN, USA

Robert E. Boykin, M.D. Steadman Philippon Research Institute, Vail, CO, USA

The Steadman Clinic, Vail, CO, USA

James P. Bradley, M.D. Burke and Bradley Orthopaedics, University of Pittsburgh Medical Center, Pittsburgh, PA, USA

Brandon Brown, M.S. Department of Bioengineering, University of Pittsburgh, Pittsburgh, PA, USA

Steven Cohen, M.D. Rothman Institute of Orthopeadics, Philadelphia, PA, USA

Mark A. Frankle, M.D. Shoulder and Elbow Service, Florida Orthopaedic Institute, Tampa, FL, USA

Erik M. Fritz, M.D. Steadman Philippon Research Institute, Vail, CO, USA

J. Gabe Horneff, M.D. Orthopedic Surgery, Thomas Jefferson University Hospital, Rothman Institute, Philadelphia, PA, USA

Seyedali R. Ghasemi, M.D. Division of Surgery, Department of Orthopaedic Surgery, The Johns Hopkins University, Baltimore, MD, USA

Aharon Z. Gladstein, M.D. Department of Orthopedics, Texas Children's Hospital, Baylor College of Medicine, Houston, TX, USA

Ashish Gupta, MBBS, MSc, FRACS, FAOrth, CIME Fowler Kennedy Sports Medicine Clinic, 3M Centre, University of Western Ontario, London, ON, Canada

Mathew J. Hamula, M.D. Division of Shoulder and Elbow Surgery, Department of Orthopaedic Surgery, NYU Langone Medical Center, NYU Hospital for Joint Diseases, New York, NY, USA

J. Christoph Katthagen, M.D. Steadman Philippon Research Institute, Vail, CO, USA

Department of Trauma, Hand, and Reconstructive Surgery, Albert-Schweitzer-Campus 1, University Hospital Muenster, Muenster, Germany

John D. A. Kelly IV, M.D. Center for Throwing Disorders and Shoulder Preservation, University of Pennsylvania, Perelman School of Medicine, Philadelphia, PA, USA

Gerhard G. Konrad, M.D. Klinikum Landkreis Erding, Erding, Germany

Thomas Kotsonis, B.S. Department of Mechanical Engineering, University of Pittsburgh, Pittsburgh, PA, USA

John E. Kuhn, M.D., M.S. Vanderbilt University Medical Center, Nashville, TN, USA

Mark D. Lazarus, M.D. Orthopedic Surgery, Thomas Jefferson University Hospital, Rothman Institute, Philadelphia, PA, USA

Edward A. Lin, M.D Kayal Orthopaedic Center, Glen Rock, NJ, USA

Robert Litchfield, M.D., F.R.C.S.C Fowler Kennedy Sports Medicine Clinic, 3M Centre, University of Western Ontario, London, ON, Canada

Edward G. McFarland, M.D. Division of Surgery, Department of Orthopaedic Surgery, The Johns Hopkins University, Baltimore, MD, USA

Patrick J. McMahon, M.D. McMahon Orthopedics and Rehabilitation, Department of Bioengineering, University of Pittsburgh, Pittsburgh, PA, USA

Peter J. Millett, M.D., M.Sc. Steadman Philippon Research Institute, Vail, CO, USA

The Steadman Clinic, Vail, CO, USA

Donavan Kip Murphy, M.D., M.B.A. San Francisco Shoulder Elbow and Hand Clinic, San Francisco, CA, USA

Surena Namdari, M.D., M.Sc. Department of Shoulder and Elbow Surgery, Rothman Institute—Thomas Jefferson University, Philadelphia, PA, USA

M. Ned Scott, D.O. Department of Orthopaedic Surgery, University of Pittsburgh Medical Center, Pittsburgh, PA, USA

Robert J. Neviaser, M.D. Department of Orthopaedic Surgery, The George Washington University School of Medicine, GWU-MFA, Washington, DC, USA

Andrew S. Neviaser, M.D. Department of Orthopaedic Surgery, The George Washington University School of Medicine, GWU-MFA, Washington, DC, USA

Gregory P. Nicholson, M.D. Department of Orthopaedic Surgery, Rush University Medical Center, Chicago, IL, USA

Tom R. Norris, M.D. San Francisco Shoulder Elbow and Hand Clinic, San Francisco, CA, USA

Loukia K. Papatheodorou, M.D., Ph.D. Department of Orthopaedic Surgery, University of Pittsburgh School of Medicine, Pittsburgh, PA, USA

Thierry Pauyo, M.D., F.R.C.S.C. University of Pittsburgh Medical Center, Pittsburgh, PA, USA

Kirsten Poehling-Monaghan, M.D. Precision Orthopedics and Sports Medicine, Silver Springs, MD, USA

Andrew S. Rokito, M.D. Division of Shoulder and Elbow Surgery, Department of Orthopaedic Surgery, NYU Langone Medical Center, NYU Hospital for Joint Diseases, New York, NY, USA

Brett Sanders, M.D. Department of Sports Medicine, Center for Sports Medicine and Orthopedics, Chattanooga, TN, USA

Christopher C. Schmidt, M.D. Department of Orthopaedic Surgery, University of Pittsburgh Medical Center, Pittsburgh, PA, USA

Dean G. Sotereanos, M.D. Department of Orthopaedic Surgery, University of Pittsburgh School of Medicine, Pittsburgh, PA, USA

Edwin E. Spencer, M.D. Shoulder and Elbow Service, Knoxville Orthopaedic Clinic, Knoxville, TN, USA

Jens Stehle, M.D. Department of Shoulder Surgery, Bodensee-Sportklinik, Friedrichshafen, Germany

Robert J. Thorsness, M.D. Department of Orthopaedic Surgery, Rush University Medical Center, Chicago, IL, USA

Justin Walden, M.D. San Francisco Shoulder Elbow and Hand Clinic, San Francisco, CA, USA

Gerald R. Williams, M.D. Department of Shoulder and Elbow Surgery, Rothman Institute–Thomas Jefferson University, Philadelphia, PA, USA

Justin C. Wong, M.D. OrthoArizona, Glendale, AZ, USA

Chapter 1
Arthroscopic Treatment of Rotator Cuff Tendonitis Including Treatment of Acromioclavicular Joint Osteoarthritis and Os Acromiale

Mathew J. Hamula and Andrew S. Rokito

Introduction

Rotator cuff tendonitis is one of the most commonly encountered shoulder pathologies, with lifetime prevalence up to 67% [1]. Also known as rotator cuff tendinopathy or "shoulder impingement syndrome (SIS)," this spectrum of disorders includes a variety of conditions such as subacromial bursitis, rotator cuff inflammation or partial tears, acromioclavicular (AC) joint pathology, and long head of the biceps tendinosis. These conditions may originate from extrinsic causes, intrinsic causes, or a combination

M.J. Hamula, M.D. (✉) • A.S. Rokito, M.D.
Division of Shoulder and Elbow Surgery, Department of Orthopaedic Surgery, NYU Langone Medical Center, NYU Hospital for Joint Diseases, New York, NY 10016, USA
e-mail: Mathew.Hamula@nyumc.org; andrew.rokito@nyumc.org

© Springer International Publishing AG 2018
P.J. McMahon (ed.), *Rotator Cuff Injuries*,
DOI 10.1007/978-3-319-63668-9_1

of both. The final common pathway is a painful shoulder that limits movement and interferes with activities of daily living.

Subacromial impingement, as described by Neer, involves the supraspinatus outlet, acromion, coracoacromial ligament, and AC joint [2]. Extrinsic causes of rotator cuff tendonitis include anatomical variants of the acromion, thickening of the coracoacromial ligament, or subacromial bursitis [3, 4]. Direct compression of the rotator cuff tendons and surrounding tissues is thought to lead to the development of rotator cuff tendonitis, degeneration, and ruptures. Conversely, intrinsic causes develop with degeneration of the rotator cuff tendons themselves. This degenerative process may have a genetic component and is exacerbated by age, vascular supply, or a history of trauma. Patients usually report shoulder pain at rest, particularly nighttime pain, or pain with overhead activity. Plain radiographs may show an os acromiale, AC degenerative changes of the AC joint or glenohumeral joint, calcium deposits, or cystic changes of the greater tuberosity. Advanced imaging such as MRI may help further delineate the extent of damage to the rotator cuff and surrounding soft tissues.

The first-line treatment of rotator cuff tendonitis is nonoperative management consisting of nonsteroidal anti-inflammatory drugs (NSAIDs), physical therapy targeting periscapular muscle strengthening, and corticosteroid injections. Surgery is reserved for patients who have failed conservative management. Several arthroscopic procedures have evolved over the past two decades to treat rotator cuff tendonitis including rotator cuff debridement, bursectomy, acromioplasty, coracoacromial ligament release, distal clavicle excision, os acromiale fixation, and biceps tenotomy or tenodesis. Arthroscopic treatment has been shown to have the benefit of fewer complications and earlier postoperative mobilization. There is currently no evidence-based consensus for the treatment of rotator cuff tendonitis. The purpose of this chapter is to review the diagnosis and arthroscopic management of rotator cuff tendonitis.

Case Presentation (Case 1—Subacromial Decompression and Distal Clavicle Resection)

A 45-year-old right-hand-dominant male presented with 6 months of worsening left shoulder pain localizing to the anterolateral and superior shoulder that was worse with overhead activity. On physical examination, he has tenderness at the anterolateral shoulder and had positive impingement signs. He also had point tenderness over the AC joint and pain with cross-chest adduction. He attempted a trial of physical therapy, NSAIDs, and one subacromial and one AC joint corticosteroid injection. His shoulder pain improved for 3 weeks following the steroid injections, physical therapy, and NSAIDs. Plain radiographs and MRI scan of the left shoulder demonstrated rotator cuff tendonitis and a fraying of the undersurface of the supraspinatus tendon and advanced joint space narrowing with associated bone marrow edema involving the AC joint (Fig. 1.1a, b).

Diagnosis

This patient presented with rotator cuff tendonitis, fraying of the undersurface of the supraspinatus tendon, and AC joint osteoarthritis. He attempted nonoperative management with

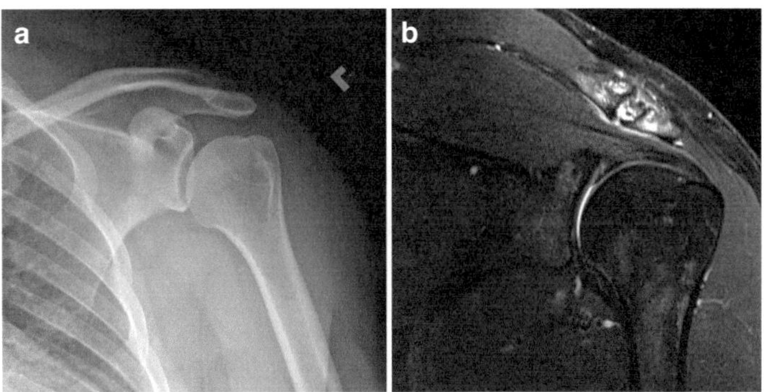

FIGURE 1.1 Plain AP radiograph (**a**) and T2 coronal MRI (**b**) demonstrating advanced joint space narrowing and bone marrow edema around the AC joint

physical therapy, NSAIDs, and steroid injections with only temporary improvement of his shoulder pain. Distinguishing AC joint pathology from rotator cuff tendonitis can be challenging. Pain localizing to the superior aspect of the shoulder, directly over the AC joint, with palpation or cross-chest adduction is typical of AC joint osteoarthritis. Conversely, pain with overhead activity or special tests such as Neer, Hawkins, or empty can (Jobe's) test localizing to the anterolateral aspect of the shoulder may indicate rotator cuff tendonitis.

Management

Our patient underwent a shoulder arthroscopy with subacromial decompression (SAD), debridement of articular sided supraspinatus tendon fraying, and arthroscopic distal clavicle resection (DCR). His immediate postoperative course was uncomplicated. He was discharged home on the day of surgery. The patient presented for follow-up and underwent a standardized physical therapy protocol, discontinuing sling immobilization within 10 days and starting active range of motion as tolerated.

Management of rotator cuff tendonitis with or without AC joint arthropathy begins with nonoperative treatment. Modalities include physical therapy, activity modification, immobilization, NSAIDs, and diagnostic or therapeutic injections. Injections into the subacromial space and/or the AC joint providing symptomatic relief are a prognostic indicator for successful surgical outcome. Physical therapy increases range of motion, flexibility, and periscapular strength [5]. It does not reliably relieve arthritis pain. A brief period of immobilization and application of ice may reduce inflammation associated with acute exacerbations of AC joint arthropathy [6].

Operative indications for rotator cuff tendonitis with or without AC joint arthropathy include continued pain and loss of shoulder function despite at least 6 months of conservative management [7]. Supraspinatus outlet impingement, which is the usual cause of rotator cuff tendonitis, typically begins with the anteroinferior aspect of the acromion and progresses to involve the AC joint. Therefore, surgical management involves adequate subacromial decompression including the subacromial bursa, coracoacromial ligament, and acromion. Specific indications for distal clavicle excision, which is a resection arthroplasty of the AC joint, include symptomatic arthritis from osteoarthritis, rheumatoid arthritis, and post-traumatic or atraumatic distal clavicle osteolysis. Absolute contraindications to SAD and DCR include active infection, while relative contraindications include neuroarthropathy, instability, and medical comorbidities precluding the patient from undergoing surgery.

Arthroscopic subacromial decompression with or without distal clavicle resection can be performed in the lateral decubitus or beach-chair position depending on surgeon preference. Our preference is lateral decubitus as it affords improved visualization and maneuverability around the subacromial space with an adjusted shoulder suspension device. The table should be placed in slight reverse Trendelenburg position to make the glenoid parallel to the floor. A bean bag is placed around the patient and suction applied to mold to the lateral position. A post on either side of the bean bag can be used to further stabilize the patient. For the lateral decubitus position, the operative arm should be placed in an apparatus consisting of a sleeve attached to a suspension of generally no more than 10 pounds. The shoulder should be in approximately 15° of forward flexion and no more than 45° abduction.

We recommend a diagnostic arthroscopy with particular attention to the supraspinatus tendon and debridement of fraying and partial-thickness tears of less than 50% of the tendon thickness in addition to subacromial decompression in the majority of patients. The most common way to approach the subacromial space and the AC joint arthroscopically is through a lateral transbursal portal located approximately 2 cm lateral to the edge of the lateral acromion as a working portal. We start the subacromial decompression by exposing the lateral and then the anterior margin of the acromion. A pilot trough is made at the anterolateral edge of the acromion using a 4 or 5.5 mm burr, and then extended across the anterior margin. We then taper the resection posteriorly over about two-thirds of the acromion undersurface using a "windshield wiper" motion. Care is taken to leave the acromion thicker as the resection proceeds posterior to minimize postoperative fracture (Fig. 1.2). For the distal clavicle excision a pilot trough is made in the anteroinferior aspect of the clavicle to guide resection. Approximately 5 mm of bone is resected, ensuring that the most posterior aspect of the clavicle is also resected (Fig. 1.2). A 4 or 5.5 mm burr is used to remove anywhere between 3 and 10 mm of distal clavicle using a "windshield wiper" motion. It can be challenging to decide how much to resect, as some authors advocate less than 5 mm of resection in the majority of cases so as not to disrupt the ligamentous structures [8, 9]. The majority of authors will agree that no more than 10 mm of distal clavicle should be resected [10–13]. The posterior inferior aspect of the AC joint may be difficult to visualize. An anterolateral portal or 70° arthroscope may help ensure that no bony contact remains between the acromion and clavicle. Care is taken to preserve the superior and posterior AC capsular ligaments to minimize anteroposterior instability and avoid release of the coracoclavicular ligaments to minimize superior instability postoperatively. To accomplish this, multiple viewing portals are used including

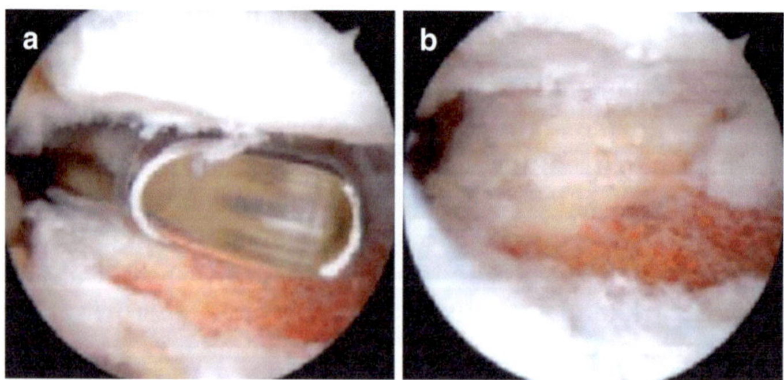

FIGURE 1.2 Arthroscopic images while performing a subacromial decompression, during (**a**) and after (**b**) distal clavicle resection

the anterior portal through the rotator interval. We do not recommend coplaning the distal clavicle by removing the inferior 25% to match the acromioplasty as has been described. We advocate beginning patients on passive range-of-motion exercises immediately postoperatively as soon as the interscalene block wears off, including pendulum exercises unless concomitant rotator cuff repair is performed. Isometric, isokinetic, and active range-of-motion exercises are begun at the first postoperative visit, typically by 7–10 days. Return to sports is generally approximately 3 months; however it may be as early as 6 weeks for non-throwing athletes.

Outcome

Our patient had complete resolution of his pain by 2 months postoperatively so he was allowed to begin advanced strength training and he returned to work. Rotator cuff tendonitis and mil partial-thickness rotator cuff tears are common findings with AC joint arthropathy as they are part of a spectrum in supraspinatus outlet impingement. In our experience, more than 5 mm of distal clavicle resection is not needed, and patient outcomes depend more on the preservation of soft tissues and early rehabilitation. The patient in this clinical vignette had improvement of their anterolateral shoulder pain with physical therapy, with persistently symptomatic AC joint arthritis. He also responded to injection of the AC joint, which is a good prognostic sign. When appropriately indicated, distal clavicle resection can improve pain and function in patients with AC joint pathology.

Literature Review

Rotator cuff tendonitis associated with subacromial impingement begins with compression of the rotator cuff tendons causing tendonitis or bursitis. Chronic inflammation may lead to degeneration and, eventually, tendon rupture [14]. Most commonly, rotator cuff fraying or partial-thickness tearing begins on the undersurface rather than the bursal side. Patients typically report pain over the anterolateral shoulder with or without radiation down the lateral humerus [15]. Neer and Hawkins test combined has a negative predictive value of 90% [16]. Subacromial decompression has long been the gold standard treatment for extrinsic impingement that has failed nonoperative management. Neer first described anterior acromioplasty in 1972. Since then, several arthroscopic techniques have been described to accomplish relieving direct compression of the rotator cuff. Ellman et al. [10] described an arthroscopic technique to resect the anterior undersurface of the acromion, bursal debridement, and coracoacromial ligament release. In contrast, McCallister et al. [17] proposed a "smooth-and-move" technique to perform extensive bursectomy and smoothing of the undersurface of the acromion without disruption of the coracoacromial ligament or avulsion of the deltoid.

Various pathologic processes can affect the AC joint, including, arthrosis, posttraumatic, or atraumatic distal clavicle osteolysis, and infections. Any resulting alteration of normal biomechanics and function of the AC joint may become symptomatic. The AC joint is also associated with subacromial impingement, originally described by Neer, as it forms the supraspinatus outlet along with the acromion and coracoacromial ligament [2]. Osteophyte formation on the inferior aspect of the AC joint has been associated with narrowing of this space and the development of rotator cuff pathology [18–20]. Additionally, AC joint pathology has been correlated with rotator cuff tears [21, 22].

Patients with AC joint arthrosis typically present with pain that localizes to the AC joint or superior shoulder exacerbated by overhead or cross-chest activity. It can sometimes be referred to the anterolateral neck, deltoid, and trapezius [6]. Mechanical symptoms may also be present, such as popping, catching, or grinding [5]. Further complicating diagnosis, concomitant injuries include rotator cuff (up to 81%), biceps (22%), or labral pathology [5, 23].

The most sensitive physical exam test is the cross-chest adduction stress test with a sensitivity of 77% while the O'Brien active compression test is the most specific exam finding with a reported specificity of up to 95% [24, 25]. Imaging of the shoulder may show degenerative changes in the AC joint, best visualized on a Zanca view with 10° to 15° cephalic tilt. An "outlet view," which is a scapular lateral projection with a 10° caudad tilt, allows visualization of inferior osteophytes emanating from the AC joint [18]. Additionally, the axillary view allows visualization of osteophytes involving the anterior or posterior aspects of the AC joint.

Although plain radiographs are sufficient to diagnose AC joint degenerative arthrosis, advanced imaging can assist in identifying other pathologies contributing to shoulder pain. A diagnostic injection can be performed, although outcome is technique dependent and is more reliably done with the use of ultrasonography [26]. A recent study by Wasserman et al. and the senior author (ASR) demonstrated that despite its superficial location, only two-thirds of in vivo AC joint injections performed were intra-articular or partial-articular [27].

Mumford in 1941 described an open resection of the distal clavicle for AC joint pathology [28]. Since the advent of shoulder arthroscopy, several techniques have evolved to perform distal clavicle resection arthroscopically. While open techniques have shown good to excellent outcomes, arthroscopic techniques are associated with accelerated recovery, decreased pain postoperatively, improved cosmesis, and preservation of vital structures such as AC ligaments, joint capsule, and deltotrapezial fascia [29].

Case Presentation (Case 2 — Os Acromiale)

A 25-year-old right-hand-dominant male presented with a 1-year history of right-shoulder pain with overhead activity that had failed nonoperative treatment including activity modification, physical therapy, nonsteroidal anti-inflammatory drugs (NSAIDs), and two subacromial corticosteroid injections. Physical examination revealed no restriction in shoulder range of motion, positive Hawkins and Neer impingement signs, point tenderness over the acromion, and pain with forward elevation. A magnetic resonance imaging (MRI)

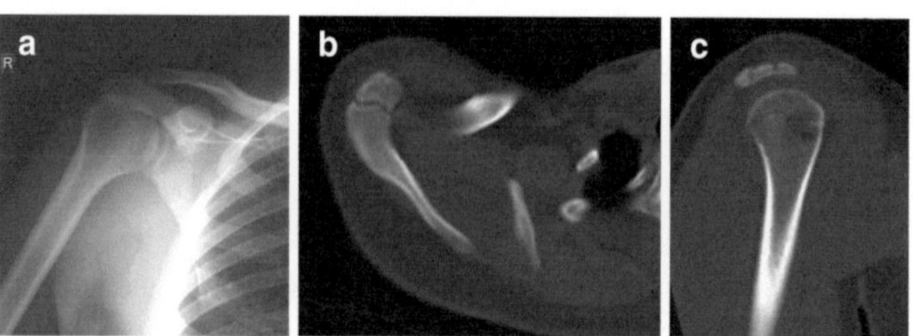

FIGURE 1.3 Plain AP radiograph (**a**) and CT scan with axial (**b**) and sagittal (**c**) views demonstrating a mesoacromion-type os acromiale

brought in by the patient demonstrated an os acromiale with associated bone marrow edema. Plain radiographs and a CT scan were also obtained and demonstrated a mesoacromion-type os acromiale (Fig. 1.3).

Diagnosis

In some cases, the underlying cause of rotator cuff tendonitis will be straightforward with a combination of clinical history, physical exam consistent with impingement, and imaging demonstrating inflammation of the tendons. In all cases, however, it is imperative to identify any and all sources of pain around the shoulder to ensure appropriate management. Shoulder pain can be difficult to localize which can be compounded by false-positive advanced imaging studies [30–32]. A thorough history and physical exam can usually lead clinicians to the correct diagnosis. Given the point tenderness over the acromion, pain with cross-chest adduction, and imaging demonstrating a mesoacromion, the patient was diagnosed with symptomatic os acromiale and underwent a trial of nonoperative management.

Management

Nonoperative management is the initial first-line treatment and standard of care for os acromiale. This consists of a physical therapy regimen for impingement and NSAIDs.

Surgical management is appropriate once an adequate attempt at nonoperative management has failed [33, 34]. Previously, authors advocated for fragment excision typically only for pre-acromion. However, there have been mixed results secondary to deltoid weakness or dysfunction following excision [35–37]. While superior results have been found with arthroscopic excision, such as those by Campbell et al. [38] demonstrating no decrease in deltoid function, excision is still typically reserved for pre-acromial subtypes. Subacromial pathology in the presence of a stable os acromiale has been treated with subacromial decompression and acromioplasty with mixed results [39, 40].

After failing conservative treatment, the patient was brought to the operating room where shoulder arthroscopy, bursectomy of the inflamed bursa, and arthroscopic assisted debridement and internal fixation of the os acromiale nonunion site using short 4 mm cannulated partially threaded screws with washers were performed. His immediate postoperative course was uncomplicated and he was discharged home on the same day.

We advocate operative management of symptomatic os acromiale that has failed nonoperative management. First, a diagnostic shoulder arthroscopy is performed to evaluate for concomitant pathology. Next, the arthroscope is directed into the subacromial space and the subacromial bursa is gently debrided. A mid-lateral acromial portal is placed and the os acromiale is marked with a spinal needle. The os acromiale fibrous nonunion is then gently debrided with small curettes and 3.5 mm shaver. A small saber incision is carried down to the subcutaneous tissue where the anterior edge of the acromion is identified and the deltoid tendon insertion is split. Using a Freer elevator, the anterior acromion is exposed and the elevator is placed in the subacromial space, marking the proper anteroposterior and mediolateral direction of the screws under fluoroscopy. Next, two 2.5 mm smooth Kirschner wires are placed and measured followed by cannulated reaming with a 2.7 mm cannulated reamer. Two short 36 mm partially cannulated 4.5 mm screws with washers are placed to achieve compression and fixation of the os acromiale non-union site (Fig. 1.4). Adequate debridement and compression of the nonunion site may obviate the need for auto- or allograft augmentation. This avoids associated donor site morbidity with procedures such as iliac crest autograft harvest.

Our postoperative protocol began with 4 weeks of sling immobilization with passive range-of-motion exercises. At 6 weeks active-assisted and active range of motion was initiated.

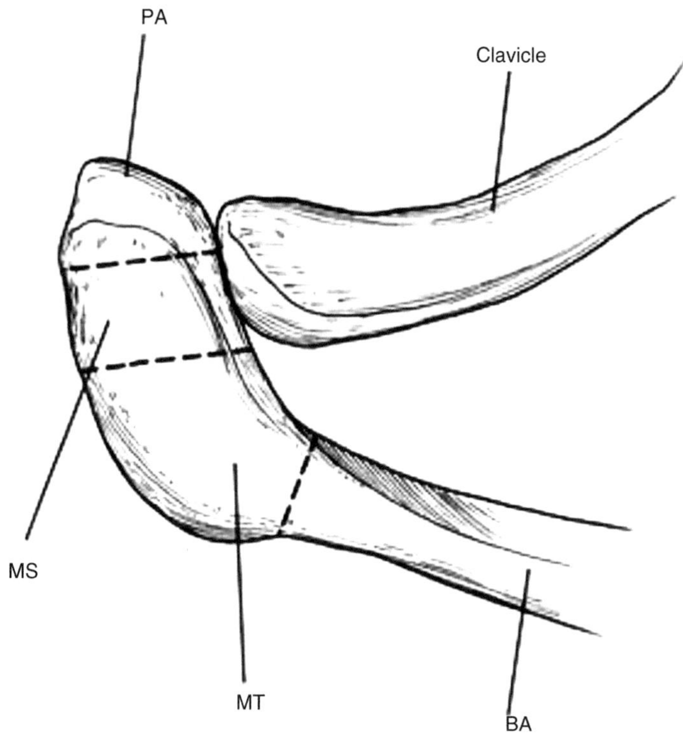

FIGURE 1.4 Types of os acromiale are based on location of failed fusion between ossification centers (*BA* basiacromion, *MT* meta-acromion, *MS* mesoacromion, *PA* preacromion). Reprinted with permission from Jon Sekiya, MD

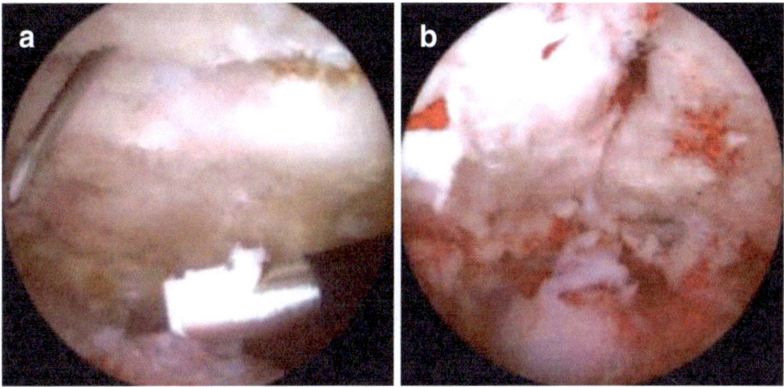

FIGURE 1.5 Arthroscopic images showing (**a**) needle localization of the nonunion prior to fixation and (**b**) nonunion site after fixation

Outcome

At the 5-week postoperative visit, our patient's pain had improved slightly, and he was counseled on continuing his course of physical therapy. Plain radiographs taken at that time demonstrated bony healing of the os acromiale (Fig. 1.5). By 3–4 months postoperatively, his pain had resolved and he began resuming advanced strength training. He reported slight limitation in forward elevation compared with the contralateral side, and aggressive range-of-motion exercises were initiated. Twelve weeks following the surgery, the patient noted dramatic improvement in his shoulder pain, and initiated the final course of PT with gradual strengthening and return to work as a photographer.

Literature Review

Os acromiale is a failure of fusion of the acromion at any of its four main ossification centers leading to a nonunion site, with some cases involving a distinct synovial joint [41]. By the age of 15–18, the acromial apophysis develops from four distinct ossification centers: basiacromion, meta-acromion, mesoacromion, and preacromion. These unite to form the acromion as late as 25 years of age [42]. The type of os acromiale is defined by the unfused segment anterior to the nonunion site (Fig. 1.6). The prevalence is between 1 and 30% in the general population and the most common manifestation is mesoacromial [35, 43]. Mudge et al. have reported on the rare double-fragment variant, typically a combination of preacromial and mesoacromial [36]. Os acromiale is often an incidental finding on standard radiographic imaging. Radiographs of the contralateral shoulder can help distinguish from a fracture. However, aberrant acromial morphology can be bilateral in up to one-third of patients with os acromiale [43]. Symptomatology can be attributed to motion

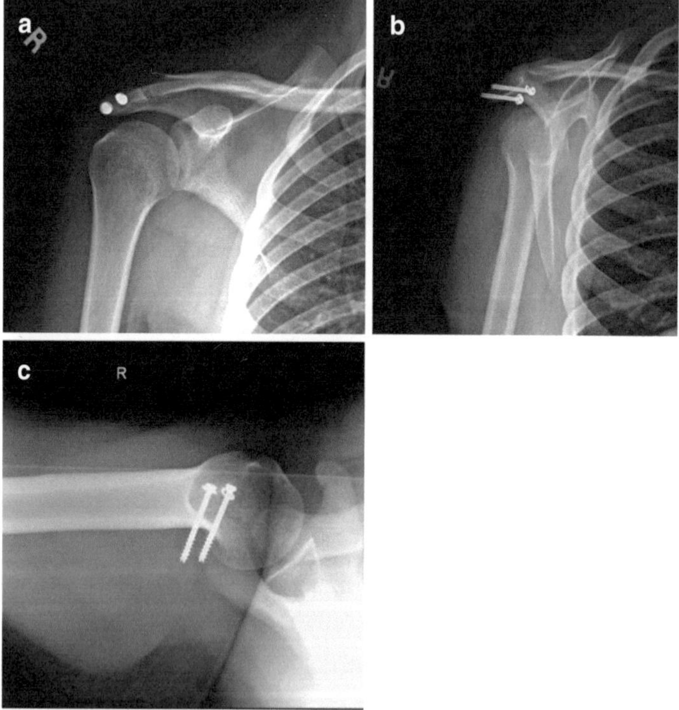

Figure 1.6 (a–c) Postoperative AP, scapular Y, and axillary radiographs of os acromiale showing interval healing

at the nonunion site or an impingement syndrome. A traumatic injury to an otherwise incidental os acromiale can produce pain by disrupting the fibrous nonunion. Symptoms of external impingement result from a reduced subacromial space and outlet resulting in rotator cuff pathology.

Advanced imaging, such as MRI or bone scans, can be helpful to identify the inflammatory response at the nonunion site [37, 44]. CT scans may further help delineate the bony anatomy. Uri et al. conducted a study of 11 MR examinations of shoulders with symptomatic os acromiale and found that while it is most easily identified on axial images, a "double-joint" appearance of the acromioclavicular joint on oblique sagittal images is a typical finding [44]. The treatment is particularly challenging when the subtype involves the mesoacromion.

Various techniques for reduction and internal fixation have been described. Sutures, screws, and tension band wire constructs have been used with or without the use of bone graft [33, 37, 45, 46]. Notably, Atoun et al. [47] reported on eight patients treated with arthroscopically assisted internal fixation. All patients had satisfactory results within 3–6 months postoperatively. However, six patients achieved union, one achieved a partial nonunion, and one failed to show evidence of union. Operative fixation can improve pain and function in patients with symptomatic os acromiale who have failed a trial of nonoperative management.

Clinical Pearls/Pitfalls

- Rotator cuff tendonitis has many sources and clinicians must make every effort to identify all sources of shoulder pain prior to pursuing nonoperative or surgical management.
- Common causes of rotator cuff tendonitis include internal or external impingement, os acromiale, AC joint arthropathy, and intrinsic degenerative changes of the tendon itself.
- Nonoperative management is the mainstay of treatment for rotator cuff tendonitis, including physical therapy, activity modification, and NSAIDs.

- Arthroscopic techniques for common causes of rotator cuff tendonitis have shown good to excellent outcomes in appropriately indicated patients.
- A well-placed lateral portal or anterior portal with a 70° arthroscope can assist in visualization of the AC joint to ensure adequate bone resection.
- Gentle debridement of an os acromiale nonunion site will help mobilize bony fragments for compression using partially threaded screws.

References

1. Luime JJ, et al. Prevalence and incidence of shoulder pain in the general population; a systematic review. Scand J Rheumatol. 2004;33(2):73–81.
2. Neer CS, Poppen NK. Supraspinatus outlet. Orthop Trans. 1987;11:234.
3. Neer CS 2nd. Anterior acromioplasty for the chronic impingement syndrome in the shoulder: a preliminary report. J Bone Joint Surg Am. 1972;54(1):41–50.
4. Seitz AL, et al. Mechanisms of rotator cuff tendinopathy: intrinsic, extrinsic, or both? Clin Biomech (Bristol, Avon). 2011;26(1):1–12.
5. Shaffer BS. Painful conditions of the acromioclavicular joint. J Am Acad Orthop Surg. 1999;7(3):176–88.
6. Mazzocca AD, Arciero RA, Bicos J. Evaluation and treatment of acromioclavicular joint injuries. Am J Sports Med. 2007;35(2):316–29.
7. Mall NA, et al. Degenerative joint disease of the acromioclavicular joint: a review. Am J Sports Med. 2013;41(11):2684–92.
8. Beitzel K, et al. Sequential resection of the distal clavicle and its effects on horizontal acromioclavicular joint translation. Am J Sports Med. 2012;40(3):681–5.
9. Stine IA, Vangsness CT Jr. Analysis of the capsule and ligament insertions about the acromioclavicular joint: a cadaveric study. Arthroscopy. 2009;25(9):968–74.
10. Ellman H. Arthroscopic subacromial decompression: analysis of one- to three-year results. Arthroscopy. 1987;3(3):173–81.
11. Esch JC, et al. Arthroscopic subacromial decompression: results according to the degree of rotator cuff tear. Arthroscopy. 1988;4(4):241–9.

12. Kay SP, Ellman H, Harris E. Arthroscopic distal clavicle excision. Technique and early results. Clin Orthop Relat Res. 1994;301:181–4.
13. Tolin BS, Snyder SJ. Our technique for the arthroscopic Mumford procedure. Orthop Clin North Am. 1993;24(1):143–51.
14. Frieman BG, Albert TJ, Fenlin JM Jr. Rotator cuff disease: a review of diagnosis, pathophysiology, and current trends in treatment. Arch Phys Med Rehabil. 1994;75(5):604–9.
15. Koester MC, George MS, Kuhn JE. Shoulder impingement syndrome. Am J Med. 2005;118(5):452–5.
16. MacDonald PB, Clark P, Sutherland K. An analysis of the diagnostic accuracy of the Hawkins and Neer subacromial impingement signs. J Shoulder Elb Surg. 2000;9(4):299–301.
17. McCallister WV, et al. Open rotator cuff repair without acromioplasty. J Bone Joint Surg Am. 2005;87(6):1278–83.
18. Chen AL, Rokito AS, Zuckerman JD. The role of the acromioclavicular joint in impingement syndrome. Clin Sports Med. 2003;22(2):343–57.
19. Kessel L, Watson M. The painful arc syndrome. Clinical classification as a guide to management. J Bone Joint Surg Br. 1977;59(2):166–72.
20. Watson M. The refractory painful arc syndrome. J Bone Joint Surg Br. 1978;60-B(4):544–6.
21. Cuomo F, et al. The influence of acromioclavicular joint morphology on rotator cuff tears. J Shoulder Elb Surg. 1998;7(6):555–9.
22. Petersson CJ, Gentz CF. Ruptures of the supraspinatus tendon. The significance of distally pointing acromioclavicular osteophytes. Clin Orthop Relat Res. 1983;174:143–8.
23. Brown JN, et al. Shoulder pathology associated with symptomatic acromioclavicular joint degeneration. J Shoulder Elb Surg. 2000;9(3):173–6.
24. Chronopoulos E, et al. Diagnostic value of physical tests for isolated chronic acromioclavicular lesions. Am J Sports Med. 2004;32(3):655–61.
25. O'Brien SJ, et al. The active compression test: a new and effective test for diagnosing labral tears and acromioclavicular joint abnormality. Am J Sports Med. 1998;26(5):610–3.
26. Bookman JS, Pereira DS. Ultrasound guidance for intra-articular knee and shoulder injections: a review. Bull Hosp Jt Dis (2013). 2014;72(4):266–70.
27. Wasserman BR, et al. Accuracy of acromioclavicular joint injections. Am J Sports Med. 2013;41(1):149–52.

28. Mumford EB. Acromioclavicular dislocation: a new operative treatment. J Bone Joint Surg Am. 1941;23:799–802.
29. Pensak M, et al. Open versus arthroscopic distal clavicle resection. Arthroscopy. 2010;26(5):697–704.
30. Bhatnagar A, Bhonsle S, Mehta S. Correlation between MRI and arthroscopy in diagnosis of shoulder pathology. J Clin Diagn Res. 2016;10(2):RC18–21.
31. Lubowitz JH. Editorial commentary: lesions of the superior labrum from anterior to posterior (SLAP) are a slap in the face to the traditional trinity of history, examination, and imaging. Arthroscopy. 2015;31(12):2470–1.
32. Rokito SE, Myers KR, Ryu RK. SLAP lesions in the overhead athlete. Sports Med Arthrosc. 2014;22(2):110–6.
33. Ortiguera CJ, Buss DD. Surgical management of the symptomatic os acromiale. J Shoulder Elb Surg. 2002;11(5):521–8.
34. Youm T, et al. Os acromiale: evaluation and treatment. Am J Orthop (Belle Mead NJ). 2005;34(6):277–83.
35. Edelson JG, Zuckerman J, Hershkovitz I. Os acromiale: anatomy and surgical implications. J Bone Joint Surg Br. 1993;75(4):551–5.
36. Mudge MK, Wood VE, Frykman GK. Rotator cuff tears associated with os acromiale. J Bone Joint Surg Am. 1984;66(3):427–9.
37. Warner JJ, Beim GM, Higgins L. The treatment of symptomatic os acromiale. J Bone Joint Surg Am. 1998;80(9):1320–6.
38. Campbell PT, Nizlan NM, Skirving AP. Arthroscopic excision of os acromiale: effects on deltoid function and strength. Orthopedics. 2012;35(11):e1601–5.
39. Abboud JA, et al. Surgical treatment of os acromiale with and without associated rotator cuff tears. J Shoulder Elb Surg. 2006;15(3):265–70.
40. Johnston PS, et al. Os acromiale: a review and an introduction of a new surgical technique for management. Orthop Clin North Am. 2013;44(4):635–44.
41. Kurtz CA, et al. Symptomatic os acromiale. J Am Acad Orthop Surg. 2006;14(1):12–9.
42. McClure JG, Raney RB. Anomalies of the scapula. Clin Orthop Relat Res. 1975;110:22–31.
43. Nicholson GP, et al. The acromion: morphologic condition and age-related changes. A study of 420 scapulas. J Shoulder Elb Surg. 1996;5(1):1–11.
44. Uri DS, Kneeland JB, Herzog R. Os acromiale: evaluation of markers for identification on sagittal and coronal oblique MR images. Skelet Radiol. 1997;26(1):31–4.

45. Hertel R, et al. Transacromial approach to obtain fusion of unstable os acromiale. J Shoulder Elb Surg. 1998;7(6):606–9.
46. Peckett WR, et al. Internal fixation of symptomatic os acromiale: a series of twenty-six cases. J Shoulder Elb Surg. 2004;13(4):381–5.
47. Atoun E, et al. Arthroscopically assisted internal fixation of the symptomatic unstable os acromiale with absorbable screws. J Shoulder Elb Surg. 2012;21(12):1740–5.

Chapter 2
Arthroscopic Management of Rotator Cuff Calcific Tendonitis

M. Ned Scott, Christopher C. Schmidt, Brandon Brown, and Thomas Kotsonis

Case Presentation

A 57-year-old female nurse presents with a 6-month history of insidious shoulder pain. She complains of pain with overhead use and activities of daily living. The discomfort wakes her from sleep. She has been treated with anti-inflammatories

M. Ned Scott, D.O.
Department of Orthopaedic Surgery,
University of Pittsburgh Medical Center, Pittsburgh, PA, USA

C.C. Schmidt, M.D. (✉)
Department of Orthopaedic Surgery,
University of Pittsburgh Medical Center,
9104 Babcock Blvd., Suite 5113, Pittsburgh, PA 15237, USA
e-mail: schmidtc@upmc.edu

B. Brown, M.S.
Department of Bioengineering,
University of Pittsburgh, Pittsburgh, PA, USA

T. Kotsonis, B.S.
Department of Mechanical Engineering,
University of Pittsburgh, Pittsburgh, PA, USA

© Springer International Publishing AG 2018
P.J. McMahon (ed.), *Rotator Cuff Injuries*,
DOI 10.1007/978-3-319-63668-9_2

and oral steroids without significant symptom relief. Her past medical history is significant for hypertension and ischemic heart disease.

Upon physical examination, the patient demonstrates painful active forward flexion of the shoulder to 10° short of the contralateral side with a shoulder shrug. Passive forward elevation and external rotation is equal to the asymptomatic side and internal rotation is short two vertebral levels. Provocative testing for signs of impingement (Neers, Hawkins, and Yocum's tests) is positive. She demonstrates 4+/5 strength of forward flexion. Biceps maneuvers are negative, as is cross-arm adduction and tenderness about the distal clavicle. Cervical spine exam shows no limitation to motion, equal reflexes, and negative provocation of myelopathy. Radiographs show a homogenous calcific body with smooth edges measuring 22 × 7 mm within the subacromial space near the insertion of the supraspinatus tendon (Fig. 2.1a–c).

The patient assents to a trial treatment of corticosteroid injection into the subacromial space and home exercises intended to strengthen the rotator cuff and stabilize the scapula. She reports back in 8 weeks with continued pain. An MRI is ordered to further assess her soft tissues and demonstrates a hypo-intense body on the bursal surface of the supraspinatus tendon that measures 19 × 6 mm. There is mass effect on the supraspinatus tendon but the rotator cuff tendons are all intact (Fig. 2.2a–c).

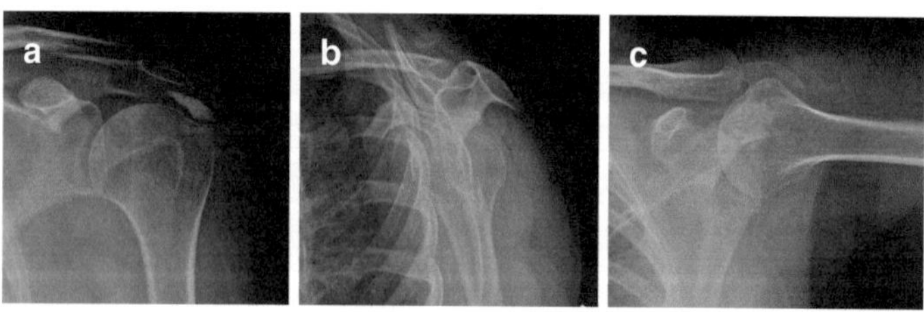

FIGURE 2.1 AP (**a**), Y view (**b**) and axillary (**c**) radiographs obtained after 6 months of shoulder pain show a large homogenous calcific deposit measuring 22 × 7 mm in the subacromial space. Compared with X-rays obtained 5 months previously, the deposit is unchanged

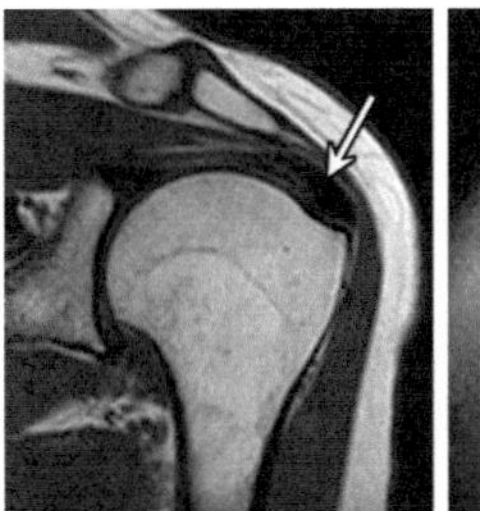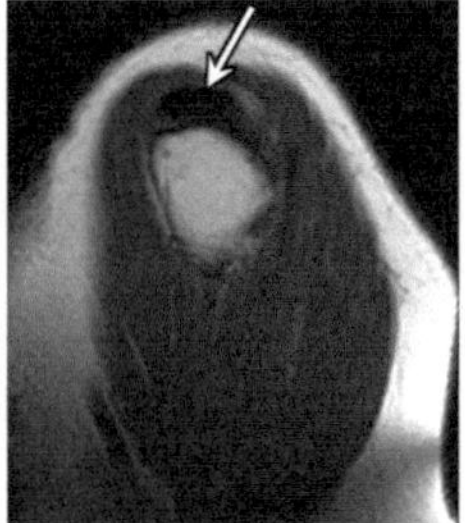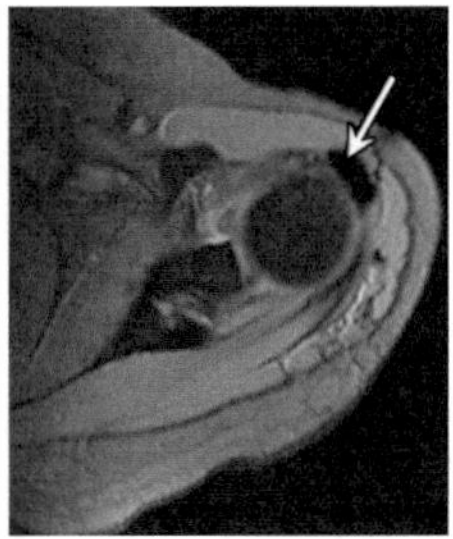

FIGURE 2.2 Coronal (**a**), sagittal (**b**), and axial (**c**) T2-weighted images demonstrate a hypo-intense, marginated mass consistent with the calcific deposit (*arrow*) on the bursal side of the rotator cuff with mass effect on the deltoid. It is impossible to tell the degree to which the calcific deposit has replaced or displaced the supraspinatus tendon

Diagnosis/Assessment

This patient presents with a classic history, physical exam, and diagnostic studies consistent with rotator cuff calcific tendonitis (RCCT), also referred to as hydroxyapatite or crystalline calcium phosphate tendon deposition. It is important to take into account the patient's symptoms, signs, and imaging findings, because not all calcific deposits cause pain [1]. The natural history of RCCT can be positive with expected improvement in clinical symptoms and possible eventual absorption of the calcific deposits. We informed our patient that people can respond to conservative treatments consisting of relative rest, anti-inflammatory medications, histamine blockers, and physical therapy and home exercise regimens [2]. Other nonsurgical but invasive management options are reviewed including therapeutic ultrasound, extracorporeal shock wave therapy, and ultrasound-guided barbotage and aspiration [3–5]. However, we also discussed that patients can fail conservative care and may continue to have unchanging pain, which would be an indication for surgical management. Level II evidence found that while radiographically inhomogeneous deposits responded well to both surgical and nonsurgical treatments, homogenous deposits responded better to arthroscopic removal [6]. The current thinking on RCCT pathogenesis and pain generators is metaplasia of tenocytes leading to cell-mediated calcification with pain mediated by swelling, neoinnervation, and neovascularization [7, 8].

Calcium deposits of the rotator cuff occur most commonly in the supraspinatus tendon, followed by the infraspinatus tendon [9]. Rarely, the deposit can occur in the subscapularis tendon [10]. The primary surgical goal is to express the calcific body to hasten the recovery process of the tendon and thus alleviate pain. Arthroscopically assisted removal of calcium deposits has largely replaced traditional open approaches to calcium removal.

Management

The patient underwent shoulder arthroscopy after 7 months of failed conservative management. Preoperatively, the patient's MRI is reviewed. Axial, sagittal, and coronal plane MRI cuts are used in conjunction to map out the location of the calcium deposit. Most deposits will be encountered on the bursal side and/or within the substance of the tendon; rarely deposits can be visualized from the articular side, but secondary changes of inflammation may be noted from the articular view [1, 11].

We position the patient in the beach chair as for standard rotator cuff-related arthroscopies. First, an arthroscopy of the glenohumeral joint is performed to evaluate for associated pathologies and to evaluate for partial articular sided or complete rotator cuff tears. If articular sided calcifications are visualized, they are tagged with a monofilament stitch outside to inside using a spinal needle that is inserted off the lateral edge of the acromion.

The arthroscope is then placed into the subacromial space. The subacromial arthroscopy is performed with anterolateral and posterolateral portals, with the arthroscope placed in the posterolateral portal and the anterolateral portal as the primary working portal. This optimizes visualization of the rotator cuff and facilitates an efficient bursectomy. After bursectomy, the calcium deposit is visualized on the bursal side of the rotator cuff tendon. Calcium deposits are detected as white or yellow patches on the cuff with surrounding areas of hyper-vascularity on the cuff, as well as hemorrhagic bursa (Fig. 2.3a, b). Most deposits present as topographic bulges

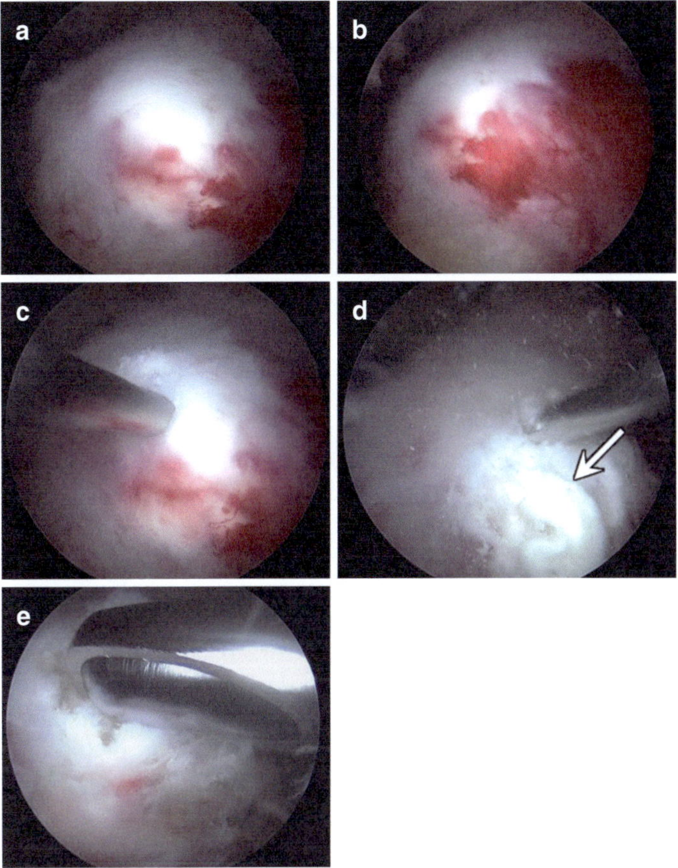

Figure 2.3 The subacromial space is viewed from the posterior lateral portal. After bursectomy, the calcific deposit is revealed as a large, white plaque bulging from the bursal side of the rotator cuff (**a**). Surrounding area of hyper-vascularity is also seen (**b**). An 18-gauge spinal needle is introduced into the deposit (**c**), and the toothpaste-like calcium initially fountains out as if under pressure (**d**) (*arrow*). The process is repeated with the spinal needle several times, re-creating several "geysers of toothpaste" and a "snowstorm" appearance in the subacromial space. Calcium hydroxyapatite is completely expressed with a blunt instrument such as a probe or Wissinger rod (**d**). The expressed deposit is collected and the surrounding abraded rotator cuff edge is trimmed and lavaged with an arthroscopic shaver (**e**)

adjacent to normal rotator cuff, but depending on their depth, hidden calcifications may also be present.

An 18-gauge needle is introduced percutaneously off the lateral edge of the acromion and the deposit is needled (Fig. 2.3c). The needle can be connected to a syringe and aspirated, but in this case the needle is withdrawn and the deposit expressed itself as stream of putty, similar to "toothpaste" (Fig. 2.3d). The paste is expressed with a Wissinger rod producing a snowstorm appearance within the subacromial space, which is removed with a shaver (Fig. 2.3e). Care is taken to preserve rotator cuff tendon at the expense of complete removal of the calcium deposits. Despite our care to maintain integrity to the cuff, a high-grade partial-thickness tear of the supraspinatus tendon was identified.

The high-grade rotator cuff tear on the bursal side is repaired with an arthroscopic Mason-Allen stitch (Fig. 2.4a–d) [12]. Antegrade passage of rotator cuff stitches with a suture lasso device through Neviaser's portal does not require takedown of intact articular sided rotator cuff fibers (Fig. 2.4b).

The need for acromioplasty is determined by the morphology of the acromion, wear on the coracoacromial (CA) ligament, condition of the bursa, and dynamic evaluation of the rotator cuff (Fig. 2.5a, b). There is abrasion of the undersurface of the CA ligament and passive elevation of the arm reveals abutment between the cuff and the lateral acromion are signs suggesting impingement and indications for acromioplasty. The subacromial decompression is performed with the use of an arthroscopic electrocautery wand and a 5.0 mm barrel burr (Fig. 2.5b). A final lavage is performed to remove any remaining bone fragments and calcium crystals.

The patient was immobilized in a sling for 4 weeks. During that time she was allowed passive supine straight-arm raises. Gentle active range of motion was started at 4 weeks and strengthening at 10 weeks following repair.

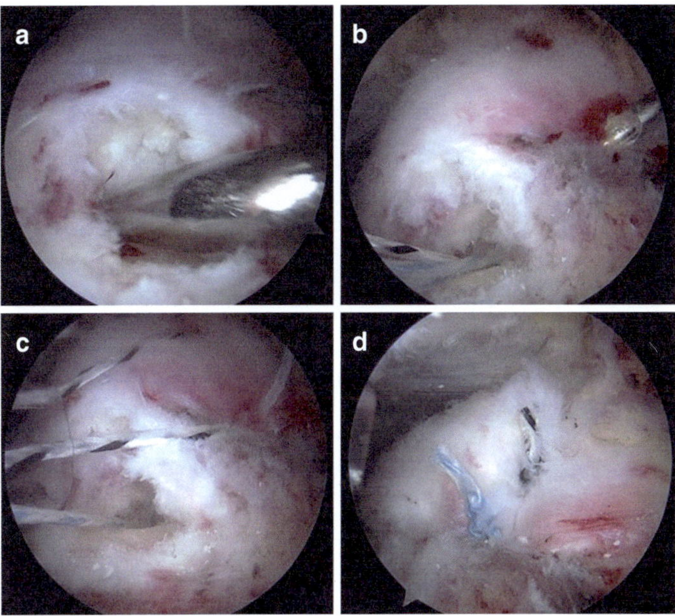

FIGURE 2.4 A high-grade bursal sided tear with intact articular supraspinatus tear is discovered after removal of the deposit from the footprint (**a**). After preparation of the denuded footprint, a 4.75 mm double-loaded anchor is placed into the tuberosity. A sturdy suture lasso (Banana SutureLasso, Arthrex, Naples, FL, USA) is used to penetrate the cuff in antegrade fashion (**b**) (*upper right corner*). Both limbs of the *black* and *white* suture and one limb of the *blue* and *white* suture are passed sequentially in a modified arthroscopic Mason-Allen configuration; in this picture the *black* and *white* suture creates a horizontal mattress after which the passed limb of the *blue* and *white* suture is thrown on the unpassed limb medial to the horizontal mattress (**c**); when tied this creates a rip-stop suture repair (**d**)

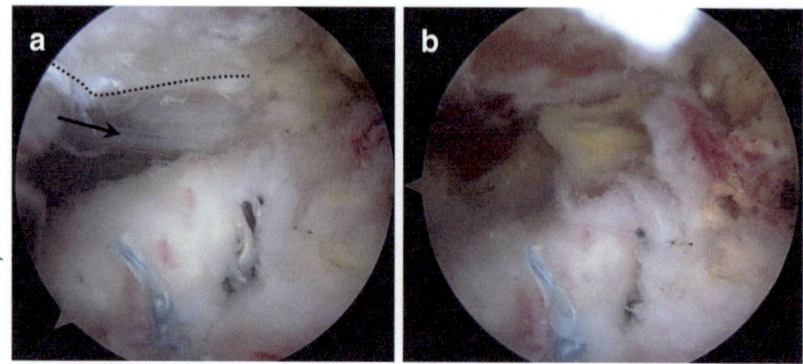

FIGURE 2.5 Arthroscopic evaluation after rotator cuff reveals a downsloping acromion (*dotted line*), which upon dynamic evaluation shows impingement on the cuff near the site of repair as well as abrasion of the coracoacromial ligament (*arrow*) suggesting signs of chronic impingement (**a**). Near-identical view after arthroscopic decompression shows impingement-free arc of rotation (**b**)

Outcome

The patient's pain resolved over the first 8 weeks and her motion returned to normal by 12 weeks. The ASES score at 4 months was 94. The patient's 2-week postoperative X-ray showed diminished but residual calcifications within the rotator cuff tendon (Fig. 2.6).

Literature Review

In a radiographic cross-sectional study, Bosworth found that the prevalence of calcific deposits was 2.7% in a group of asymptomatic patients [13]. The finding emphasizes the need to methodically rule out other sources of pain such as adhesive capsulitis, biceps tendinopathy, and rotator cuff dysfunction. The disease is more common in middle-aged women, and those with a history of diabetes mellitus, thyroid disorders, hypertension, and heart disease, but it is not associated with calcium or phosphate disorders [9, 14]. It is important to distinguish calcific tendinitis from dystrophic calcification of

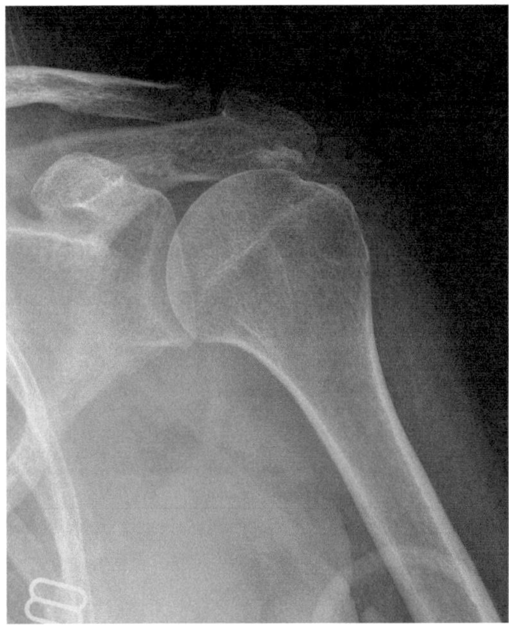

FIGURE 2.6 AP X-ray obtained at the 2-week postoperative visit shows residual calcification

the rotator cuff as the latter is age related and not generally a painful finding. Louwerens and coworkers compared the prevalence of calcifications of the rotator cuff in an asymptomatic cohort with another group of patients with impingement symptoms. The asymptomatic group had a lower overall rate of calcifications present (7.8% versus 42.5%), and the symptomatic group had larger deposits [9]. These authors did not distinguish between dystrophic and reactive calcifications. The history and physical exam of RCCT match those of subacromial impingement, but pain with RCCT is typically more severe and may resemble gout or other reactive arthritis. Past authors have suggested that there are different stages of calcification, which have different radiographic and clinical characteristics [1, 15].

However, a patient may fail nonoperative treatment at any point along the continuum of disease [1, 12, 15, 16]. It is our opinion that staging the disease is not as important as clinically correlating the disease to the patient's symptoms, treating with appropriate conservative measures, and offering surgery to those who have failed a course of conservative care.

It is important to remember that RCCT may occur with other disorders of the shoulder. Orthogonal X-rays are adequate to make the diagnosis of RCCT when combined with physical exam. Advanced imaging is useful for identifying the location of the deposit and associated disorders, particularly of the rotator cuff. MRI is a readily available diagnostic test that is useful for evaluation of the entire shoulder joint. Ultrasound is another diagnostic tool that has distinct advantages for RCCT, (1) Doppler signals within calcific deposits have been shown to correlate with pain [17], and (2) ultrasound can be used to guide therapeutic injections or attempt aspiration of the calcium deposits, and for dynamic evaluation of associated subacromial impingement.

Originally, the surgical management of calcific tendinitis consisted of open subacromial decompression and removal of the calcific bodies with a longitudinal incision in the rotator cuff. Arthroscopic surgery facilitates the same goals with less damage to the deltoid muscle and potentially with improved visualization of the calcific deposit, theoretically limiting damage to the rotator cuff. Numerous studies show significant improvement with arthroscopic treatment of painful calcium deposits [11, 16, 18–21].

For optimal recovery, the arthroscopist must confront a few controversies when approaching RCCT surgically. Considerations are (1) whether one must completely remove all the calcific deposits and in doing so possibly damaging intact rotator cuff; (2) if, in removing a calcific body, a complete or an incomplete rotator cuff tear is encountered, should this be fixed at that time of removal; and (3) should one routinely perform subacromial decompression as part of the procedure.

The question of how much of the calcific deposit needs to be removed is unanswered. Two studies in particular question the need for any removal of calcific deposits [15, 22].

In contrast, in a 2-year follow-up review of arthroscopically removed deposits, Porcellini found that patients' Constant scores were correlated to the amount of residual calcifications seen on follow-up X-rays [16]. The average 2-year follow-up Constant score of patients with no calcifications was 96.8, compared to 84.4 for patients with microcalcifications and 79 for calcifications measuring <10 mm ($p < 0.01$). Maier and associates evaluated for residual calcifications on X-rays in the immediate postoperative period. Eighty-two patients had complete removal; 17 had residual calcifications visualized [20]. At final follow-up, there was no difference in average Constant score (89.6 versus 86.1, $p > 0.05$). Furthermore, only 3 of 17 patients with residual calcifications showed continued calcifications at final follow-up. Based on equivalent results in patients with residual calcifications seen on X-ray, Seil et al. speculated that residual calcifications correspond to a shell of the deposit and lesion decompression relieves the pain [11]. Softer collections of crystalline calcium are easier to express than firm deposits [20]. Based on the results of others and our own experience, our recommendation is that the calcific deposits should be unroofed and soft deposits thoroughly expressed using blunt instruments, while firm calcifications within the rotator cuff do not need to be completely removed. Clinical improvement can be slower than expected whether or not the calcifications are completely removed.

Inevitably, removal of some calcium deposits will result in partial and even complete rotator cuff defects in many cases. Neer commented that in cases of RCCT the residual cuff does not need to be sutured [23]. Other authors have reported side-to-side repairs and anchored repairs for defects left in the cuff [16, 19, 21]. In Porcellini et al.'s study, all longitudinal tears <1 cm had no rotator cuff defects seen at follow-up ultrasound done at a minimum of 2 years. It is worth noting that none of the 63 patients followed in this study had a postoperative rotator cuff tear diagnosed by ultrasound in the postoperative period. In a study of 54 patients undergoing arthroscopic excision of deposits, El Shewy used a less aggressive technique to remove the deposit in order to maintain integrity of the rotator cuff, leaving partial-thickness tears (up to 50% thickness) unrepaired [19]. Two of the 54 cuffs (3.7%) required revision surgery for rotator cuff repair. Overall, the patients in this study had good outcomes with average ASES score of 95, but patients were not subclassified into treatment arms by degree of damage to the rotator cuff. Yoo et al. shared the experience of 35 consecutive calcific deposits having undergone arthroscopic removal, commenting that following thorough debridement of calcific deposits as well as local degenerative tissue (82% having no residual calcification on immediate follow-up X-ray), most rotator tendons were left with defects [21]. Low-grade tears were simply debrided or stitched in a side-to-side manner, and high-grade tears were fixed to bone with suture anchors. There was no statistical difference between those in the low-grade versus high-grade treatment arms of the study (mean Constant score 87 versus 86.2). Ten patients experienced postoperative stiffness, but there was no difference in the suture anchor group versus the non-suture anchor group. A prospective study of 17 patients reviewing the results of needling without repair reported that 13/17 (76%) of the patients had rotator cuff defects and 5/17 (29%) were full-thickness tears at 1 year following surgery [24]. Keener prospectively observed 56 partial-thickness tears over 5 years, and 44% of partial-thickness tears showed progression of the tear [25]. When we debride calcific lesion that results in a defect of the rotator cuff, we treat the defect as we normally treat rotator cuff tears; low-grade defects are left alone and high-grade or complete tears are treated with suture anchor fixation to bone [12].

The role of subacromial decompression for RCCT has been debated, with the focus of arguments for and against having focused on the pathogenesis and pain generators. Just as these factors are undecided, so too is the answer as to whether or not to perform subacromial decompression. The sheer volume of hydroxyapatite, along with swelling and local invasion of blood vessels, may predispose the patient to subacromial impingement. Recent histologic work by Hackett shows that the calcific deposit results in a substantial inflammatory response, which suggests that pain is intrinsic to the rotator cuff [7]. In 1998, Tillander and Norlin published the results of 25 patients with calcific deposits who underwent simple arthroscopic subacromial decompression leaving the calcific deposits intact [15]. Seventy-nine percent of the calcifications had disappeared or diminished on follow-up X-ray. Furthermore, there was no clinical difference between patients who had radiographic resolution and those who did not (average Constant score 78 versus 75). Balke and coworkers retrospectively compared shoulders with arthroscopic removal of calcific deposits and subacromial decompression with those who did not have subacromial decompression [18]. The decision whether or not to perform subacromial decompression was based on preoperative X-ray and findings of scuffing on the undersurface of the coracoacromial ligament. There was no statistically significant difference in improvement of shoulder scores at final follow-up between subacromial decompression and not as the Constant score was 74.8 versus 79.4. However, subitem evaluation pain was significantly better in the subacromial decompression group (11.4 versus 12.9, $p = 0.048$). The authors attributed this to possible selection bias as the study was not randomized and decompression was performed on patients with arthroscopically evident signs of impingement. While the question of the need for calcium removal remains, and if subacromial decompression alone is sufficient, the reason why subacromial decompression alone is successful remains unclear [16, 22]. Marder and coworkers retrospectively compared 25 shoulders that had arthroscopic removal of calcifications with subacromial decompression with 25 that did not [26]. At a mean of 5-year follow-up, quick DASH (11.1 versus 6.3, $p = 0.191$) and UCLA scores (32.4 versus 32, $p = 0.678$) showed no statistical difference. Contrary to the findings of Balke et al., these authors found that patients who underwent removal of the calcific body alone had earlier reduction of pain and return to normal activity (mean 11 weeks versus 18 weeks, $p < 0.006$). Given the body of evidence, we recommend that calcific deposits be removed along with subacromial decompression if there is impingement on physical examination, or radiographic evidence of a hooked acromion (i.e., type III). We end up doing a subacromial decompression in the majority of cases as we also perform it if we think that the RCCT is a risk factor predisposing the patient to impingement.

Clinical Pearls and Pitfalls

- Most patients presenting with acute RCCT can be treated with time, rehabilitation, and subacromial injection of steroids, but patients may require surgery if there is impingement after 3–6 months of debilitating symptoms.
- At arthroscopy the calcific deposits do not need to be completely removed, but can be decompressed by needling and expressing with blunt instruments.
- Small partial-thickness rotator cuff tears that can be debrided and high-grade tears (>50% of the thickness) should be repaired as in standard arthroscopy to limit the chance of tear progression. Patients should be counseled preoperatively about the possibility of rotator cuff repair and the differences in postoperative rehabilitation compared to debridement alone.
- One should consider the patient with calcific deposits as at risk for impingement. However, subacromial decompression can be performed on a case-by-case basis, if there are impingement signs on physical examination, a hooked (i.e., grade 3) acromial undersurface on preoperative imaging, scuffing on the undersurface of the coracoacromial ligament, or a rotator cuff tear that needs repair after calcium removal and we think that the tear is from impingement.
- Patients should be counseled that clinical improvement and radiographic resolution happens over a course of a year.

References

1. Uhthoff HK, Loehr JW. Calcific tendinopathy of the rotator cuff: pathogenesis, diagnosis, and management. J Am Acad Orthop Surg. 1997;5:183–91.

2. Greis AC, Derrington SM, Mcauliffe M. Evaluation and nonsurgical management of rotator cuff calcific tendinopathy. Orthop Clin North Am. 2015;46:293–302.
3. Gatt DL, Charalambous CP. Ultrasound-guided barbotage for calcific tendonitis of the shoulder: a systematic review including 908 patients. Arthroscopy. 2014;30:1166–72.
4. Gerdesmeyer L, Wagenpfeil S, Haake M, Maier M, Loew M, Wortler K, Lampe R, Seil R, Handle G, Gassel S, Rompe JD. Extracorporeal shock wave therapy for the treatment of chronic calcifying tendonitis of the rotator cuff: a randomized controlled trial. JAMA. 2003;290:2573–80.
5. Kim YS, Lee HJ, Kim YV, Kong CG. Which method is more effective in treatment of calcific tendinitis in the shoulder? Prospective randomized comparison between ultrasound-guided needling and extracorporeal shock wave therapy. J Shoulder Elb Surg. 2014;23:1640–6.
6. Rompe JD, Zoellner J, Nafe B. Shock wave therapy versus conventional surgery in the treatment of calcifying tendinitis of the shoulder. Clin Orthop Relat Res. 2001;387:72–82.
7. Hackett L, Millar NL, Lam P, Murrell GA. Are the symptoms of calcific tendinitis due to neoinnervation and/or neovascularization? J Bone Joint Surg Am. 2016;98:186–92.
8. Uhthoff HK, Sarkar K, Maynard JA. Calcifying tendinitis: a new concept of its pathogenesis. Clin Orthop Relat Res. 1976;118:164–8.
9. Louwerens JK, Sierevelt IN, Van Hove RP, Van Den Bekerom MP, Van Noort A. Prevalence of calcific deposits within the rotator cuff tendons in adults with and without subacromial pain syndrome: clinical and radiologic analysis of 1219 patients. J Shoulder Elb Surg. 2015;24:1588–93.
10. Arrigoni P, Brady PC, Burkhart SS. Calcific tendonitis of the subscapularis tendon causing subcoracoid stenosis and coracoid impingement. Arthroscopy. 2006;22(1139):e1–3.
11. Seil R, Litzenburger II, Kohn D, Rupp S. Arthroscopic treatment of chronically painful calcifying tendinitis of the supraspinatus tendon. Arthroscopy. 2006;22:521–7.
12. Jarrett CD, Schmidt CC. Arthroscopic treatment of rotator cuff disease. J Hand Surg Am. 2011;36:1541–52. quiz 1552
13. Bosworth BM. Calcium deposits in the shoulder and subacromial bursitis. JAMA. 1941;116:2477–88.
14. Speed CA, Hazleman BL. Calcific tendinitis of the shoulder. N Engl J Med. 1999;340:1582–4.

15. Tillander BM, Norlin RO. Changes of calcifications after arthroscopic subacromial decompression. J Shoulder Elb Surg. 1998;7:213–7.
16. Porcellini G, Paladini P, Campi F, Paganelli M. Arthroscopic treatment of calcifying tendinitis of the shoulder: clinical and ultrasonographic follow-up findings at two to five years. J Shoulder Elb Surg. 2004;13:503–8.
17. Le Goff B, Berthelot JM, Guillot P, Glemarec J, Maugars Y. Assessment of calcific tendonitis of rotator cuff by ultrasonography: comparison between symptomatic and asymptomatic shoulders. Joint Bone Spine. 2010;77:258–63.
18. Balke M, Bielefeld R, Schmidt C, Dedy N, Liem D. Calcifying tendinitis of the shoulder: midterm results after arthroscopic treatment. Am J Sports Med. 2012;40:657–61.
19. El Shewy MT. Arthroscopic removal of calcium deposits of the rotator cuff: a 7-year follow-up. Am J Sports Med. 2011;39:1302–5.
20. Maier D, Jaeger M, Izadpanah K, Bornebusch L, Suedkamp NP, Ogon P. Rotator cuff preservation in arthroscopic treatment of calcific tendinitis. Arthroscopy. 2013;29:824–31.
21. Yoo JC, Park WH, Koh KH, Kim SM. Arthroscopic treatment of chronic calcific tendinitis with complete removal and rotator cuff tendon repair. Knee Surg Sports Traumatol Arthrosc. 2010;18:1694–9.
22. Hofstee DJ, Gosens T, Bonnet M, De Waal Malefijt J. Calcifications in the cuff: take it or leave it? Br J Sports Med. 2007;41:832–5.
23. Neer CS, Marberry TA. Calcium deposits: shoulder reconstruction. Philadelphia: Saunders; 1990.
24. Verhaegen F, Brys P, Debeer P. Rotator cuff healing after needling of a calcific deposit using platelet-rich plasma augmentation: a randomized, prospective clinical trial. J Shoulder Elb Surg. 2016;25:169–73.
25. Keener JD, Galatz LM, Teefey SA, Middleton WD, Steger-May K, Stobbs-Cucchi G, Patton R, Yamaguchi K. A prospective evaluation of survivorship of asymptomatic degenerative rotator cuff tears. J Bone Joint Surg Am. 2015;97:89–98.
26. Marder RA, Heiden EA, Kim S. Calcific tendonitis of the shoulder: is subacromial decompression in combination with removal of the calcific deposit beneficial? J Shoulder Elb Surg. 2011;20:955–60.

Chapter 3
Arthroscopic Repair of Partial-Thickness Articular Sided Rotator Cuff Tendon Tears

Patrick J. McMahon

Case Presentation

The patient is a 62-year-old male lineman for an electric company with an 8-month history of persistent right shoulder pain. He reports that while working overhead in a bucket truck he pulled with this previously asymptomatic dominant right shoulder and felt a sudden tearing sensation and pain. For a few months he continued to work with light duty restrictions including avoidance of overhead activities and he took Ibuprofen and did a home exercise program of stretching and strengthening. Persistent moderate, achy occasional shoulder pain that radiated to the lateral upper arm was worse with overhead activities and awakened him at night

P.J. McMahon, M.D.
Orthopedics and Rehabilitation,
Department of Bioengineering, University of Pittsburgh,
2100 Jane St., Pittsburgh, PA 15203-2076, USA
e-mail: mcmahonp@upmc.edu

© Springer International Publishing AG 2018
P.J. McMahon (ed.), *Rotator Cuff Injuries*,
DOI 10.1007/978-3-319-63668-9_3

resulting in his being treated with physical therapy and two cortisone injections in the subacromial space. Each resulted in diminished pain for 5–6 weeks but then the pain recurred and resulted in difficulty working and sleeping.

On physical examination, the patient stood 6 feet tall and weighed 200 pounds. He had full range of motion of the right shoulder with pain in the mid arc of motion and the scapula moved the same as the left asymptomatic side without scapula winging. There was tenderness at the greater tuberosity and none at the bicipital groove or the acromioclavicular and sternoclavicular joints. The right shoulder strength was diminished in abduction, rated as 4/5 with pain, and was normal in internal and external rotation at 5/5. He had positive Hawkins and Neer impingement signs and no pain with cross-body motion. There were no signs of shoulder instability as he had negative apprehension and relocation tests and the O'Brien's test was negative as well.

The true lateral (i.e., Grashey) (Fig. 3.1a), axillary lateral (Fig. 3.1b), supraspinatus outlet (Fig. 3.1c), and acromioclaviclular, also called Zanca view (Fig. 3.1d), radiographs of the patient's right shoulder were normal except for moderate AC joint osteoarthritis. An MRI was ordered and revealed rotator cuff tendonitis and a small partial-thickness anterior supraspinatus tendon avulsion (PASTA) tear (Fig. 3.2) and moderate AC joint osteoarthritis. As the patient had failed nonsurgical treatment, and was substantially limited by his pain, he was interested in shoulder arthroscopy and rotator cuff repair. We also discussed the chance of the tearing healing without surgery and the risks of the tear getting worse over time.

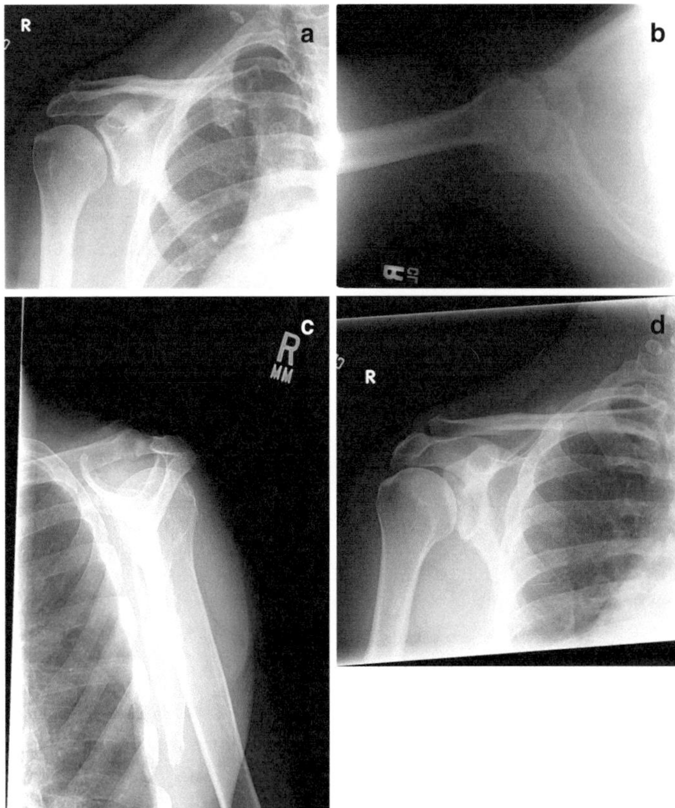

FIGURE 3.1 (**a–d**) Radiographs of the shoulder including true lateral (i.e., Grashey), axillary lateral, supraspinatus outlet, and acromioclaviclular (i.e., Zanca) views were normal except for moderate AC joint osteoarthritis

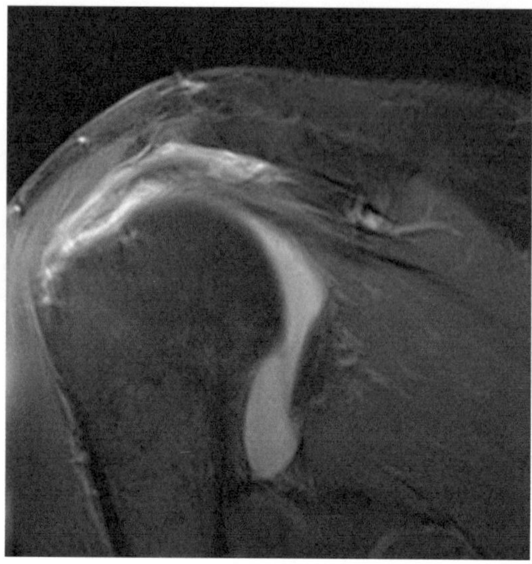

FIGURE 3.2 The MRI revealed rotator cuff tendonitis and a small partial-thickness anterior supraspinatus tendon tear

Diagnosis/Assessment

The patient's history, physical, and imaging findings are consistent with the diagnosis of symptomatic partial-thickness rotator cuff tear. Initial treatment was nonoperative including rehabilitation, NSAIDs, and avoidance of overhead activities. The symptoms persisted so a subacromial injection of lidocaine and cortisone that resulted in immediate diminished pain that persisted for several weeks was important in ruling out other causes of shoulder pain such as cervical radiculopathy and malingering. This is important because rotator cuff tears are prevalent, especially in the elderly and even in athletes but are not always the cause of a patient's shoulder pain [1]. I read the shoulder MRI myself to guide the patient in the expected postoperative treatments. I debride tears of less than 50% of the tendon thickness and allow early range of motion and I repair those involving more than 50% as this much of the tendon has to be torn before there is sufficient tendon tissue to hold a suture. When the intact tendon overlying the articular sided tear appears normal, as with this patient, I perform the repair without completing the tear. Only when the intact tendon is damaged do I complete the tear before doing the repair. When there is AC joint osteoarthritis as with this patient, some physicians prefer to routinely excise the distal clavicle. I have been successful using the absence of tenderness at the AC joint and the absence of pain at the AC joint with cross-body motion in leaving the AC joint alone. However, it has been my experience that these signs are commonly found in worker's compensation cases.

Partial-thickness rotator cuff tears can be treated with an arthroscopic repair without completing the tear by utilizing the following techniques: (1) making a small longitudinal incision over the tear in the intact portion of the tendon; (2) while viewing the articular side of the tendon, making multiple passes with a small instrument, such as an 18 g spinal needle through the intact margin of the torn tendon; (3) tying the sutures on the bursal side of the tendon; and (4) performing a subacromial decompression if the surgeon thinks it is helpful. Each case must be taken on an individual basis, as the findings at arthroscopy direct the surgeon through the best method of repair. For example, the intact tendon at the location of the partial-thickness tear is often robust and there is little retraction of the torn tendon making it amenable to repair without completing the tear (Fig. 3.3a, b). But if the intact tendon is stretched, such that there is excessive retraction of the tear, then excising the stretched tendon, known as completing the tear, and using techniques detailed in Chap. 4 is the best course.

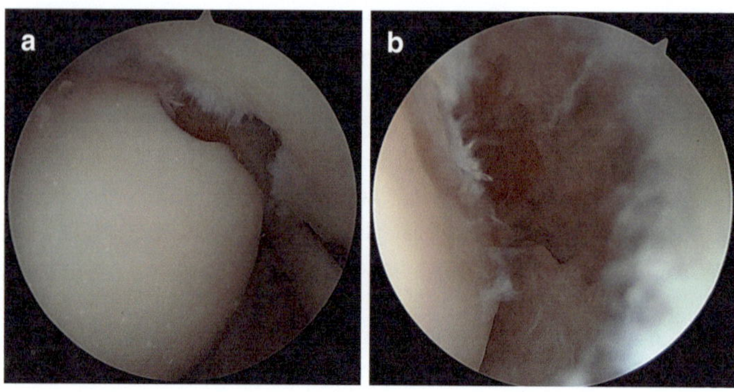

FIGURE 3.3 (**a**) Arthroscopic picture of the partial-thickness rotator cuff tear with a robust intact portion of the tendon and little retraction that is amenable to repair without completion of the tear. (**b**) Arthroscopic close-up picture of the partial-thickness rotator cuff tear and little retraction of the tendon that is amenable to repair without completion of the tear

Management

With the patient in a lateral decubitus position and the arm suspended in about 45° of abduction and 15° of forward flexion, a standard posterior portal is made for viewing. The articular surfaces, labrum, biceps tendon, subscapularis tendon, and infraspinatus tendon are normal. A standard anterior portal is also made lateral to the coracoid and entering the joint between the biceps and subscapularis tendons. There is a 15 mm partial-thickness anterior supraspinatus tendon tear of about 60% of the tendon thickness (Fig. 3.4). The determination of the percent of the supraspinatus tendon tear is assessed by looking at the width of exposed tuberosity and knowing the average footprint is about a centimeter and a half in thickness and not by looking at the tendon as fraying and retraction make this difficult. For example for an average-sized person if 9 mm of the greater tuberosity width is exposed, then 60% of the tendon thickness is torn. The surgeon then has the choice of doing the repair or going into

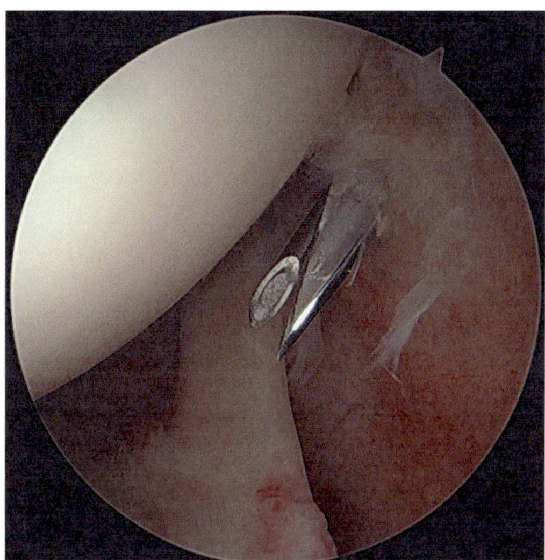

FIGURE 3.4 The intact tendon over the partial-thickness rotator cuff tear is longitudinally incised in line with the collagen fibers with the spine needle in place that was used to localize the tear

the subacromial space and doing a bursectomy to make it easier to find the sutures in the subacromial space after the repair. I usually do the former as doing the bursectomy often makes it difficult to see the tear afterwards.

I plan to make a portal about 2 cm off the lateral acromion. I start by using an 18 g spinal needle in this location that I then place into the tear as a guide. Adjacent to the needle I make an incision in the skin for a portal with a #11 scalpel and also make a longitudinal incision in line with the fibers of the supraspinatus tendon through the intact portion of tendon over the PASTA lesion (Fig. 3.4). A 6 mm cannula is placed into the joint and I debride the torn tendon with a shaver and greater tuberosity with a burr (Fig. 3.5). This portal is not usually good for placing the anchor as trying to do so would skive the humeral head. A portal about 3 mm in size, just large enough for placing an anchor loaded with two

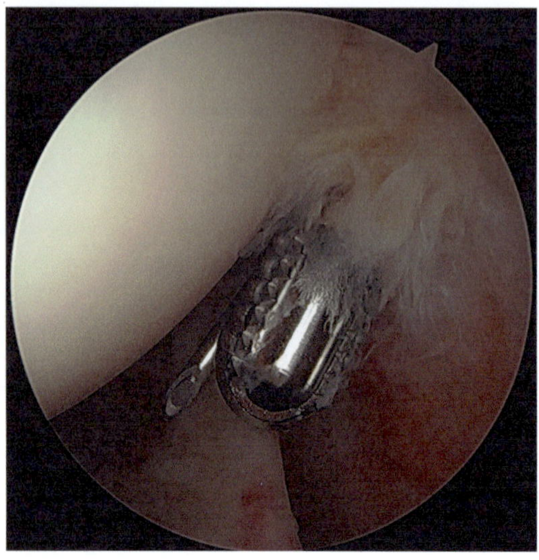

FIGURE 3.5 The edges of the torn tendon are debrided with a shaver. The greater tuberosity is then burred

sutures, is made adjacent to the lateral acromion. I once again use an 18 g spinal needle as a guide starting in this location and placing it into the tear. If the anchor is placed without a cannula, as I do, it can be a challenging part of the procedure. More than one anchor can usually be placed without additional incisions in the anterior and posterior greater tuberosity by holding the arm in either external or internal rotation, respectively. The edges of the torn tendon are debrided (Fig. 3.6) with a shaver and the exposed tuberosity is burred (Fig. 3.7). The sutures are then pushed into the joint with a suture passer so that they will be easy to retrieve though the anterior portal (Fig. 3.8). An 18 g spinal needle is placed through the anterolateral shoulder and into the anterior, intact portion of the tendon about 5–7 mm medial to the edge of the tear. A suture relay is passed through the 18 g spinal needle and retrieved out of the anterior portal along with one

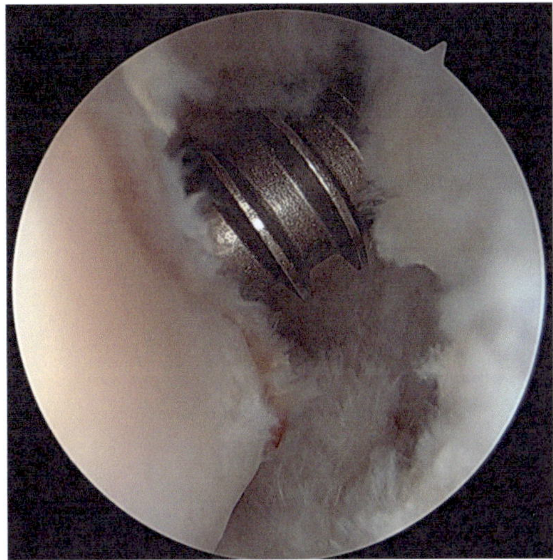

FIGURE 3.6 The greater tuberosity is then tapped

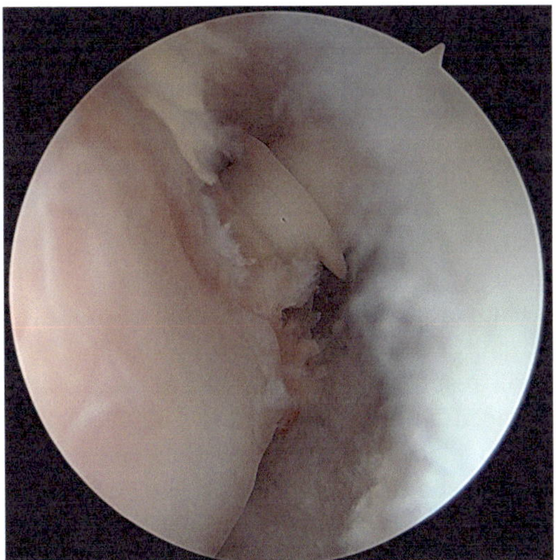

FIGURE 3.7 The anchor is placed

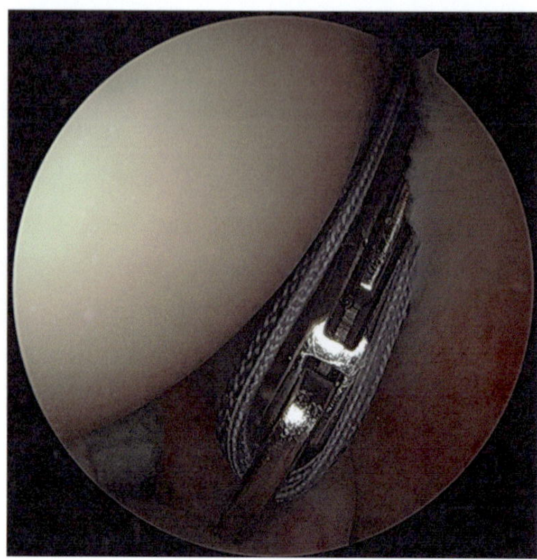

FIGURE 3.8 The sutures are then pushed into the joint to ease retrieving them one at a time out the anterior portal

limb of one of the sutures (Fig. 3.9). The suture is placed into the suture relay and shuttled out the anterolateral shoulder (Fig. 3.10). The 18 g spinal needle is again placed through the anterolateral shoulder about 7 mm anterior to the first suture into the intact portion of the tendon. The suture relay is passed through the 18 g spinal needle and retrieved out of the anterior portal along with the other limb of the suture that is then again shuttled out the anterolateral shoulder that is then tied and will result in a mattress suture. A second mattress suture is placed anterior to the first (Fig. 3.11). The arthroscope is then placed in the subacromial space and if the sutures can be seen they are retrieved and tied. If they cannot be seen then a bursectomy must be done very carefully so as not to cut the sutures! To avoid doing so I start the bursectomy in the subdeltoid space, lateral to the sutures and move posterior first (Fig. 3.12). My assistant pulls on the sutures to make them taut and before starting the bursectomy I use the shaver as a probe, with the blade not moving, to give me an idea of where the sutures are. I can usually find the sutures

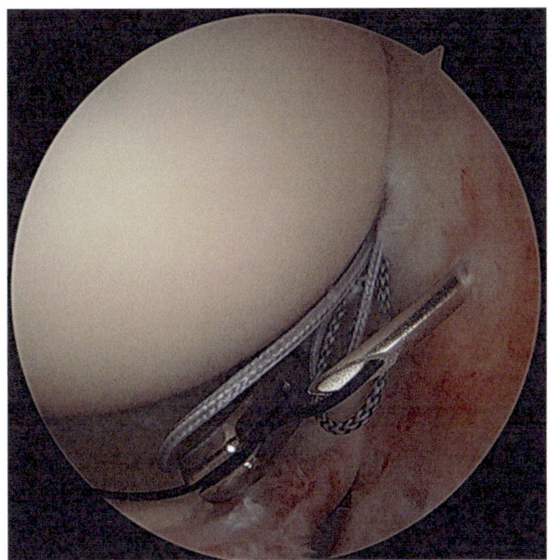

FIGURE 3.9 A spinal needle is placed about 5–7 mm medial to the edge of the torn tendon. The suture relay is passed through the tendon and grasped. The spinal needle is removed and the suture relay is retrieved out the anterior portal. In this case it was suture in the posterior part of the tear

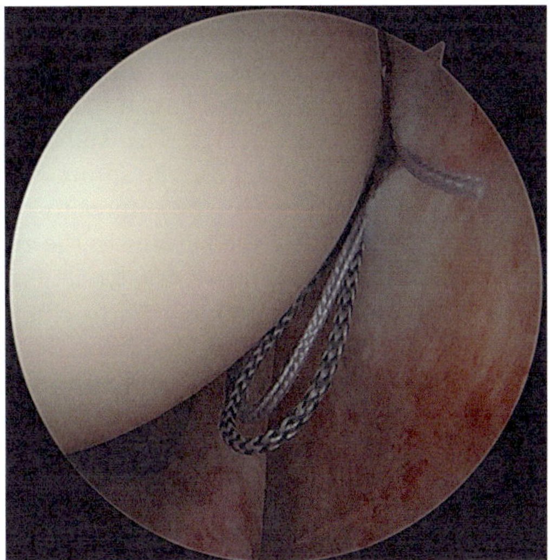

FIGURE 3.10 The suture was passed back through to complete that suture passing

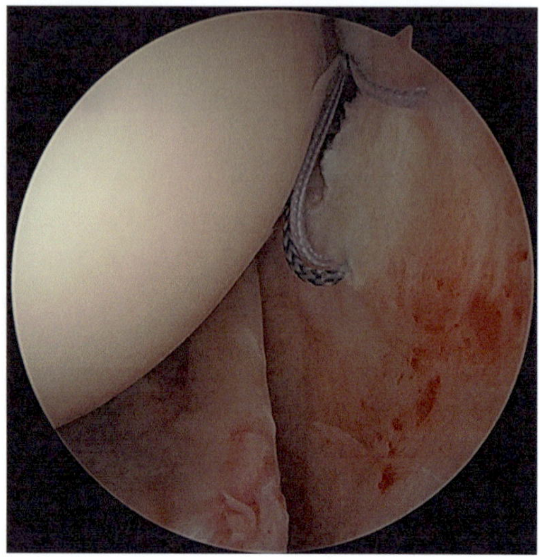

FIGURE 3.11 A view from the articular side of the tendon after the two mattress sutures have been completed. Both limbs of the posterior suture and only one limb of the anterior suture can be seen. The other limb of the anterior suture is through the intact tendon that is behind the humeral head

after clearing the subdeltoid space (Fig. 3.13). On rare occasions I will debride some of the subacromial space around the sutures to better expose them (Figs. 3.14 and 3.15). More commonly if I cannot find them, I use the suture retriever as a probe while my assistant pulls on the sutures to keep them taut and this helps me to find the sutures in the remaining bursa. Once I find one and determine which one it is, it helps me to find the rest. I then tie the sutures to complete the repair (Fig. 3.16), and then complete the bursectomy of the subacromial space and then do a subacromial decompression. The necessity of subacromial decompression with rotator cuff repair is controversial. Lastly, the arthroscope is placed into the joint to assess the repair (Fig. 3.17).

Supervising the rehabilitation is important for a successful outcome. The patient's arm stays in a sling for 4–6 weeks postoperative depending on the size of the tear and the

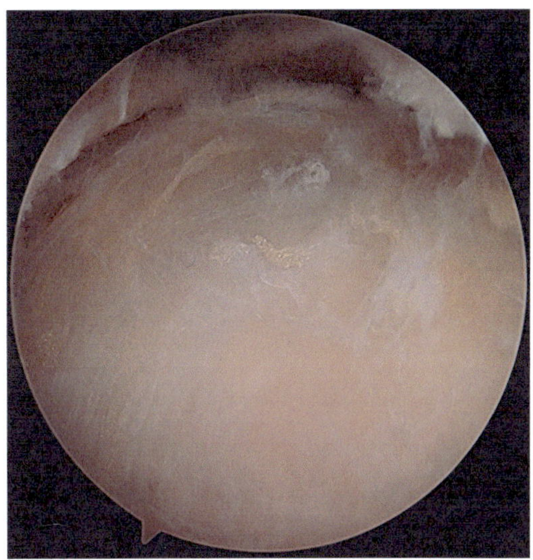

FIGURE 3.12 A view from the bursa side showing the bursectomy starting in the subdeltoid bursa and not the subacromial bursa to avoid the sutures

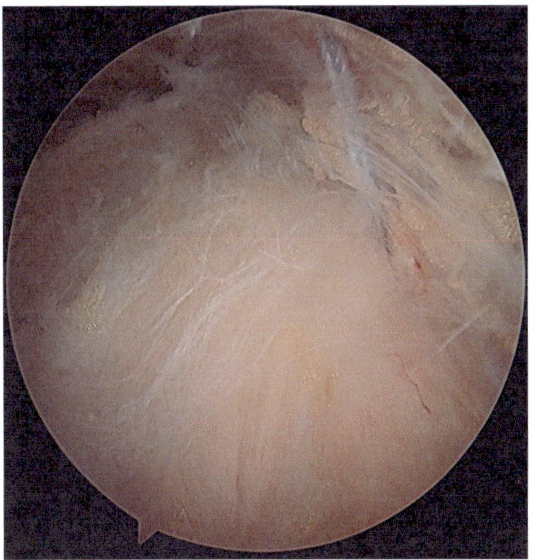

FIGURE 3.13 This usually reveals the sutures so that they can be retrieved

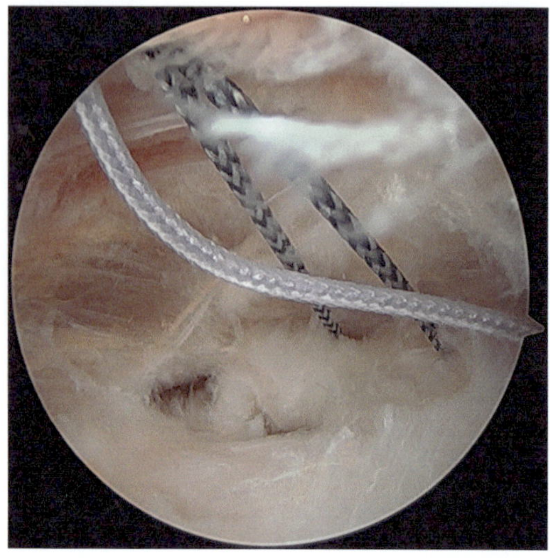

FIGURE 3.14 The subacromial bursa can then be debrided if needed without damaging the sutures, if needed

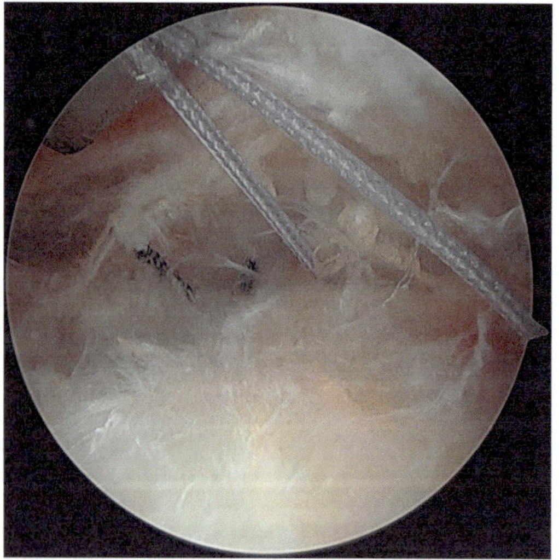

FIGURE 3.15 The sutures can then be retrieved and tied

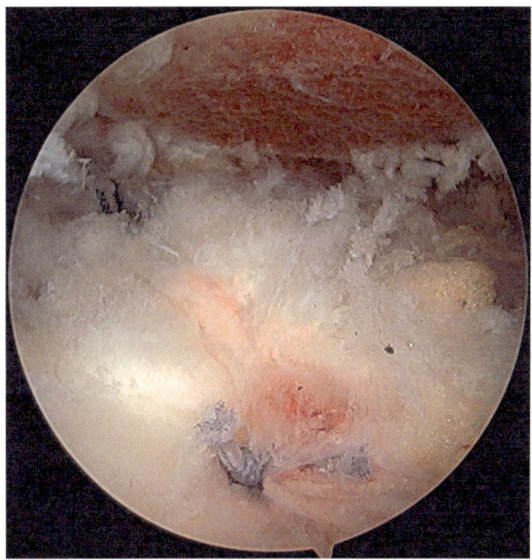

FIGURE 3.16 View from the bursal side of the completed repair

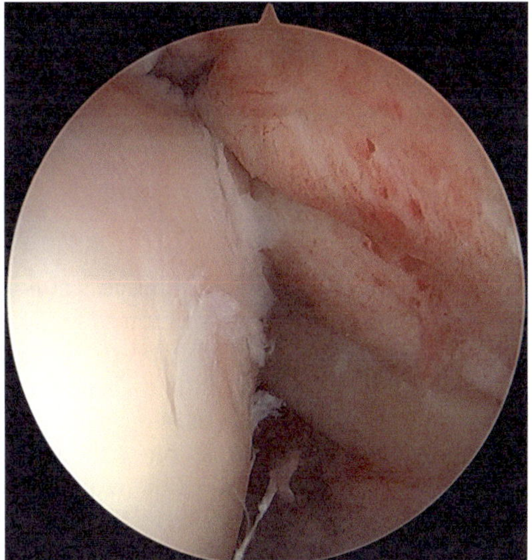

FIGURE 3.17 View from the articular side of the completed repair

patient does pendulum exercises. If only one anchor is used for the repair as is often the case then 4 weeks is sufficient but if two or three anchors are used then the arm stays in the sling for 6 weeks. After this time the patient begins active ROM and stretching to diminish stiffness. Strengthening is begun 3 months postoperative and return to work as a laborer is about 5 months postoperative. Recurrence is most likely in the first 3–6 months after the repair which may be failure of the tear to heal rather than recurrent tearing [2, 3]. Failure of partial-thickness rotator cuff repair has been reported as being a full-thickness tear as well [4, 5]. Patient satisfaction is over 90% [6, 7].

Outcome

This 62-year-old gentleman with a partial-thickness rotator cuff tear that was repaired without completion of the tear recovered uneventfully. At 4 months postoperative, he had no pain and was sleeping normally. He had full range of motion with forward flexion to 150°, external rotation with the arm at the side to 40° and internal rotation to L1, and normal strength of 5/5 to these motions. He returned to work as a lineman 5 months after the surgery.

Literature Review

Initial treatment of most rotator cuff injuries is nonoperative. The usual indication for surgery is symptoms that persist over several months of nonoperative treatments. In addition to patient age, the onset being traumatic or insidious, and the duration being acute or chronic, the management of partial rotator cuff tears includes consideration of the tear size and the extent of tendon involvement, prior treatment, and the patient's physical limitations. Partial-thickness rotator cuff tears can be bursal, intratendinous, or as in this case articular. Factors that may be associated with less favorable outcomes following partial-thickness rotator cuff repair include greater tear size, greater duration, abnormalities of the rotator cuff muscles, worker's compensation status, and earlier mobilization after surgery. Another consideration is the chance of the tear becoming larger over time, and while less likely than with full-thickness tears, this can over several years' time [8, 9]. It occurs more often in patients with persistent symptoms. The rotator cuff muscles can also atrophy and develop fatty changes over time [8]. Patients with a worker's compensation claim have functional improvement after rotator cuff repair that is less robust than other patients [10]. And, several weeks of immobilization before initiating active range of motion and several months before strengthening results in the best outcomes. When surgery is done, arthroscopic repair of partial-thickness rotator cuff tears without completing the tear results in high patient satisfaction and about 80% can be expected to heal [11] which is similar to that for small full-thickness rotator cuff tears.

Clinical Pearls/Pitfalls

- The key to the management of a partial-thickness rotator cuff tear without completing the tear is making a small longitudinal incision in the intact portion of the cuff at the location of the tear for anchor placement. More than one anchor can usually be placed without additional incisions in the anterior and posterior greater tuberosity by holding the arm in either external or internal rotation, respectively.
- For the lateral portal that is used to place anchors there arc small disposable cannulas or reusable guides to ease anchor placement.
- More sutures are better and I like to place mattress suture ties over about 7 mm of tendon. Not much space, only a mm or 2 is needed between the mattress sutures.
- Place the arthroscope into the GH joint at the end of the procedure to assess the repair after the sutures are tied in a subacromial space.

References

1. McMahon PJ, Prasad A, Francis KA. What is the prevalence of senior-athlete rotator cuff injuries and are they associated with pain and dysfunction? Clin Orthop Relat Res. 2014;472(8):2427–32. doi:10.1007/s11999-014-3560-7. PMID: 24619795
2. Miller BS, et al. When do rotator cuffs fail? Serial ultrasound examination after arthroscopic repair of large and massive rotator cuff tears. Am J Sports Med. 2011;39(10):2064–70.
3. Iannotti JP, Deutsch A, Green A, Rudicel S, Christensen J, Marraffino S, Rodeo S. Time to failure after rotator cuff repair: a prospective imaging study. J Bone Joint Surg Am. 2013;95(11):965–71. doi:10.2106/JBJS.L.00708. PMID: 23780533
4. Kim YS, Lee HJ, Bae SH, Jin H, Song HS. Outcome comparison between in situ repair versus tear completion repair for partial thickness rotator cuff tears. Arthroscopy. 2015;31(11):2191–8. doi:10.1016/j.arthro.2015.05.016. Epub 2015 Jul 15. PMID: 26188786
5. Weber SC. Arthroscopic debridement and acromioplasty versus mini-open repair in the treatment of significant partial-thickness rotator cuff tears. Arthroscopy. 1999;15(2):126–31. doi:10.1053/ar.1999.v15.0150121.
6. Mazzocca AD, Rincon LM, O'Connor RW, et al. Intra-articular partial-thickness rotator cuff tears: analysis of injured and repaired strain behavior. Am J Sports Med. 2008;36(1):110–6. doi:10.1177/0363546507307502.
7. Matthewson G, Beach CJ, Nelson AA, Woodmass JM, Ono Y, Boorman RS, Lo IK, Thornton GM. Partial thickness rotator cuff tears: current concepts. Adv Orthop. 2015;2015:458786. doi:10.1155/2015/458786. Epub 2015 Jun 11. Review. PMID: 26171251
8. Keener JD, Galatz LM, Teefey SA, Middleton WD, Steger-May K, Stobbs-Cucchi G, Patton R, Yamaguchi K. A prospective evaluation of survivorship of asymptomatic degenerative rotator cuff tears. J Bone Joint Surg Am. 2015;97(2):89–98. doi: 10.2106/JBJS.N.00099. PMID: 25609434
9. Kim YS, Kim SE, Bae SH, Lee HJ, Jee WH, Park CK. Tear progression of symptomatic full-thickness and partial-thickness rotator cuff tears as measured by repeated MRI. Knee Surg Sports Traumatol Arthrosc. 2016 [Epub ahead of print]. doi: 10.1007/s00167-016-4388-3. PMID: 27904936

10. Henn RF 3rd, Kang L, Tashjian RZ, Green A. Patients with workers' compensation claims have worse outcomes after rotator cuff repair. J Bone Joint Surg Am. 2008;90(10):2105–13. PMID: 18829907
11. Xiao J, Cui G. Clinical and structural results of arthroscopic repair of bursal-side partial-thickness rotator cuff tears. J Shoulder Elb Surg. 2015;24(2):e41–6. doi:10.1016/j.jse.2014.07.008. PMID: 25240814

Chapter 4
Arthroscopic Repair of Full-Thickness Small-to-Moderate Rotator Cuff Tears

Justin C. Wong, J. Gabe Horneff, and Mark D. Lazarus

Case Presentation

The patient is a 60-year-old left-hand-dominant male dye setter at the U.S. Mint who presents with 6 weeks of pain and weakness of the left shoulder, particularly with overhead activity. He reports a specific injury when reaching overhead to grab a dye tool. He felt and heard a pop with associated onset of pain in his lateral shoulder. He thought that the pain would subside with modification of his activities, but the pain has persisted. He reports nighttime shoulder discomfort, lateral shoulder pain, and weakness with overhead reaching activity and feels that he is unable to perform his usual job

J.C. Wong, M.D.
OrthoArizona, 20325 North 51st Avenue, Bldg 4, Suite 124, Glendale, AZ 85308, USA

J. Gabe Horneff, M.D. • M.D. Lazarus, M.D. (✉)
Orthopedic Surgery, Thomas Jefferson
University Hospital, Rothman Institute,
925 Chestnut Street, Philadelphia, PA 19107, USA
e-mail: shoulderdoc@comcast.net

© Springer International Publishing AG 2018
P.J. McMahon (ed.), *Rotator Cuff Injuries*,
DOI 10.1007/978-3-319-63668-9_4

with his current level of pain and shoulder dysfunction. His treatment to date has included nonsteroidal anti-inflammatory medication as well as a short course of physical therapy. He has no neck pain or radicular symptoms. He denies any history of prior shoulder discomfort or injury. His worker's compensation physician obtained an MRI of his left shoulder because of his lack of improvement with physical therapy and now he presents for further evaluation and management.

On physical examination, he is 5′10″ and 202 lbs. He has full cervical range of motion and a negative Spurling's maneuver. His shoulder girdle does not demonstrate any signs of atrophy. Palpation of the shoulder girdle shows that his acromioclavicular (AC) and sternoclavicular joints are non-tender, but he does have tenderness in the anterior and lateral subacromial region. His active shoulder range of motion in forward elevation and abduction is limited secondary to pain. Passively, his range of motion in forward elevation, abduction, and arm-at-side external rotation is normal and symmetric with the contralateral shoulder. Resisted strength testing of the shoulder reveals 4/5 strength with supraspinatus testing but preserved 5/5 strength with resisted external and internal rotation with the arm at the side and a negative abdominal compression test.

Radiographs of his left shoulder revealed a concentrically located glenohumeral joint with no evidence of glenohumeral joint arthritis and no proximal humeral migration (Fig. 4.1). Magnetic resonance imaging of the left shoulder revealed a moderate-sized rotator cuff tear involving the supraspinatus and the anterior portion of the infraspinatus with no evidence of muscle belly atrophy or fat infiltration (Fig. 4.2).

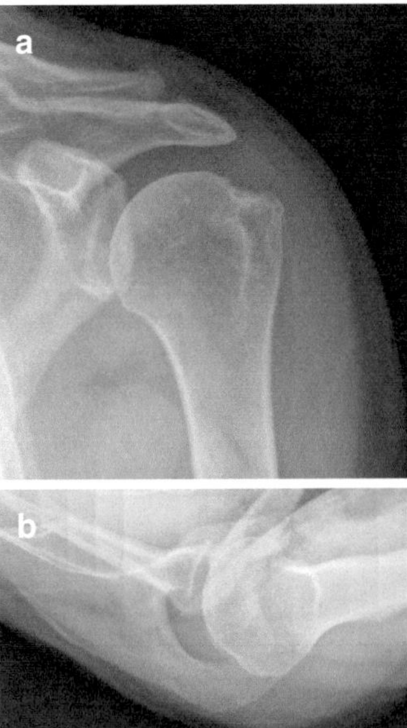

FIGURE 4.1 Radiographs of shoulder. (**a**) AP view and (**b**) axillary view of left shoulder demonstrate concentric glenohumeral joint with no evidence of glenohumeral arthritis or proximal humeral migration

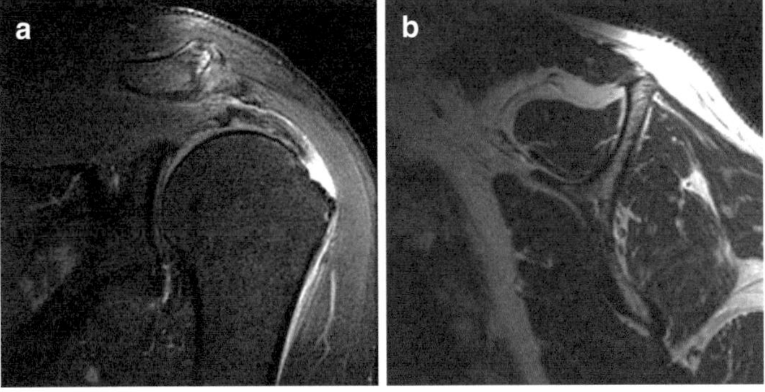

FIGURE 4.2 MRI of shoulder. (**a**) Coronal T2 image demonstrates full-thickness rotator cuff tear. The tear involved supraspinatus and the anterior portion of the infraspinatus. (**b**) Sagittal T1 image demonstrates no evidence of rotator cuff atrophy or fatty infiltration

Diagnosis/Assessment

The patient's history, physical examination, and diagnostic imaging are consistent with an acute symptomatic full-thickness rotator cuff tear. This was discussed with the patient including options for continued nonoperative treatment or consideration of rotator cuff repair. With regard to pursuing nonoperative treatment, the risks of tear-size progression and specifically possible progression of a repairable tear to an irreparable tear and possible development of irreversible muscle atrophy and fat infiltration were discussed. With regard to pursuing operative treatment, risks of infection, stiffness, and failure of rotator cuff repair were discussed. Based upon the patient's age, occupation, acute onset of injury, and failure of improvement with prior nonoperative treatment, he opted to proceed with rotator cuff repair.

Management

Our preferred surgical technique for repair of small, medium, large, and even massive full-thickness rotator cuff tears, which can be appropriately mobilized to the anatomic footprint, is to utilize an all-arthroscopic suture-passing device that enables the surgeon to pass sutures transosseously via a tunnel between medial based and lateral based holes in the greater tuberosity (Tornier © Arthrotunneler device (Amsterdam, The Netherlands)) (Fig. 4.3). Each tunnel can accommodate three to four sutures. With the sutures placed transosseously, the surgeon can then proceed with passage of suture limbs through the rotator cuff tendon, followed by securely tying down the tendon to the greater tuberosity footprint, thus generating a true-transosseous rotator cuff repair.

We perform arthroscopic rotator cuff repair in the beach-chair position under general anesthesia with a regional block. The operative arm is held with a pole (McConnell Orthopedic Manufacturing, Greenville, TX) that is utilized to support the arm in various ranges of shoulder abduction and external

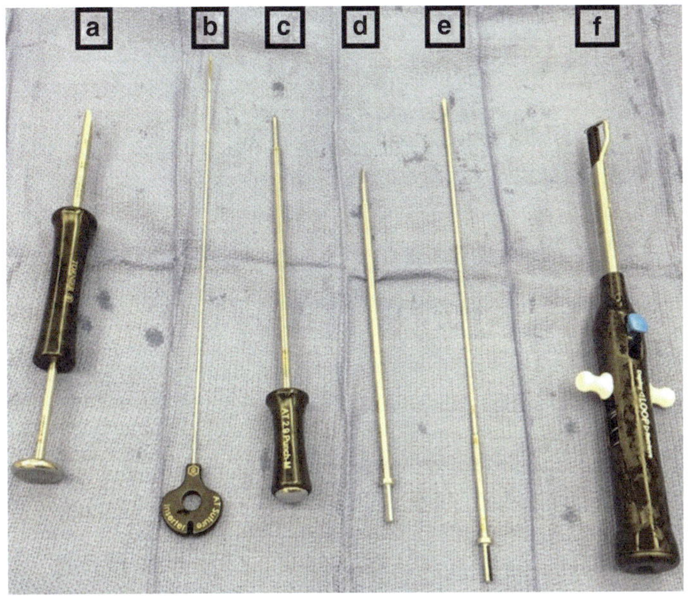

FIGURE 4.3 Image of tunneler instrumentation. (**a**) Drill guide and trocar—used for drilling medial tunnel holes, (**b**) stick suture passer, (**c**) awl with hard stop, (**d**) drill for medial hole with hard stop, (**e**) drill for lateral hole, (**f**) tunneler

rotation to bring different areas of the greater tuberosity into view and in-line with the trajectory of instruments during the surgery.

We begin with a standard posterior portal and a diagnostic arthroscopy to evaluate the condition of the glenohumeral joint. Careful attention is paid to the subscapularis tendon, and if repair is indicated, it is performed prior to transitioning the scope to the subacromial bursa. After completion of the diagnostic arthroscopy and any possible biceps tendon, subscapularis, or other glenohumeral joint treatment, the scope is directed into the subacromial bursa. Once in the subacromial bursa, a spinal needle allows for localization of the lateral portal, which is made horizontal. It is critical that the superior-to-inferior height of the lateral portal is not too high, or it can make the use of the arthrotunneler device more difficult. Our preference is that a spinal needle, held in a horizontal position, should just skim the top surface of the greater tuberosity, when the shoulder is in a neutral position.

The next phase of the operation is obtaining optimal visualization of the rotator cuff tear to allow for assessment of tear size and configuration. The subacromial bursa is resected with a combination of shaver and electrocautery devices; acromioplasty is not routinely performed. The footprint of the rotator cuff is debrided and lightly decorticated with the use of an arthroscopic burr to help stimulate a healing response. Although tendon mobilization is not typically a problem for small- to moderate-sized tears, it is important to perform appropriate releases for retracted tears to allow for maximal tendon excursion and to minimize tension on the repair. The anterior-to-posterior size of the rotator cuff tear is utilized as a guide for the number of tunnels to be placed. In general, a "two-tunnel" suture configuration is utilized for tears 1–2 cm in anterior-to-posterior size. For larger tears, additional tunnels can be utilized with a repeating pattern of suture organization and configuration.

In our two-tunnel rotator cuff repair, each tunnel contains three nonabsorbable #2 sutures; two of the sutures are utilized in a simple suture configuration, while the third suture is utilized to create a "rip-stop stitch" by creating a box suture configuration when paired with a suture from the adjacent tunnel (Fig. 4.4). For suture management purposes, we typically utilize black-striped, blue-striped, and solid-colored sutures in each tunnel. For larger tears requiring three or more tunnels, the approach is the same: the most anterior and most posterior tunnel contains three nonabsorbable sutures, and each of the central tunnels contains four nonabsorbable sutures. In cases of utilizing three or more tunnels, the more central tunnel contains an additional nonabsorbable suture to allow for a rip-stop box suture configuration to be created with a suture from the adjacent tunnel anterior and posterior to it.

A posterolateral viewing portal is created prior to beginning the next phase of the operation and allows for good

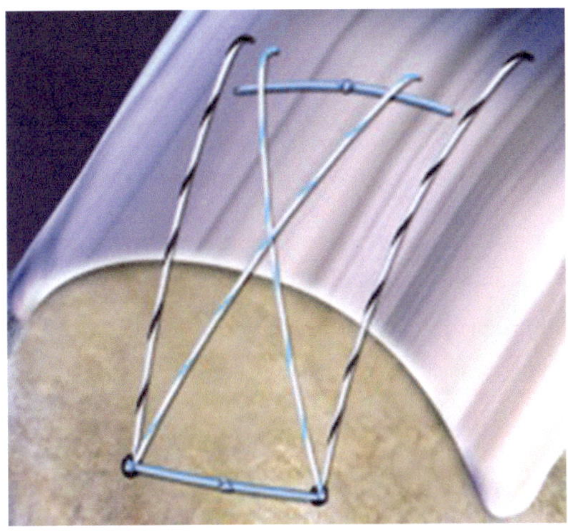

FIGURE 4.4 A two-tunnel repair. A two-tunnel repair schematic, a lateral box stitch (*blue suture*) is created to serve as a rip stop for the simple sutures (*blue-striped* and *black-striped*)

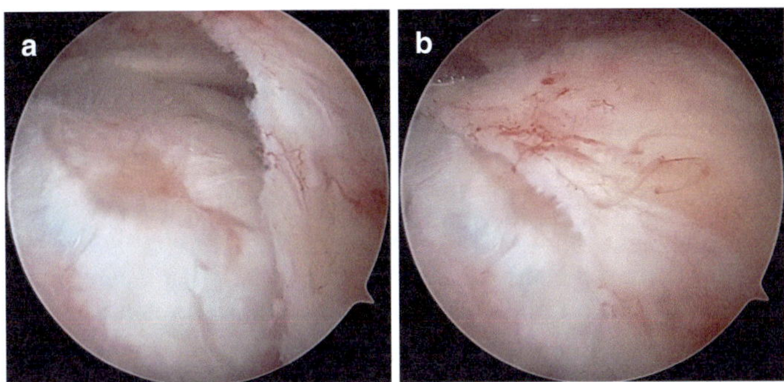

FIGURE 4.5 Rotator cuff tear before and after being reduced. Left shoulder, posterolateral viewing portal showing the rotator cuff tear (**a**) and it reduced on the greater tuberosity with a grasper (**b**)

visualization of the rotator cuff tear (Fig. 4.5) so that we can understand the size, retraction, and pattern of the tear as this aids us in how it will be repaired (Fig. 4.5b). A spinal needle is typically inserted into the subacromial spacer along the

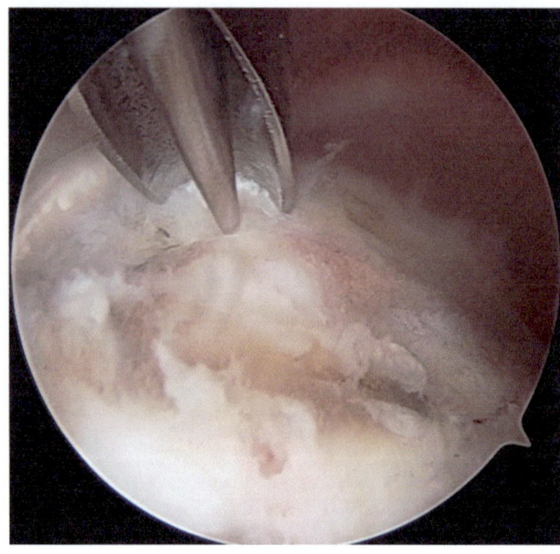

FIGURE 4.6 Tunneler medial hole drilling. Left shoulder, posterolateral viewing portal; drill guide utilized to place medial drill hole, drill is advanced to a hard stop

lateral edge of the acromion to help estimate the number and placement of the medial based tunnel holes. The process for passing the sutures transosseously begins with the use of a drill and drill guide to create the medial based holes in the greater tuberosity. This is performed through an accessory anterolateral portal with a trajectory that is roughly 70–80° upright from the footprint of the tuberosity. The placement of this portal should allow for access to create all of the medial holes by simply externally or internally rotating the arm. The drill guide is positioned on the medial edge of the footprint and the drill is advanced until the hard stop of the drill (Fig. 4.6). An awl with a hard stop is then utilized to increase the diameter of the hole and be sure that it is the appropriate depth. All of the medial holes can be placed successively before moving to the next step of passing transosseous sutures.

Once all of the medial holes have been created, the lateral portal is lengthened to about 1.5 cm in length, which allows

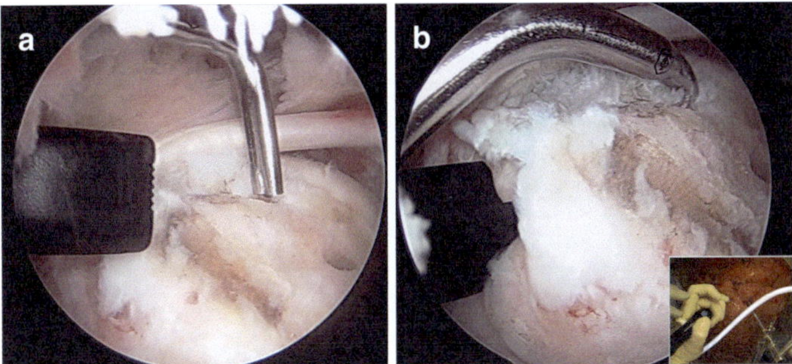

FIGURE 4.7 Tunneler position and seated on medial hole. Left shoulder, posterolateral viewing portal with the tunneler guided into position (**a**) and the tunneler seated into medial drill hole and held flush to greater tuberosity with the inset being the external view of hand positioning for the tunneler (**b**)

for introduction of the arthrotunneler device into the subacromial space. Beginning with the most anterior tunnel and working posteriorly, the arthrotunneler device is seated into the most anterior of the medial holes and held firmly against the tuberosity (Fig. 4.7b). It is important to properly position the tunneler such that the lateral drill holes are adequately spaced from one another. A second drill is utilized to create a horizontal hole in the lateral aspect of the greater tuberosity that intersects with the tip of the arthrotunneler device medially. A wire loop can be deployed and acts as a capture device to ensure that the two holes intersect. The wire loop is left in the deployed position and the drill is withdrawn with care not to disrupt the orientation of the arthrotunneler. Next, a suture passer with a passing stitch is then placed down the barrel of the arthrotunneler and captured with the wire loop. The suture passer is gently removed to allow the wire loop to securely hold the passing suture when the tunneler is removed.

At this point, the tunneler device is withdrawn, keeping the looped end of the passing suture captured by the wire loop. This leaves a passing suture through the tunnel which can be used to shuttle sutures of different size, type, and color

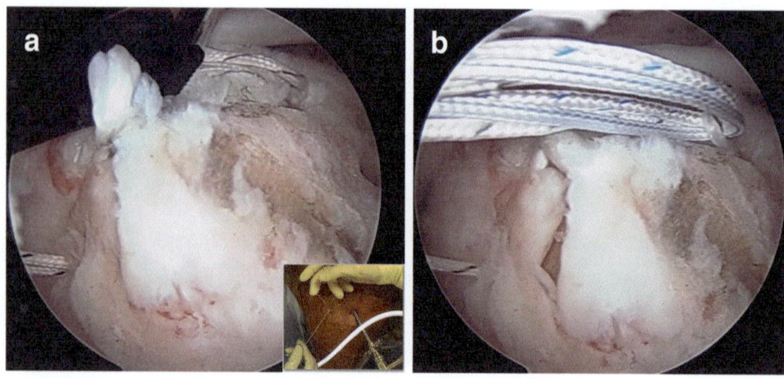

FIGURE 4.8 Suture passing stitch. Left shoulder, posterolateral viewing portal with the tunneler retrieving a looped passing stitch and the inset being after the looped passing stitch is placed so that three or four sutures to be utilized in the repair can be passed (**a**) and the looped passing stitch is being used to pass a set of sutures into the tunnel (**b**)

according to the surgeon's preference (Fig. 4.8a, b). For the most anterior tunnel, three nonabsorbable #2 sutures are passed with the looped passing suture. The medial and lateral tails of these nonabsorbable sutures are successively brought out of an anterior portal and tagged with hemostats. We prefer to tag the medial limbs with a single hemostat and the lateral limbs with two hemostats. Since the operation requires multiple tunnels and multiple sets of sutures for each tunnel, we use color-coded hemostats for suture management. The tunneling process and suture passage process are repeated as needed (Fig. 4.9). For the most posterior tunnel the sutures are brought out through the posterior portal.

The medial limbs of the sutures in each tunnel are then passed in successive fashion through the cuff tendon tissue. We prefer to pass the sutures beginning with the most posterior tunnel. The hemostat is removed from the medial limb sutures and the blue-striped suture is retrieved and passed through an appropriate posteromedial location in the tendon utilizing a jawed suture passer. Next the medial limb of the solid suture is retrieved and passed—just anterior and slightly lateral to the placement of the previous striped suture.

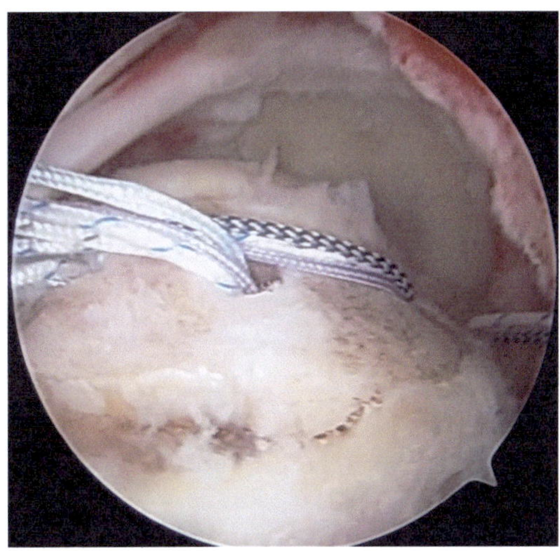

Figure 4.9 All sutures passed into tunnels. Left shoulder, postero-lateral viewing portal; all sets of sutures have been passed through their corresponding tunnels. This view shows the medial tunnel holes with their corresponding sutures. This particular example is a four-tunnel repair, where most of the anterior and most posterior tunnels each contain three sutures, while the middle two tunnels contain four sutures

The black-striped suture is next passed more anteriorly (in-line with the blue-striped suture, with regard to medial-to-lateral placement) (Fig. 4.10). This process is repeated with the set of sutures from the anterior tunnel, again placing the solid suture a few millimeters lateral to the placement of the striped sutures. The pair of solid sutures from each tunnel will be utilized to create the rip-stop box suture configuration.

After all of the medial limbs are passed, we begin tying the sutures by creating the rip-stop box suture configuration. To do this, the medial limbs of the solid sutures in both the anterior and posterior tunnel are retrieved through an anterior cannula. These medial suture limbs are tied together with square knots and tested to ensure that the knots do not slide. The medial tails are cut with a 1 cm tail. Subsequently, their

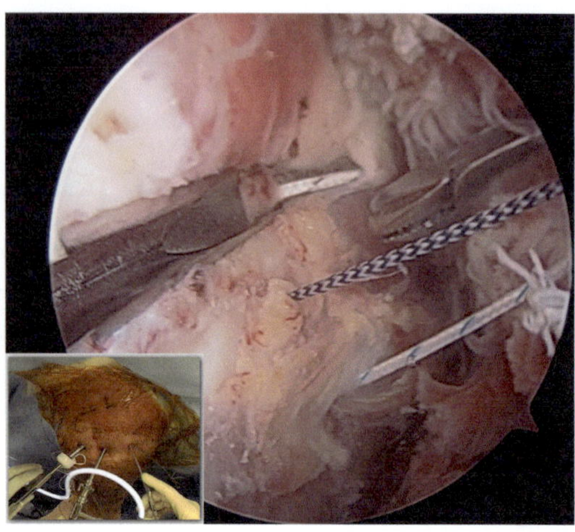

FIGURE 4.10 Medial suture limbs passed through tendon. Left shoulder, posterolateral viewing portal; medial limbs of sutures are being passed through the tendon. Of note, the middle suture shown will be utilized to form the lateral box rip stop, by pairing with a similar suture from the adjacent tunnel. These rip-stop sutures are placed 1–2 mm more lateral than the sutures that will be utilized in a simple-suture configuration. *Inset*—external view of instrument orientation

lateral based counterparts are retrieved from the lateral portal. As the lateral limbs of the solid sutures are tensioned down, the medial knot is pulled into the shoulder and sits atop the rotator cuff. An arthroscopic grasper can be utilized to pull on the tendon edge and aid in this process. The lateral limbs are tensioned and tied against the lateral aspect of the greater tuberosity with non-sliding knots. This creates the rip-stop box suture configuration, and this horizontal mattress suture also serves as medial row fixation. The remaining suture limbs are retrieved and tied in successive fashion with a simple suture configuration (Figs. 4.11 and 4.12). The same process can be applied for larger tears with three or more tunnels, noting that a rip-stop box suture configuration is created between each adjacent tunnel.

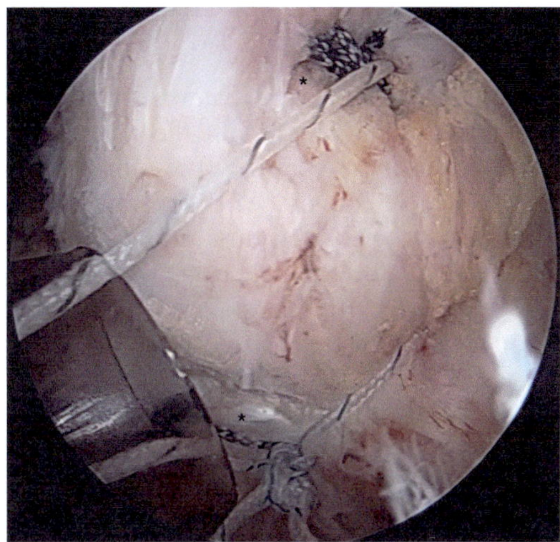

FIGURE 4.11 Tying sutures. Left shoulder, posterolateral viewing portal; tying of simple suture over box rip-stop suture. Box rip-stop suture depicted by *asterisk*

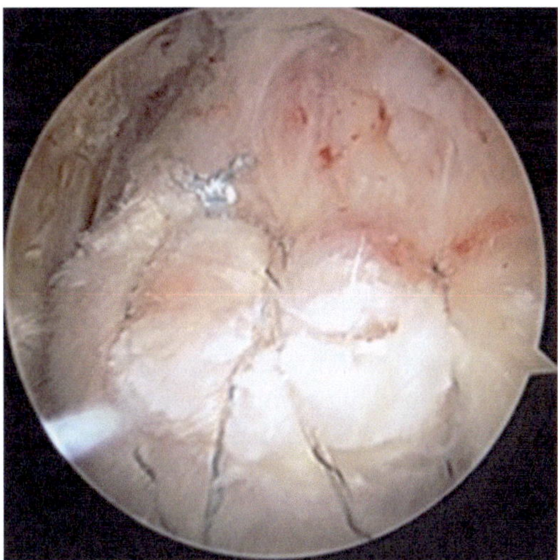

FIGURE 4.12 Final repair construct. Left shoulder, posterolateral viewing portal; example of final two-tunnel rotator cuff repair — simple sutures (striped sutures) tied over the box rip-stop sutures

Postoperative Rehabilitation

Our patient wore a sling and abduction pillow for 4 weeks. Then he was permitted to discontinue the sling and abduction pillow and begin a passive range-of-motion home-exercise program consisting of forward elevation and external rotation. Exercises were performed three to five times a day. He was instructed to avoid reaching, pushing, or pulling with the operative arm. Weight-lifting limits are that of a coffee cup and all use of the arm should be performed with the elbow against the side of the torso and forearm directly in front of them. At 2 months postoperatively, passive range of motion was assessed. If passive range of motion is adequate, he would continue with the same home-exercise program for another 4 weeks. If there was substantial shoulder stiffness defined as passive forward elevation <100° he would be encouraged and directed to perform the home-exercise program hourly. He was permitted to use the operative arm for light activities but is instructed to avoid lifting objects greater than a few pounds. At 3 months postoperatively he began active strengthening of the rotator cuff and continued with therapy for several more months. He was released to full activity at about 6 months.

Outcome

Our patient remained out of work for the initial 2-month postoperative period and then was transitioned to a modified-duty job with restrictions to not use the operative side for any lifting, pulling, and pushing. At 3 months he began formal physical therapy with rotator cuff strengthening. From 3 to 6 months he continued to demonstrate improvement in rotator cuff strength. He was released to his regular duties at work 6 months after the surgery.

Literature Review

Rotator cuff tears are a common shoulder condition for middle-aged and older patients and often occur as a result of age-related degenerative attrition [1–5]. The prevalence of asymptomatic full-thickness rotator cuff tears may be 20% in the general population, but increases with patient age—more than 50% of patients over age 80 may have an asymptomatic full-thickness rotator cuff tear [1]. Over time, asymptomatic rotator cuff tears may cross over to becoming symptomatic rotator cuff tears, which may be heralded by the development of pain, weakness, and functional limitations [6]. In the appropriate scenario, repair of a full-thickness rotator cuff tear is indicated when a patient continues to have limitations despite a trial of nonoperative management or when an active patient presents acutely with a traumatic rotator cuff tear.

In the absence of significant symptoms, the role for repair of full-thickness rotator cuff tears is less well defined. In these cases, the decision for operative or nonoperative management will include consideration of patient age, occupation, short-term and long-term activity requirements, as well as the potential risk for progression in size of the rotator cuff tear, fat infiltration, and muscle atrophy. Recent longitudinal observational studies of asymptomatic partial and full-thickness rotator cuff tears have documented the risk of tear progression as ranging from 36 to 67% within 3 years [7–9]. Full-thickness tears have a higher risk of tear progression and, in general, tear progression is associated with the development of pain symptoms [8]. Patient age, gender, and smoking status have not been shown to correlate significantly with risk of tear progression [9]. In one study of small symptomatic full-thickness tears in younger patients treated nonoperatively, the risk of tear progression was 25% at 3-year follow-up and no tear progressed to becoming irreparable over that time period [10]. For patients with known full-thickness rotator cuff tears that are being treated nonoperatively, there is a role for surveillance imaging with the goal of detecting patients who develop tear progression and may be at risk of further progression with continued nonoperative treatment [11, 12]. Although the ideal timing of surveillance imaging is not well defined, we consider follow-up imaging 12 months from the initial imaging study or earlier if a patient begins developing symptoms.

The primary goal of rotator cuff repair is to reestablish the mechanical link between the rotator cuff tendon and its bony insertion, in order to allow for improved function, strength, and pain relief. Principles for rotator cuff repair include adequate tendon mobilization to permit a tension-free repair with sufficient time-zero repair integrity to allow for tendon healing [13–16]. Overall, arthroscopic or open rotator cuff repair typically results in significant improvement in pain and function for the majority of patients [17–21]. Retear rates average around 21–26% but can vary according to tear size, chronicity, and repair technique; retear rates as high as 91% have been reported for large-to-massive tears [22, 23]. Despite relatively predictable improvements in pain relief, improvements in strength are more predictable in patients for whom rotator cuff repair leads to tendon-to-bone healing [18, 21, 24]. A number of factors can contribute to the healing potential of the torn rotator cuff, including patient age and comorbidities, tear size and chronicity, presence of fat infiltration of the muscle belly, and repair technique [24–28].

Repair Construct: Single Row vs. Double Row vs. Transosseous

In an attempt to improve the tendon-to-bone interface of rotator cuff repair, surgical techniques have transitioned through a number of different methods since the first open transosseous repair. Arthroscopic technique alone has changed to include arthroscopic single-row anchored repair, arthroscopic double-row anchored repair, arthroscopic transosseous equivalent, and arthroscopic anchorless transosseous repairs [25, 29–32]. These variations in arthroscopic techniques have been developed with the intention of achieving improved tendon-to-bone construct fixation and improved tendon-to-bone contact area for maximal healing potential.

The anatomical footprint of the supraspinatus tendon averages 12.7 mm from medial to lateral and 16.3 mm from anterior to posterior [33]. Relative to the anatomical footprint, single-row anchor repair constructs may only restore 46% of the normal tendon-bone interface compared with

71% for simple transosseous repair and 100% for double-row suture anchor repairs [34]. One study found that a transosseous-equivalent repair using four-suture bridge technique demonstrated over 90% more contact area and 42% greater contact pressure at the insertion site over a double-row repair ([35, 36], Part 1). Along with improved contact area, double-row repairs have demonstrated greater ultimate tensile loads compared with single-row repairs, decreased gap formation, and less strain at the repair site [35–38].

When comparing transosseous equivalent and arthroscopic anchorless transosseous techniques, one cadaveric study demonstrated that the transosseous equivalent technique had greater average load to failure (558 N vs. 291 N) and decreased average gap formation (5 mm vs. 8 mm) compared to transosseous anchorless repair [39]. However, when the authors modified the suture orientation of the anchorless transosseous repair to have an "X-Box" configuration, the average load to failure increased to 388 N. Whether these biomechanical strength differences in the cadaverics lead to changes in clinical outcome is unclear. Based upon rotator cuff cross-sectional area, Burkhart has calculated that the typical maximal physiologic load that a two-tendon rotator cuff repair site may be subject to is roughly 302 N [13]. Considering that many surgeons utilize passive range-of-motion or complete immobilization protocols in the early postoperative phase, it is even less clear what level of biomechanical strength is necessary to prevent construct failure in vivo.

In general, the type of rotator cuff fixation utilized has not demonstrated significant differences in patient functional outcomes [40–43]. Some systematic reviews have found an increased rate of partial- and full-thickness retears in patients undergoing single-row fixation compared to double-row fixation [26, 44] although functional differences were not detectable. Given that the functional outcomes may not be detectable between single-row and double-row or transosseous equivalent techniques, there is some debate as to whether routine use of a double-row anchor or transosseous equivalent surgical technique is justifiable. Our opinion is that arthroscopic anchorless transosseous surgical technique offers the benefits of improved rotator cuff repair contact area compared with single-row, while also being less costly when compared to double-row or transosseous equivalent techniques. One study, evaluating the cost of transosseous equivalent technique versus anchorless transosseous technique, showed that anchorless transosseous technique was on average $336 less expensive per case with no difference in surgical time [45]. This difference in cost was more substantial for larger rotator cuff tears where transosseous equivalent technique required additional suture anchors (Fig. 4.13).

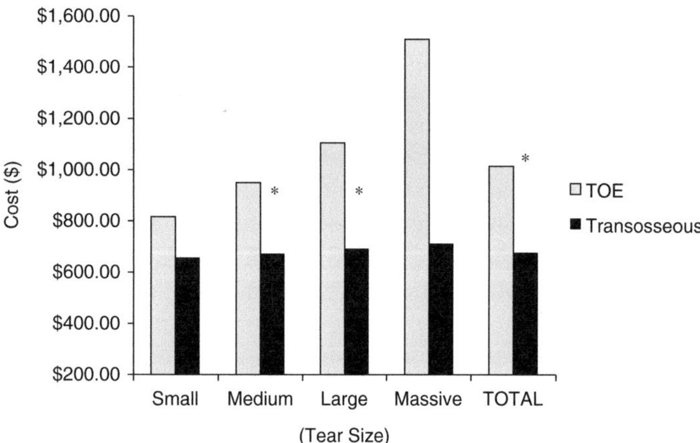

FIGURE 4.13 Cost of arthroscopic anchorless transosseous vs. transosseous equivalent depending upon rotator cuff tear size. TOE—transosseous equivalent; *Asterisk* denotes *p*-value <0.0001. *Note:* Authors felt that statistical significance was not reached in the small and massive tears because of smaller sample sizes in those two groups (with permission from Black EM, Austin LS, Narzikul et al. Comparison of implant cost and surgical time in arthroscopic transosseous and transosseous equivalent rotator cuff repair. J Shoulder Elbow Surg. 2016;25(9):1449–56 (Epub: S1058–2746(16)0026-4))

Role of Subacromial Decompression and Acromioplasty

The premise of subacromial decompression and acromioplasty is based upon the concept of extrinsic compression of the rotator cuff leading to rotator cuff impingement and development of subsequent tearing [46, 47]. Prior studies have classified acromial morphology into three shapes (straight, curved, and hooked) and linked these morphologies with varying prevalence to rotator cuff pathology [48, 49]. Neer advocated anterior acromioplasty to decompress the subacromial space for patients with impingement syndrome [46, 47]. However, this may have deleterious effects in the setting of a rotator cuff tear by releasing the coracoacromial ligament and destabilizing the coracoacromial arch. Such destabilization may allow for anterosuperior escape if the rotator cuff repair fails [50, 51]. Additional complications of acromioplasty include potential acromial fracture as well as disruption of the deltoid origin [52, 53].

There are several studies to suggest that the routine use of acromioplasty with rotator cuff repair may not be necessary [54–59]. Gartsman and O'Connor conducted a prospective randomized study in patients with isolated full-thickness tears of the supraspinatus tendon and a type 2 acromion [56]. Patients were randomized to receive or not receive subacromial decompression with rotator cuff repair. At a minimum of 1-year follow-up, there was no difference in American Shoulder and Elbow Surgeons (ASES) scores. Similarly, Abrams et al. performed a prospective study and randomized patients undergoing arthroscopic rotator cuff repair to acromioplasty and non-acromioplasty groups [55]. At 2 years, both groups demonstrated significant improvements in functional outcome scores with no difference between the acromioplasty and non-acromioplasty groups in regard to ASES and Constant scores. Given the lack of evidence to support the routine use of arthroscopic acromioplasty, we rarely perform it with rotator cuff repair.

Clinical Pearls/Pitfalls

- There is no minimum anterior-to-posterior distance between the medial holes of the bone tunnels created by the drill and awl. This is because the bone bridge for the simple sutures is length of bone from medial hole to lateral hole for each tunnel and medially the rip-stop suture does not need a bone bridge.
- In contrast to the medial tunnel holes, the lateral tunnel holes require a bone bridge between tunnels. With the tunneler device sitting flush in the medial hole, attention must be paid to the spacing of the lateral holes that will be drilled. We recommend a minimum anterior-posterior distance of 5–10 mm between adjacent lateral tunnel holes. If these lateral tunnel holes are placed too closely and converge, then the later step of tying the lateral limbs of the rip-stop suture can be compromised.
- If integrity of the lateral cortical bone in the greater tuberosity is in question, the transosseous tunnels can be reinforced by placing tunnel augment implants (Tornier © TunnelPro). We use them infrequently.
- After passing sutures into their respective tunnels, it is imperative that the medial and lateral limbs of the suture be organized because only the medial limbs of the suture will eventually be passed through the rotator cuff tendon. We prefer to use color-coordinated hemostats—one hemostat on the medial suture limbs and two hemostats on the lateral suture limbs. Each color corresponds to a separate tunnel and its corresponding sutures.
- When tying sutures, the rip-stop sutures from adjacent tunnels should be tied prior to tying the simple sutures. By doing so, the rip-stop suture helps with reduction of the rotator cuff tear and also sits beneath the simple sutures.

References

1. Templehof S, Rupp S, Seil R. Age-related prevalence of rotator cuff tears in asymptomatic shoulders. J Shoulder Elb Surg. 1999;8:296–9.

  2. Yamamoto A, Takagishi K, Osawa T, et al. Prevalence and risk factors of a rotator cuff tear in the general population. J Shoulder Elb Surg. 2010;19(1):116–20.
  3. Kim HM, Teefey SA, Zelig A, et al. Shoulder strength in asymptomatic individuals with intact compared with torn rotator cuffs. J Bone Joint Surg Am. 2009;91(2):289–96.
  4. Yamaguchi K, Ditsios K, Middleton WD, et al. The demographic and morphological features of rotator cuff disease. A comparison of asymptomatic and symptomatic shoulders. J Bone Joint Surg Am. 2006a;88(8):1699–704.
  5. Yamaguchi K, Ditsios K, Middleton WD, et al. The demographic and morphologic features of rotator cuff disease: a comparison of symptomatic and asymptomatic shoulders. J Bone Joint Surg Am. 2006b;88A:1699–704.
  6. Yamaguchi K, Tetro AM, Blam O, et al. Natural history of asymptomatic rotator cuff tears: a longitudinal analysis of asymptomatic tears detected sonographically. J Shoulder Elb Surg. 2001;10(3):199–203.
  7. Moosmayer S, Tariq R, Stiris M, Smith HJ. The natural history of asymptomatic rotator cuff tears: a three-year follow-up of fifty cases. J Bone Joint Surg Am. 2013;95(14):1249–55.
  8. Keener JD, Hsu JE, Steger-May K, et al. Patterns of tear progression for asymptomatic degenerative rotator cuff tears. J Shoulder Elb Surg. 2015a;24(12):1845–51.
  9. Keener JD, Galatz LM, Teefey SA, et al. A prospective evaluation of survivorship of asymptomatic degenerative rotator cuff tears. J Bone Joint Surg Am. 2015b;97(2):89–98.
10. Fucentese SF, von Roll AL, Pfirrmann CW, et al. Evolution of nonoperatively treated symptomatic isolated full-thickness supraspinatus tears. J Bone Joint Surg Am. 2012;94(9):801–8.
11. Tashjian RZ. Risk of tear progression in nonoperatively treated small full-thickness rotator cuff tears: commentary on article by Sandro F. Fucentses, MD et al: "Evolution of nonoperatively treated symptomatic isolated full-thickness supraspinatus tears". J Bone Joint Surg Am. 2012;94(9):e61.
12. Keener JD. Surveillance of conservatively treated rotator cuff tears is warranted. Commentary on an article by Stefan Mossmayer, MD, PhD, et al. "The natural history of asymptomatic rotator cuff tears. A three-year follow-up of fifty cases". J Bone Joint Surg Am. 2013;95(14):e101–2.
13. Burkhart SS. A stepwise approach to arthroscopic rotator cuff repair based on biomechanical principles. Arthroscopy. 2000;16:82–90.

14. Blaine TA, Freehill MQ, Bigliani LU. Technique of open rotator cuff repair. Instr Course Lect. 2001;50:43–52.
15. Ahmad CS, Steward AM, Izquierdo R, et al. Tendon-bone interface motion in transosseous suture and suture anchor rotator cuff repair techniques. Am J Sports Med. 2005;33:1667–71.
16. Gerber C, Schneeberger AG, Beck M, et al. Mechanical strength of repairs of the rotator cuff. J Bone Joint Surg Br. 1994;76:371–80.
17. Ellman H, Kay SP, Wirth M. Arthroscopic treatment of full-thickness rotator cuff tears: 2- to 7-year follow-up study. Arthroscopy. 1993;9(2):195–200.
18. Harryman DT, Mack LA, Wang KY, et al. Repairs of the rotator cuff. Correlation of functional results with integrity of the rotator cuff. J Bone Joint Surg Am. 1991;73A:982–9.
19. Hawkins RJ, Misamore GW, Hobeika PE. Surgery for full-thickness rotator-cuff tears. J Bone Joint Surg Am. 1985;67(9):1349–55.
20. Lee E, Bishop JY, Braman JP, et al. Outcomes after arthroscopic rotator cuff repairs. J Shoulder Elbow Surg. 2007;16(1):1–5. Epub
21. Galatz LM, Griggs S, Cameron BD, et al. Prospective longitudinal analysis of postoperative shoulder function: a ten-year follow-up study of full-thickness rotator cuff tears. J Bone Joint Surg Am. 2001;83A(7):102–1056.
22. Galatz LM, Ball CM, Teefey SA, et al. The outcomes and repair integrity of completely arthroscopically repaired large and massive rotator cuff tears. J Bone Joint Surg Am. 2004;83A:1052–6.
23. Hein J, Reilly JM, Chae J, et al. Retear rates after arthroscopic single-row, double-row and suture bridge rotator cuff repair at a minimum of 1 year of imaging follow-up: a systematic review. Arthroscopy. 2015;31(11):2274–81.
24. Boileau P, Brassart N, Watkinson DJ, et al. Arthroscopic repairs of full-thickness rotator tears of the supraspinatus: dose the tendon really heal? J Bone Joint Surg Am. 2005;15:290–9.
25. Matsen FA III, Fehringer EV, Lippitt SB, et al. Rotator cuff. In: Rockwood Jr CA, Matsen III FA, editors. The shoulder. 4th ed. Philadelphia: Saunders; 2009. p. 771–880.
26. Saridakis P, Jones G. Outcomes of single-row and double-row arthroscopic rotator cuff repair: a systematic review. J Bone Joint Surg Am. 2010;92(3):732–42.
27. Tashjian RZ, Hollins AM, Kim HM, et al. Factors affecting healing rates after arthroscopic double-row rotator cuff repair. Am J Sports Med. 2010;38(12):2435–42.

28. Goutallier D, Postel JM, Gleyze P, et al. Influence of cuff muscle fatty degeneration on anatomic and functional outcomes after simple suture of full-thickness tears. J Shoulder Elb Surg. 2003;12(6):550–4.
29. Lo IK, Burkhart SS. Double-row arthroscopic rotator cuff repair: reestablishing the footprint of the rotator cuff. Arthroscopy. 2003;19(9):1035–42.
30. Park MC, ElAttrache NS, Ahmad CS, et al. "Transosseous equivalent" rotator cuff repair technique. Arthroscopy. 2006;22(1360):e1–5.
31. Garofalo R, Castagna A, Borroni M, Krishnan SG. Arthroscopic transosseous (anchorless) rotator cuff repair. Knee Surg Sports Traumatol Arthrosc. 2012;20(6):1031–5.
32. Garrigues GE, Lazarus MD. Arthroscopic bone tunnel augmentation for rotator cuff repair. Orthopedics. 2012;35(5):392–7.
33. Dugas JR, Campbell DA, Warren RF, et al. Anatomy and dimensions of rotator cuff insertions. J Shoulder Elb Surg. 2002;11:498–503.
34. Meier SW, Meier JD. Rotator cuff repair: the effect of double-row fixation on three-dimensional repair site. J Shoulder Elb Surg. 2006;15(6):691–6.
35. Park MC, ElAttrache NS, Tibone JE, et al. Part I: footprint contact characteristics for a transosseous-equivalent rotator cuff repair technique compared with a double-row technique. J Shoulder Elb Surg. 2007a;16(4):461–8.
36. Park MC, Tibone JE, ElAttrache NS, et al. Part II: biomechanical assessment for a footprint-restoring transosseous-equivalent rotator cuff repair technique compared with a double-row repair technique. J Shoulder Elb Surg. 2007b;16(4):469–76.
37. Ma CB, Comerford L, Wilson J, et al. Biomechanical evaluation of arthroscopic rotator cuff repairs: double-row compared with single-row fixation. J Bone Joint Surg Am. 2006;88A:403–10.
38. Kim DH, ElAttrache NS, Tibone JE, et al. Biomechanical comparison of single-row versus double-row suture anchor technique for rotator cuff repair. Am J Sports Med. 2006;34:407–14.
39. Salata MJ, Sherman SL, Lin EC, et al. Biomechanical evaluation of transosseous rotator cuff repair: do anchors really matter? Am J Sports Med. 2013;41(2):283–90.
40. Suguya H, Maeda K, Matsuki K, et al. Functional and structural outcome after arthroscopic full-thickness rotator cuff repair: single-row versus double-row fixation. Arthroscopy. 2005;21(1):1307–16.

41. Wall LB, Keener JD, Brophy RH. Clinical outcomes of double-row versus single-row rotator cuff repairs. Arthroscopy. 2009;25(11):1312–8.
42. Francheschi F, Ruzzini L, Longo UG, et al. Equivalent clinical results of arthroscopic single-row and double-row suture anchor repair for rotator cuff repairs: a randomized controlled trial. Am J Sports Med. 2007;35:1254–60.
43. Grasso A, Milano G, Salvatore M, et al. Single-row versus double-row arthroscopic rotator cuff repair: a prospective randomized clinical study. Arthroscopy. 2009;25:4–12.
44. Millet PJ, Warth RJ, Dornan GJ, et al. Clinical and structural outcomes after arthroscopic single-row versus double-row rotator cuff repair: a systematic review and meta-analysis of level I randomized clinical trials. J Shoulder Elb Surg. 2014;23(4):586–97.
45. Black EM, Austin LS, Narzikul A, et al. Comparison of implant cost and surgical time in arthroscopic transosseous and transosseous equivalent rotator cuff repair. J Shoulder Elbow Surg. 2016;25(9):1449–56. Epub: S1058–2746(16)0026-4.
46. Neer CS. Anterior acromioplasty for the chronic impingement syndrome in the shoulder: a preliminary report. J Bone Joint Surg Am. 1972a;54(1):41–50.
47. Neer CS. Anterior acromioplasty for the chronic impingement syndrome in the shoulder: a preliminary report. J Bone Joint Surg Am. 1972b;54A:141–50.
48. Bigliani LU, Morrison DS, April EW. The morphology of the acromion and its relationship to rotator cuff tears. Orthop Trans. 1986;10:228.
49. Bigliani LU, Ticker JB, Flatow EL, et al. The relationship of acromial architecture to rotator cuff disease. Clin Sports Med. 1991;10(4):823–38.
50. Su WR, Budoff JE, Luo ZP. The effect of coracoacromial ligament excision and acromioplasty on superior and anterosuperior glenohumeral stability. Arthroscopy. 2009;25(1):13–8.
51. Shi LL, Edwards TB. The role of acromioplasty for management of rotator cuff problems: where is the evidence? Adv Orthop. 2012;2012:467–571.
52. Green A, Griggs S, Labrador D. Anterior acromial anatomy: relevate to arthroscopic acromioplasty. Arthroscopy. 2004;20(10):1050–4.
53. Matthews LS, Burkhead WZ, Gordon S, et al. Acromial fracture: a complication of arthroscopic subacromial decompression. J Shoulder Elb Surg. 1994;3:256–61.

54. Goldberg BA, Lippitt SB, Matsen FA III. Improvement in comfort and function after cuff repair without acromioplasty. Clin Orthop. 2001;390:142–50.
55. Abrams GD, Gupta AK, Hussey KE, et al. Arthroscopic repair of full-thickness rotator cuff tears with and without acromioplasty: a randomized prospective trial with 2-year follow-up. Am J Sports Med. 2014;42(6):1296–303.
56. Gartsman GM, O'Connor DP. Arthroscopic rotator cuff repair with and without arthroscopic subacromial decompression: a prospective, randomized study of one-year outcomes. J Shoulder Elb Surg. 2004;13(4):424–6.
57. MacDonald P, McRae S, Leiter J, Mascarenhas R, Lapner R. Arthroscopic rotator cuff repair with and without acromioplasty in the treatment of full-thickness rotator cuff tears: a multi-center, randomized controlled trial. J Bone Joint Surg Am. 2011;93(21):1953–60.
58. Milano G, Grasso A, Salvatore M, et al. Arthroscopic rotator cuff repair with and without subacromial decompression: a prospective randomized study. Arthroscopy. 2007;23(1):81–8.
59. Shin SJ, Oh JH, Chung SW, Song MH. The efficacy of acromioplasty in the arthroscopic repair of small-to-medium-sized rotator cuff tears without acromial spur: a prospective comparative study. Arthroscopy. 2012;28(5):628–35.

Chapter 5
Open Rotator Cuff Repair

Ashish Gupta and Robert Litchfield

Case Presentation

A 61-year-old right-hand-dominant office worker presented with a 3-month history of a painful right shoulder. The pain was present throughout the day and was aggravated by activity. He complained of night pain, which disturbed his sleep, and he was taking NSAIDs and acetaminophen regularly. He also complained of significant weakness of his shoulder, which was affecting the activities of daily living such that he was unable to lift overhead and unable to carry weights with his right arm. There was no history of trauma. The patient did not smoke tobacco and he denied any medical comorbidities. A subacromial injection provided temporary pain relief and numerous sessions of physiotherapy had yielded no clinical improvement. He had a prior arthroscopic rotator cuff repair of the supraspinatus tendon with a biceps tenodesis 3 years ago with a normal postoperative recovery and return to full function.

A. Gupta, MBBS, MSc, FRACS, FAOrth, CIME
R. Litchfield, M.D., F.R.C.S.C (✉)
Fowler Kennedy Sports Medicine Clinic, 3M Centre, University of Western Ontario, London, ON, Canada
e-mail: rlitchf@uwo.ca

© Springer International Publishing AG 2018
P.J. McMahon (ed.), *Rotator Cuff Injuries*,
DOI 10.1007/978-3-319-63668-9_5

Physical examination demonstrated forward elevation to 160°, abduction to 160°, internal rotation to L3, and external rotation to 40°. Strength testing revealed severe weakness in abduction and external rotation with the arm at the side. He had normal strength in internal rotation and external rotation with the arm at 90° of abduction. There was no tenderness of the bicipital groove or the AC joint.

True anteroposterior (Grashey) axillary lateral and supraspinatus outlet radiographs (Figs. 5.1, 5.2, and 5.3) revealed no osteoarthritis of the glenohumeral joint, moderate osteoarthritis of the acromioclavicular (AC) joint, a mildly curved acromial undersurface, and metal suture anchors in the greater tuberosity. An ultrasound demonstrated a 2.7 × 3 cm supraspinatus tendon tear with retraction to the glenoid. The

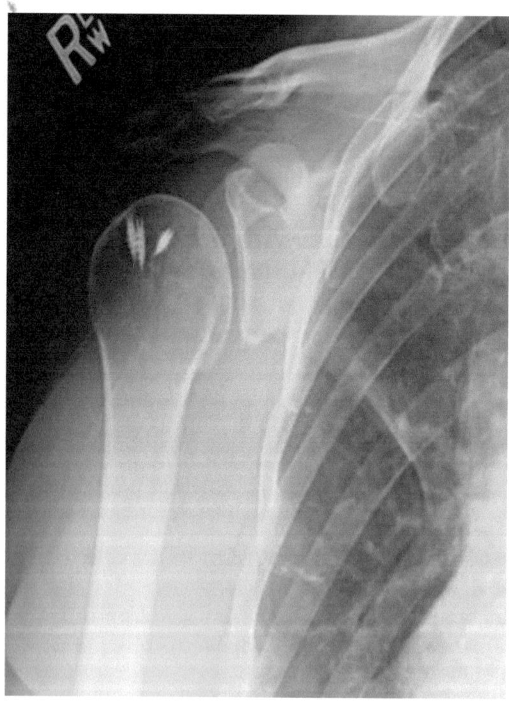

FIGURE 5.1 AP Shoulder

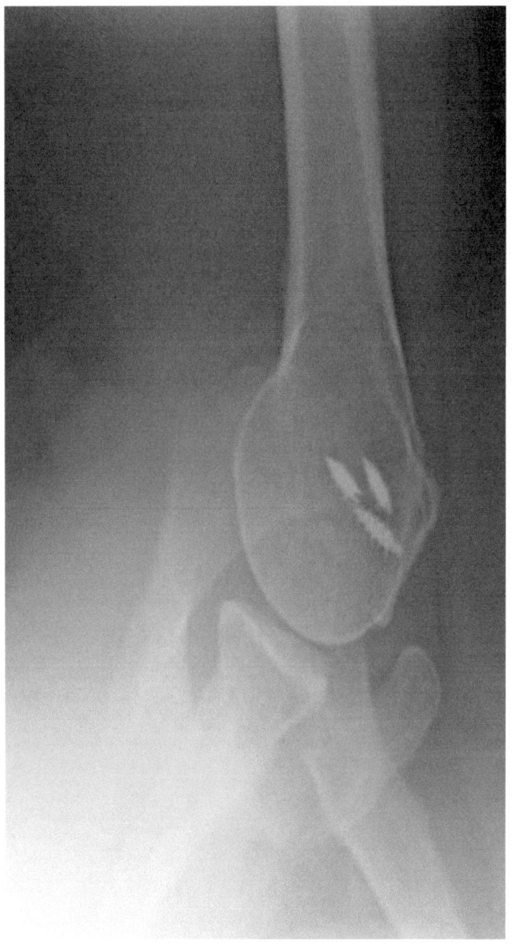

Figure 5.2 Axillary Lateral

tear was noted to extend into the anterior 1/3 of the infraspinatus tendon. The supraspinatus and infraspinatus muscle bellies had normal echogenicity. The subscapularis tendon was intact.

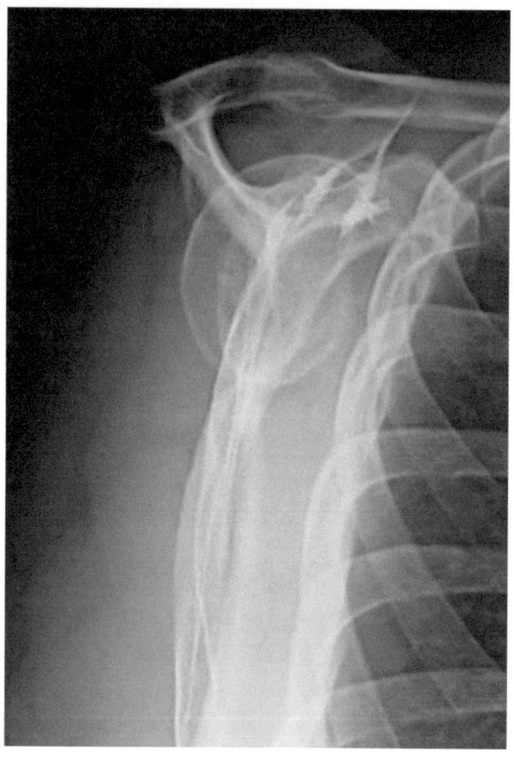

Figure 5.3 Lateral Scapular View

Diagnosis/Assessment

The patient was diagnosed with a symptomatic, recurrent moderate-sized full-thickness rotator cuff tear. We had a lengthy chat discussing the risks and results of a revision rotator cuff repair including the possibility of partial cuff repair or the cuff being nonrepairable. The patient was very keen to proceed with surgery and he consented to an open cuff repair. We prefer the use of an open approach in the case of a revision cuff repair. This approach in our hands gives us the flexibility of grafting defects or performing transfers if needed.

Management

The anesthetist administered an ultrasound-guided intrascalene nerve block in the preanesthetic area. The block has several advantages. It minimizes the need for intraoperative and postoperative opioid analgesia. As the patient is relatively pain free during the procedure, the anesthetist can often control the blood pressure more accurately, as pain causes sympathetic stimulation that in turn leads to an increase in the blood pressure, and this minimizes intraoperative bleeding and improves the surgeon's view of the field.

The patient was administered a general anesthetic and a second-generation cephalosporin. The patient was positioned in the beach-chair position, at 45° of inclination with a shoulder positioner (T-max®, Smith and Nephew, USA) (Fig. 5.4). All the bony prominences are padded. The upper extremity was prepped and draped in a sterile fashion and the patient's arm was held by a pneumatic articulating arm (Spider®, Smith and Nephew, USA).

The surface anatomy was marked on the skin including the clavicle, acromion, acromioclavicular joint, and coracoid and the skin incision was marked with a line from the posterior margin of the AC joint to the anterolateral edge of the acromion and extending another 3 cm distally. This results in a total incision length of about 5 cm (Fig. 5.5).

Five milliliters of Marcaine with adrenaline was injected in the subcutaneous tissue and the skin incision was made. The skin and subcutaneous tissue were retracted so we could see the deltoid muscle. The junction of the anterior and middle portions of the deltoid is the raphe identified by a fat streak (Fig. 5.6) and split so as to minimize trauma to the deltoid muscle. The deltoid origin was dissected off the superior

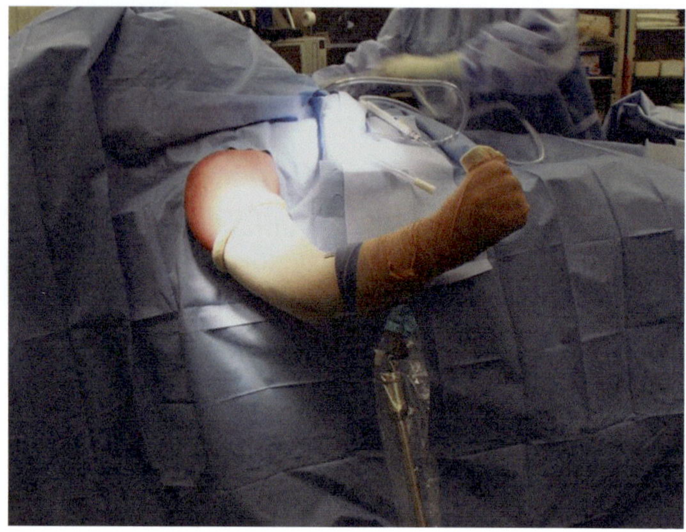

Figure 5.4 Beach-chair position

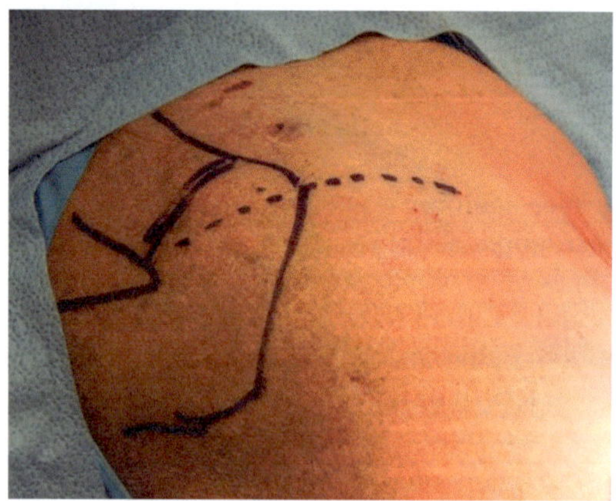

Figure 5.5 The skin incision is marked

surface of the acromion with anterior and posterior flaps. Care must be taken during this step to elevate about 2 cm of the anterior deltoid along with the periosteum as a single layer.

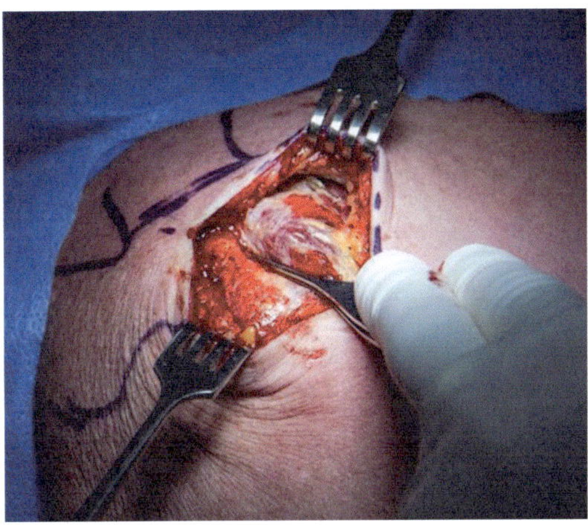

FIGURE 5.6 The deltoid raphe

The coracoacromial ligament was incised off the acromion and the underlying artery that bleeds copiously was coagulated. The posterior deltoid flap was 1 cm in length and also included its periosteum. While we do not routinely perform a subacromial decompression, our indication being impingement signs on physical examination and radiographs with a type II or type III acromion, in this case the subacromial decompression began with a Cobb's elevator being inserted into the subacromial space and the humeral head being depressed. The anterior 1/3 of the undersurface of the acromion was excised with the aid of a 1 cm wide osteotome. An oscillating saw can alternatively be used. The undersurface was flattened with a rasp. At the end of the subacromial decompression the surgeon can easily insert the tip of the index finger under the acromion with the arm in minimal traction. Next the thick subacromial bursa was excised along with the bursa from under the anterior, lateral, and posterior deltoid. This is easier with external and internal rotation of the flexed shoulder.

The rotator cuff tear size, pattern, and retraction were next determined. This was made easier by placing multiple traction stitches with 1.0 Vicryl suture into the edge of the tendon (Figs. 5.7 and 5.8) so that the best repair could be planned. We identified each rotator cuff tendon. First the subscapularis was inspected. The biceps tendon was retracted posteriorly and the arm was internally rotated and flexed to 90° to take the tension off the subscapularis. The subscapularis tendon is better seen after the rotator interval is opened and the rotator interval tissue is excised. An anteriorly subluxed biceps tendon or a biceps tendon which subluxes with internal rotation of the humeral head (Sentinel sign) is highly suggestive

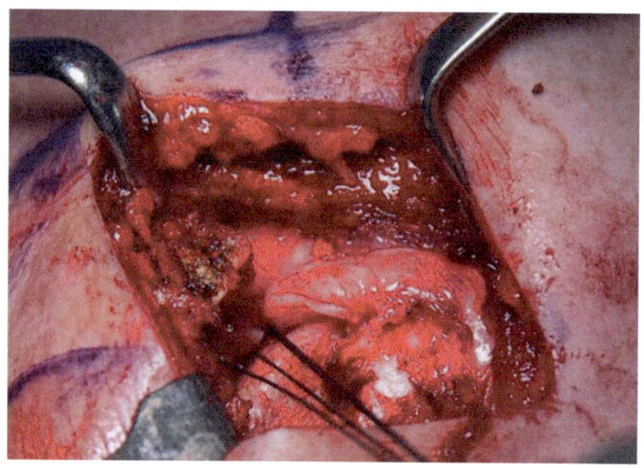

FIGURE 5.7 Supraspinatus traction suture

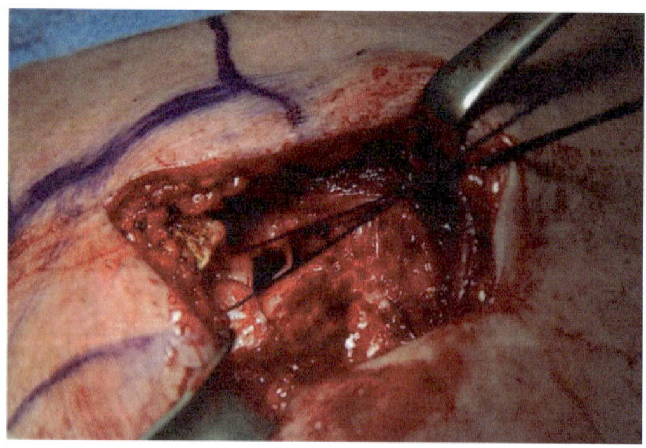

FIGURE 5.8 Infraspinatus traction suture

of a subscapularis tendon tear. Next was the supraspinatus. The size, pattern, and retraction of the tear were noted. Retraction was classified according to the Patte classification. Stage 1 is the torn tendon edge being close to its bony insertion. Stage 2 is the torn tendon edge at the level of humeral head. Stage 3 is the torn tendon edge at the glenoid. Delamination of the tendon was also noted. In cases of chronic rupture where the tendon is retracted to the glenoid rim it may be difficult to delineate the tendon from the superior labrum as the tendon is stuck down to it. Lastly the infraspinatus and teres minor were inspected. The arm was placed besides the thorax and maximally internally rotated. Traction was applied to the posterior cuff so that the extent of the tear could be seen. To do so, the posterior subdeltoid bursa needs to be totally excised, and as it is usually very vascular, the use of electrocautery is preferred.

Most important in large-to-massive chronic cuff tears, we also performed a systematic cuff mobilization for our moderate-sized tear. This was performed in an anterior-to-posterior direction and for large-to-massive retracted tears we prefer a general anesthetic with muscle relaxation. First the coracohumeral ligament was incised medially close to its origin from the coracoid while traction was applied to the torn edge of the supraspinatus tendon. This usually results in a sudden increase in the excursion of the tendon. Then the subacromial adhesions to the supraspinatus were excised with the use of Mayo scissors to the spine of the scapula, which is palpable posteriorly. The undersurface of the supraspinatus was released off its adhesions to the glenoid labrum. A No. 15 blade can be used to incise the interval between the labrum and the supraspinatus. This window was then utilized and a Mayo scissors or a Cobb elevator was used to release the medial undersurface of the supraspinatus. Care must be taken to avoid injury to the infraspinatus branch of the supra-scapular nerve which lies 1 cm medial to the glenoid surface. If the tendon is delaminated, traction is applied to the inferior leaflet while the release is done.

Now the quality of tendon, and its excursion, was evaluated with the patient under a general anesthetic under complete paralysis. It must be noted that a premature evaluation of the cuff mobility may misguide the surgeon and lead to a cuff repair under excessive tension. Three situations may now arise. First, the rotator cuff can be mobilized to the lateral edge of the cuff footprint. This is the ideal scenario where the cuff mobilization is complete and a double-row repair can be performed. This is our preferred technique. Second, there can be incomplete mobilization of the cuff to the osteochondral junction or the medial edge of the footprint. In this scenario, the rotator cuff is repaired medial to the footprint with a single-row technique. This repair may be augmented with a synthetic or an allogenic graft or patch. Lastly, there can be mobilization medial to the humeral head. For these irreparable rotator cuff tears the options include a subacromial decompression and lysis of adhesions or a muscle transfer procedure such as a latissimus dorsi transfer. The decision is based upon the patient's age, function, as well as extent of glenohumeral arthrosis. An older patient with retracted irreparable cuff tear would be a candidate for a reverse total shoulder arthroplasty.

There is a fine balance between cuff mobilization and cuff damage. We caution against performing large interval slides and excessive cuff debridement as this may result in denervation of the muscle or compromise the blood supply.

For our transosseous repair (Figs. 5.9, 5.10, and 5.11) four strands of #5 Ethibond were passed through the greater tuberosity from lateral to medial with 2 cm bone bridges, exiting near the articular margin. Drill holes were avoided as we think this weakens the bone and we want to minimize suture cut out as often the bone is osteopenic. The next step is to bring the torn edge of the anterior supraspinatus to its location on the greater tuberosity just posterolateral to the biceps groove. The sutures were passed through the rotator cuff about 1.5 cm medial to the rotator cable with the Mason-Allen technique. The result was a horizontal suture configuration medially that provided traction to the cuff and a vertical transosseous suture configuration laterally that compressed the cuff onto the footprint of the greater tuberosity for minimal gap forming between the tendon and the bone. This technique maximizes contact across the footprint and

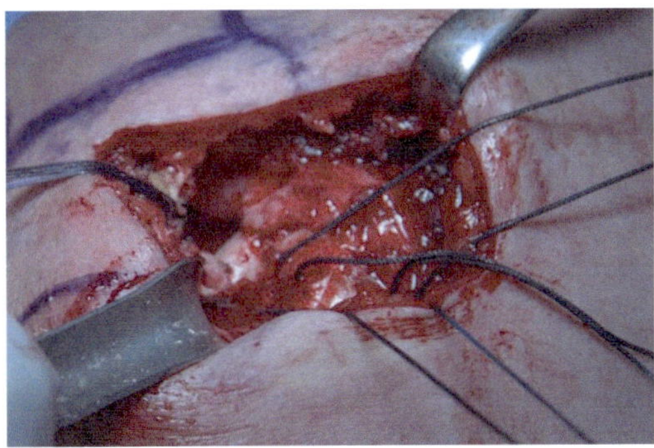

FIGURE 5.9 Double-row transosseous sutures into the greater tuberosity

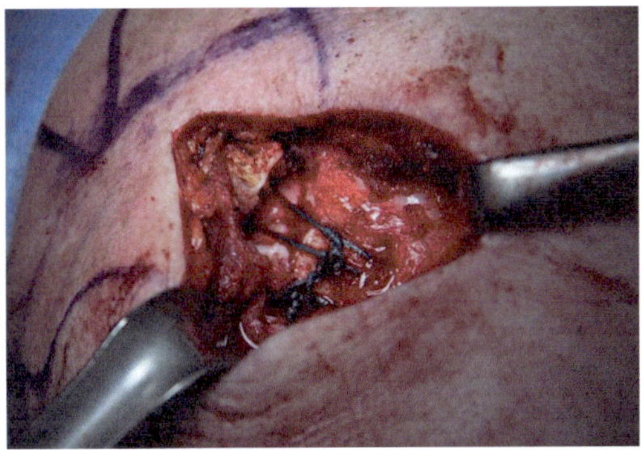

FIGURE 5.10 Transosseous cuff repair

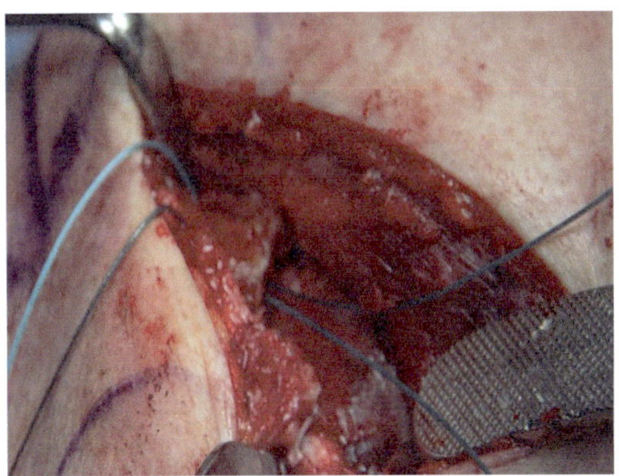

FIGURE 5.11 Transosseous No. 2 Ethibond®

reproduces in essence a double-row repair. Prior to tying down the transosseous sutures consider closing any defects in the intervals with side-to-side sutures; these sutures can take considerable tension off the primary repair.

Although not used in this case as it is a revision procedure, the senior author often performs a double-row repair with double-loaded medial row anchors and knotless lateral row anchors as described below.

We prefer the transosseous technique for revision surgery but often use a double-row cuff repair with other open rotator cuff repairs. In this repair all of the torn tendon and scar tissue are debrided off of the footprint on the greater tuberosity with a rongeur and a small osteotome until there is punctate bleeding. Care must be taken not to excessively debride the cortical bone as in elderly patients the underlying cancellous bone may be osteopenic. Depending upon the tear size 1–3 double-loaded suture anchors are placed at the osteochondral junction of the humerus. The author prefers a plastic anchor as there is less artifact compared to a metal anchor if a postoperative MRI is done. An anchor must be positioned just posterior to the biceps so that when sutures are then passed through the cuff with a Mason-Allen configuration the torn edge of the anterior supraspinatus is repaired to its location on the greater tuberosity just posterolateral to the biceps groove. Care must be taken that the sutures are passed through both the superficial and the deep layer of the cuff especially if it is delaminated. More anchors are placed and sutures are passed sequentially posterior. Sutures are passed medial to the rotator cuff cable but not yet tied. Albeit tempting, the surgeon must resist making the transverse limb of the suture too broad as this causes more devascularization of the cuff and more movement of the repair that may be a cause of failure. Once all the sutures are passed, traction is applied to all the sutures to evaluate the final cuff positioning. Some of the tear can usually be repaired with side-to-side suturing with nonabsorbable sutures. Remember not to cut your medial row sutures after tying them so that they may be used for the lateral row repair. Performing a side-to-side repair prior to tying the sutures down results in better distribution of forces and prevents dog ear formation. [Authors, is this something you want to include in the transosseous technique or do you only do it in the double-row repair? ADDED] The sutures are now tied down starting posterior and going anterior. This enables the cuff to be brought forward as it is brought lateral as often the supraspinatus is pulled posteriorly by its infraspinatus connections. By the end of this step the cuff must be well positioned and repaired to the footprint. Before the lateral row anchor insertion every other suture end is cut off leaving four suture ends. The anterior and the posterior anchor must have one suture each for the lateral row repair. Alternatively two lateral row anchors can be used allowing incorporation of additional medial sutures. The arm is now abducted and internally rotated to expose the lateral aspect of the greater tuberosity, which is then debrided, and one or two double-row anchors with two to four sutures each are inserted to attain a crisscross suture configuration. The anchors are tapped into place with the sutures under tension. Care must be taken to avoid excessive tension on the sutures. At the end the humeral head and greater tuberosity should be covered by the repaired rotator cuff. The shoulder is than taken through a complete range of rotation to ascertain that a complete repair is attained. The wound is irrigated with copious amounts of saline and hemostasis is attained.

In our case the deltoid was reattached by placing sutures through the acromion (Fig. 5.12) with two sutures of #2 Ethibond® suture on a cutting needle placed in each the posterior and anterior limb of the deltoid. The remainder or the deltoid is closed in a side-to-side fashion with #1 absorbable suture. [Authors, I do not understand what you mean by the "medial free edges of each limb" (Removed)] A layered skin closure was performed. The wound was dressed with a waterproof dressing and the arm was immobilized in a broad arm sling with an abduction pillow for comfort.

Most of our patients go home the same day as the procedure. Our patient was instructed to take a long-acting opiod

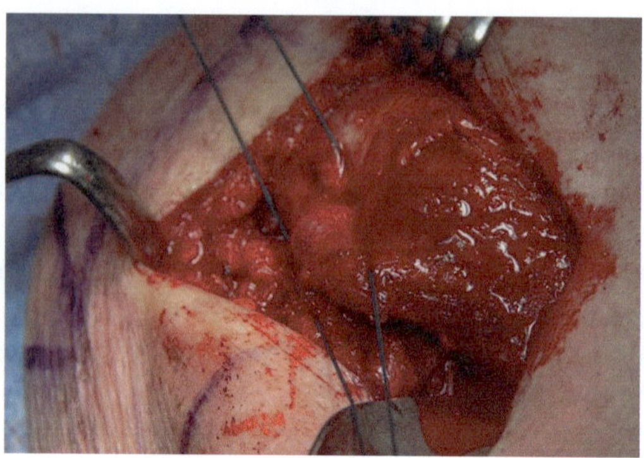

FIGURE 5.12 Deltoid repair transosseous acromial sutures

before going to bed even if he was not yet in pain to avoid the sudden onset of pain in the early hours of the morning when the interscalene block wore off.

Our patient began active motion of the wrist and elbow on day 1 and gentle pendulum exercises of the shoulder on day 2. He was advised against lifting anything heavier than a coffee mug for 4 weeks. The rehabilitation then consisted of four phases. Phase 1 from 0 to 6 weeks was passive range of motion (ROM). The aims of this phase are to maintain posture, enhance comfort of the arm in the sling, reduce pain and swelling, encourage controlled passive range of motion within pain toleration, avoid stiffness of the joint, and avoid active muscle contraction. The patient was encouraged to wear the sling day and night for the first 4 weeks and nighttime only for the next 2 weeks. Phase 2 from 6 to 12 weeks began with active assist and progressed to active range of motion as tolerated. The aim of this phase was diminished stiffness of the glenohumeral joint with a goal of 90–120° of motion at the glenohumeral joint in both flexion and abduction. We want to restore ROM without scapular compensation. The resting pain considerably decreased. HE started functional activities and activities of daily living and proprioception exercises below shoulder height. Phase 3 from 12 to

18 weeks was resisted exercises for strengthening, and we addressed specific strength deficits. He progressed with functional activities and heavier activities of daily living below shoulder height and specifically he increased external rotation strength and endurance. There was now satisfactory range of movement in flexion and external rotation that was to 160° and external rotation at the side was 45° and in abduction was 90°. Phase 4 began at 16 weeks and consisted of advanced strengthening and dynamic stability. The patient had full pain-free active ROM and continued to improve in strength, stability, and endurance and there was specifically continued emphasis on external rotation strength. Functional activities with activities of daily living above shoulder height were initiated. He lastly advanced in strengthening with plyometric training as he desired to return to overhead sports. The program would have been the same had he been a laborer and wanted to return to such an occupation.

Outcome

Our experience with the open transosseous cuff repair technique is very satisfying. The tendon can be repaired anatomically and securely utilizing the techniques described. In a revision situation the expectations are tempered with respect to range of motion and strength but an improvement in pain is generally achieved. We tell all patients that the recovery is at best 10% a month so that they understand the realistic recovery timeline. With careful patient selection, tissue management, and use of antibiotic prophylaxis the infection and wound complication rates should be very low.

Literature Review

Even though the arthroscopic rotator cuff repair is now a common procedure, open rotator cuff repair has stood the test of time. The simplicity of the procedure with minimal equipment ensures that an orthopedic surgeon can safely perform it. Our aim with all of our rotator cuff repairs is four-fold, to attain anatomic and tension-free fixation with minimal gap formation, ensure mechanical stability while the tendon is loaded during rehabilitation, optimize bone tendon healing, and minimize the incidence of re-rupture. Mochizuki and coworkers [1] in a study of 113 cadaveric shoulders demonstrated that the supraspinatus tendon insertion was triangular with an average measurement of 6.9 mm in the mediolateral direction and 12.6 mm in the AP direction. Its insertion is the anterior most part of the highest point of the greater tuberosity. The infraspinatus tendon has a trapezoidal footprint with an average measurement of 10.2 mm in the mediolateral direction and 32.7 mm in the AP direction. It has a broad insertion that curves anteriorly to the anterolateral part of the greater tuberosity.

In a histological study of the cuff insertion Fallon and coworkers [2] found that the medial part of the supraspinatus tendon consists of horizontally aligned collagen fibers known as the rotator cable and then in the lateral part of the tendon the collagen fibers convert to a multidirectional weave interdigitating with fibrocartilage as they insert into the greater tuberosity. The densely packed unidirectional collagen fibers of the rotator cable extend from the coracohumeral ligament anteriorly to the infraspinatus tendon posteriorly, coursing both superficial and deep to the tendon. The capsule is composed of thin collagen sheets each with uniform fiber alignment that differ slightly between sheets. This creates a specialized tendon capable of internally compensating for changing joint angles by the fascicles which are structurally independent and can slide relative to one another. The tendon insertion is adapted to disperse tension and compression. The forces in the rotator cuff greatly vary and depend upon the arm position [3–5]. The supraspinatus tendon experiences forces ranging from 43 to 350 N and with abduction the maximal force is concentrated at its insertion with more load on the articular than the bursal surface. The infraspinatus tendon experiences forces ranging from 55 to 900 N. Since maximal force in the rotator cuff is at its insertion, we think a repair with a medial row is important.

Biomechanical studies have highlighted the superiority of a double-row repair in recreating the anatomy of the footprint, reducing gap formation, and providing initial stability to allow for cuff healing [6–9]. Despite this, the clinical outcomes of some studies have shown that double-row and single-row repair techniques are the same [10, 11]. Others have found the single-row repair to be inferior. In a recent meta-analysis, Millet and coworkers [12] reported that the single-row repair had a higher retear rate of 25.9% compared to 14.2% for the double-row repair (relative risk of 1.76). Hein and coworkers [13] evaluated retear rates between single-row and double-row and suture bridge techniques. They analyzed small (<1 cm), medium (1–3 cm), large (3–5 cm), and massive (>5 cm) tears. With all tear sizes the single-row repair had a higher retear rate compared to double-row and suture bridge techniques ($p = 0.024$, relative risk 1.07, 95% confidence interval 1.01–1.14). Of note after repair of the large and massive tears there was a retear rate of 48 and 34% (611 tears) after single-row repair and 78% vs. 40% (161 tears) after double-row repair, respectively. No difference was found in the retear rates between double-row and suture bridge techniques.

There has been considerable debate of the superiority of the mini open technique and the arthroscopic cuff repair. The mini open technique has the advantage of being an easier procedure to learn but has more complications of deltoid detachment, postoperative scarring, and infection. The arthroscopic technique enables better visualization and repair of all types of rotator cuff tears with small incisions; however it is harder to learn. Ji and coworkers [14] performed a meta-analysis of five level 1 randomized control trials comparing arthroscopic and mini open cuff repair and found no difference in surgery time, functional outcome score, pain with the visual analog scale, and range of motion. Van der Zwaal and coworkers [15] found no difference in clinical outcome, range of motion, pain, and complications between arthroscopic and mini open rotator cuff repairs at 1 year of follow-up in 100 patients. However, patients had the benefits of diminished pain and improved range of motion sooner, after 6 weeks, with an arthroscopic repair. In the end however, both techniques have similar outcomes.

Clinical Pearls/Pitfalls

- Regional anesthetic provides excellent perioperative pain relief and enables the anesthetist to control the blood pressure, which in turn results in less bleeding within the surgical field.
- The deltoid should be elevated along with its periosteum as a single layer and anterior and posterior flaps created.
- Acromion resection should not be the same in all cases; significant variation exists in the thickness of the acromion. Care must be taken not to resect too much bone, as it may result in an acromion fracture. Care must also be taken to identify an os acromiale and resect the acro-, meta-, and meso-type and fix the baso-type os acromiale. [Authors, do you agree? YES]
- The rotator cuff can be tagged with traction sutures so that the tear pattern, size, retraction, and tissue quality can be best evaluated.
- Systematic sequential cuff releases are performed from the anterior to the posterior direction. The subacromial and intra-articular adhesions are released.
- Cuff mobility is tested. With large-to-massive chronic rotator cuff repairs complete muscle paralysis aids in determining cuff mobility.
- Small cuff tears are repaired with a single-row technique and more severe tears are repaired with a double-row or a transosseous technique.
- The deltoid is reattached with transosseous sutures passing through the acromion using No. 5 Ethibond®.
- A graduated and physician-supervised rehabilitation program is followed.

References

1. Mochizuki T, Sugaya H, Uomizu M, et al. Humeral insertion of the supraspinatus and infraspinatus. New anatomical findings regarding the footprint of the rotator cuff. J Bone Joint Surg Am. 2008;90:962–9.
2. Fallon J, Blevins FT, Vogel K, Trotter J. Functional morphology of the supraspinatus tendon. J Orthop Res. 2002;20:920–6.
3. Cole BJ, ElAttrache NS, Anbari A. Arthroscopic rotator cuff repairs: an anatomic and biomechanical rationale for different suture-anchor repair configurations. Arthroscopy. 2007;23:662–9.
4. Wakabayashi I, Itoi E, Sano H, et al. Mechanical environment of the supraspinatus tendon: a two-dimensional finite element model analysis. J Shoulder Elb Surg. 2003;12:612–7.
5. Juul-Kristensen B, Bojsen-Moller F, Finsen L, et al. Muscle sizes and moment arms of rotator cuff muscles determined by magnetic resonance imaging. Cells Tissues Organs. 2000;167:214–22.
6. Mazzocca AD, Millett PJ, Guanche CA, Santangelo SA, Arciero RA. Arthroscopic single-row versus double-row suture anchor rotator cuff repair. Am J Sports Med. 2005;33:1861–8.
7. Kim DH, Elattrache NS, Tibone JE, et al. Biomechanical comparison of a single-row versus double-row suture anchor technique for rotator cuff repair. Am J Sports Med. 2006;34:407–14.
8. Ma CB, Comerford L, Wilson J, Puttlitz CM. Biomechanical evaluation of arthroscopic rotator cuff repairs: double-row compared with single-row fixation. J Bone Joint Surg Am. 2006;88:403–10.
9. Wall LB, Keener JD, Brophy RH. Double-row vs single-row rotator cuff repair: a review of the biomechanical evidence. J Shoulder Elb Surg. 2009;18:933–41.
10. Wall LB, Keener JD, Brophy RH. Clinical outcomes of double-row versus single-row rotator cuff repairs. Arthroscopy. 2009;25:1312–8.
11. DeHaan AM, Axelrad TW, Kaye E, Silvestri L, Puskas B, Foster TE. Does double-row rotator cuff repair improve functional outcome of patients compared with single-row technique? A systematic review. Am J Sports Med. 2012;40:1176–85.
12. Millett PJ, Warth RJ, Dornan GJ, Lee JT, Spiegl UJ. Clinical and structural outcomes after arthroscopic single-row versus

double-row rotator cuff repair: a systematic review and meta-analysis of level I randomized clinical trials. J Shoulder Elb Surg. 2014;23:586–97.

13. Hein J, Reilly JM, Chae J, Maerz T, Anderson K. Retear rates after arthroscopic single-row, double-row, and suture bridge rotator cuff repair at a minimum of 1 year of imaging follow-up: a systematic review. Arthroscopy. 2015;31:2274–81.
14. Ji X, Bi C, Wang F, Wang Q. Arthroscopic versus mini-open rotator cuff repair: an up-to-date meta-analysis of randomized controlled trials. Arthroscopy. 2015;31:118–24.
15. van der Zwaal P, Thomassen BJ, Nieuwenhuijse MJ, Lindenburg R, Swen JW, van Arkel ER. Clinical outcome in all-arthroscopic versus mini-open rotator cuff repair in small to medium-sized tears: a randomized controlled trial in 100 patients with 1-year follow-up. Arthroscopy. 2013;29:266–73.

Chapter 6
Arthroscopic Repair of Subscapularis Tendon Tears

Gerhard G. Konrad

Case Presentation

A 46-year-old patient suffered forced external rotation of the right shoulder without luxation, due to a fall in the workplace. Immediately after the trauma, the patient experienced anterior shoulder pain, movement restriction, and reduced force with abduction and internal rotation. Compared with other rotator cuff tears, pain and tenderness related to subscapularis pathology are more often anterior than superior or lateral. At the clinical examination, there was pain on internal rotation against resistance and also a positive liftoff test. For this test, the dorsum of the hand is placed on the back with the arm rotated inwards, and the patient then attempts to raise the dorsum of the hand from the back. In the presence of a subscapularis tendon rupture, the patient is unable to do so. In the belly-press test, the patient's hand is pressed against

G.G. Konrad, M.D.
Klinikum Landkreis Erding,
Bajuwarenstrasse 5, 85435 Erding, Germany
e-mail: ggkonrad@aol.com

© Springer International Publishing AG 2018
P.J. McMahon (ed.), *Rotator Cuff Injuries*,
DOI 10.1007/978-3-319-63668-9_6

the abdomen, and the elbow is positioned anterior to the midcoronal line. Inability to maintain the elbow and hand in this position is a positive test. We believe that the bear-hug test is the most sensitive examination maneuver for subscapularis insufficiency. For this test, the patient places the palm of the affected side on the superior aspect of the contralateral shoulder, with the elbow in a flexed and elevated position. The examiner then tries to lift the hand off the shoulder, perpendicular to the plane of the forearm. If the patient cannot resist, the examination is positive, indicating at least a partial subscapularis tear. In our patient, all three of these tests were positive.

Radiographs of the patient's shoulder were normal but magnetic resonance imaging revealed a rupture with retraction of the cranial portion of the subscapularis tendon. The supraspinatus and infraspinatus tendons were intact. In addition, an effusion was visible in the subdeltoid bursa and in the subcoracoid recess, as well as fluid along the course of the long biceps tendon (Fig. 6.1).

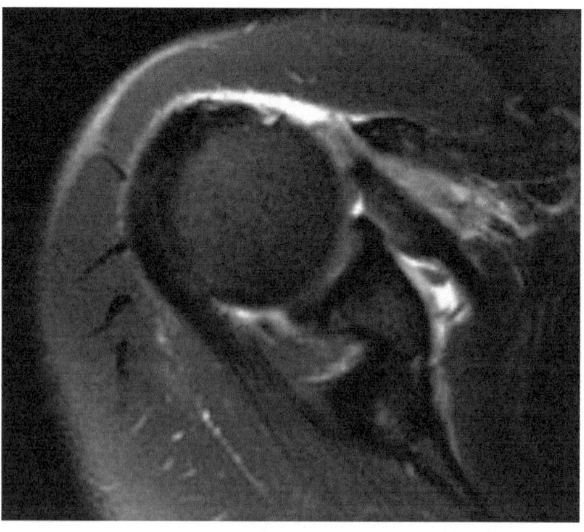

FIGURE 6.1 Tendon rupture with retraction of the cranial parts of the subscapularis muscle on axial image o f the MRI

Diagnosis/Assessment

The patient's history, physical, and imaging findings are consistent with the diagnosis of symptomatic full-thickness tear of the superior portion of the subscapularis tendon of the rotator cuff. The management of subscapularis tears is aimed to restore the fundamental role of this muscle in the kinematics of the shoulder. Operative management of our patient is indicated since it is the only treatment option to allow restoration of subscapularis function. We believe that especially in a young patient who is working physically on a high demand operative reconstruction of a partial subscapularis tear will provide better long-term results compared to conservative treatment.

Management

With the patient in the beach-chair position, the bony landmarks (clavicle, acromioclavicular joint, acromion, coracoid process) and the planned positions of the portals were marked. The standard practice for arthroscopic subscapular repair is to use three portals:

- A posterior standard portal using the "soft spot," approximately 2 cm below and 2 cm medial to the posterolateral acromial angle.
- An anterosuperior working access portal, ventral to the acromioclavicular (AC) joint. This portal is used for anchor placement and for passing and tying sutures using the knot pusher. A cannula that is at least 7 mm in diameter is required to allow passage of a suture-passing device. An 8.25 mm cannula can also be used because it can help to retract the soft tissue of the anterior capsule.
- An anterolateral portal, at the anterior edge of the long biceps tendon: Using this portal, temporary tension sutures are introduced to test the required tendon mobilization, the bony base at the lesser tubercle is dissected, and tenodesis of the biceps tendon is carried out if needed.

In cases of complete rupture, a lateral portal can also be created so that the inferior edge of the rupture can be demonstrated. The marked portal positions are injected with local anesthetic (Suprarenin® 2% in 5 mL; 1–2 ampules), and diagnostic arthroscopy follows via the standard dorsal portal. The entire rotator cuff, articular cartilage, and capsuloligamentous structures are inspected. In most cases a 30° arthroscope can be used, but in some cases, especially with retraction of the subscapularis tendon, a 70° arthroscope may be beneficial.

The subscapularis tendon is best assessed in a neutral position and with slight abduction and internal rotation of the arm. Articular sided ruptures near the insertion can be recognized by seeing the footprint. In addition to inspection of the remaining cuff, a precise examination of the biceps tendon and pulley system is carried out. The integrity and function of the medial and lateral slings are checked. Internal and external rotation can be used to assess the stability of the long biceps tendon in the pulley sling. The long biceps tendon is examined for partial lesions and irritation of the tenosynovium. When the subscapularis tendon avulses from the lesser tubercle, with tearing of the anteromedial pulley sling, it may dislocate medially into the joint. Pulling the extra-articular part of the long biceps tendon out of the sulcus and into the joint may reveal areas of tendon thickening that are obstructing the sliding process.

Subscapularis lesions are divided into four types arthroscopically using the Fox and Romeo classification [1]:

- Type 1: articular sided partial lesion
- Type 2: complete rupture affecting the upper 25% of the tendon
- Type 3: complete rupture affecting the upper 50% of the tendon
- Type 4: complete rupture affecting more than the upper 50% of the tendon

With internal rotation and slight abduction of the arm, the insertion of the subscapularis tendon can be easily followed in the caudal direction, and about 50% of the craniocaudal diameter of the tendon can be visualized. Partial ruptures and complete tendon avulsions from the lesser tubercle can be diagnosed in this way. With complete tendon avulsion, the subscapularis tendon footprint on the lesser tubercle is bare. In this case, the tendon is usually retracted medially and is adherent to the capsuloligamentous structures and the coracoid. Residual fibers from the pulley sling, the superior glenohumeral ligament and coracohumeral ligament complex, are often torn at the same time and form scar tissue adherent to the superolateral edge of the SSC tendon, known as the "comma sign" [2]. This sign can be used as an orienting structure to locate the superior and lateral edges of the tendon and must not be wrongly interpreted as an intact tendon insertion.

In our case there was a type 3 rupture of the subscapularis tendon as seen in Figs. 6.2 and 6.3.

With intra-articular visualization, correct portal placement was determined with a spinal needle and then with a small incision translucent twist-in cannulas were used to maintain water pressure and retract the soft tissues. If there is a lesion on the long head of the biceps tendon or there is a torn pulley system, a long biceps tenotomy or tenodesis is carried out with an

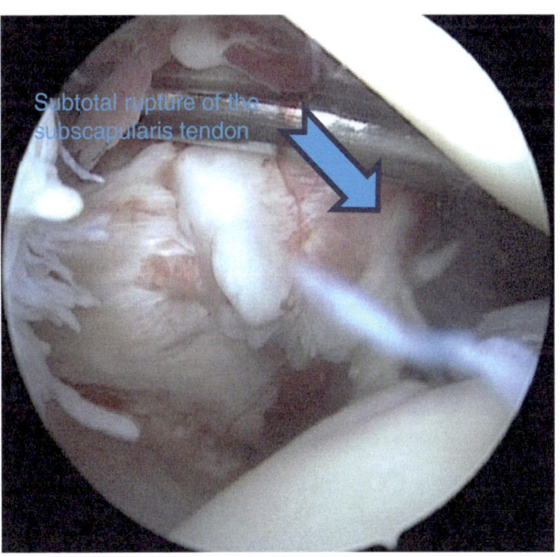

FIGURE 6.2 Subtotal subscapularis tendon rupture, type Fox and Romeo 3 (view from dorsal)

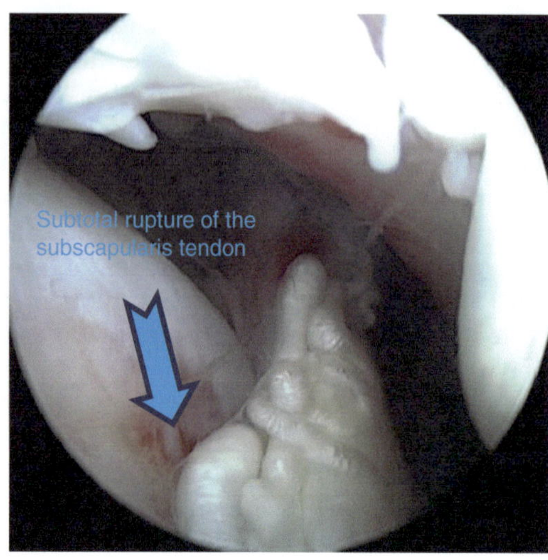

FIGURE 6.3 Subtotal subscapularis tendon rupture, type Fox and Romeo 3 (view from lateral)

electrothermal device or arthroscopic scissors via the antero-superior portal, before the subscapularis tendon is addressed. An unstable biceps tendon would put later reattachment of the subscapularis tendon at risk, due to medial subluxation or luxation. After tenotomy of the long biceps tendon, visualization of the SSC tendon was substantially better. The extent of the mobilization of the tendon that was necessary was assessed by grabbing the tendon with tissue-grasping forceps and pulling it lateral to reposition it on the lesser tubercle (Fig. 6.4). Alternatively tension sutures can be introduced with a perforating instrument and led out via the anterolateral portal.

Mobilization of the tendon was also carried out medially using a soft-tissue shaver or an electrothermal device to release capsular adhesions, particularly with the MGHL and adhesions to the coracoids and by detaching the coracohumeral ligament.

In complete ruptures, the "comma sign" serves as an orienting structure indicating the actual edge of the tendon. To facilitate debridement of adhesions to the subscapularis tendon, a tension suture can be placed through the tendon as a lasso-loop (Fig. 6.5).

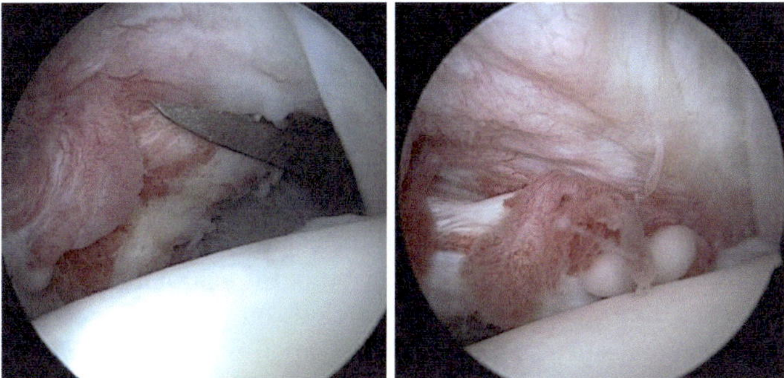

FIGURE 6.4 Assessing the mediolateral translation of the subscapularis tendon using tissue-grasping forces (view from dorsal)

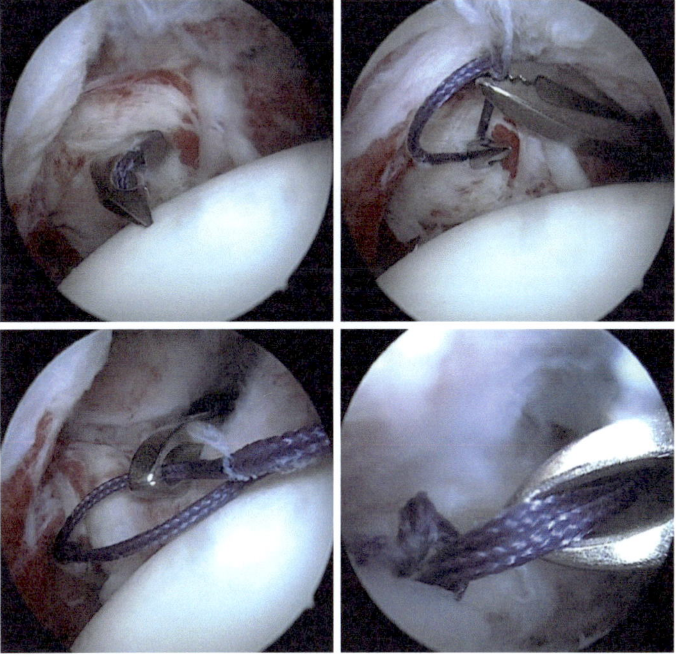

FIGURE 6.5 Placing of a suture through the subscapularis tendon to facilitate mobilization and debridement of adhesions to the tendon (view from dorsal)

While tension is being applied to the tendon using the introduced tension sutures, a 270° release of the tendon (anterior, superior, and posterior) was carried out while protecting the axillary nerve at the inferior edge of the tendon and the musculocutaneous nerve that was medial to the coracoid.

If the inferior edge of the rupture can be seen and there is no humeral avulsion of the glenohumeral ligaments (HAGL lesion), then repair can be carried out arthroscopically. Arthroscopic subscapularis tendon repair is best done immediately after identification of a complete rupture since visualization of the anterior part of the joint deteriorates during the operation as a result of increasing swelling [2, 3].

Following adequate tendon mobilization, dissection of the insertion site at the lesser tubercle, or with slight medialization at the cartilage–bone transition, was carried out. To do this, the bone was debrided with a shaver until bleeding started (Fig. 6.6).

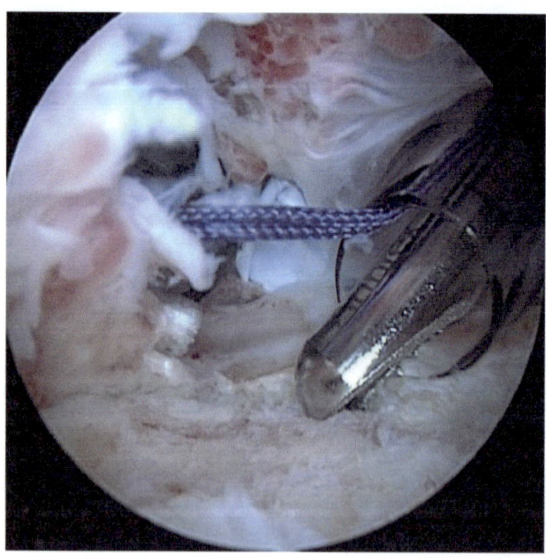

FIGURE 6.6 Debridement of the insertion site at the lesser tubercle using a shaver (dorsal view)

One to four anchors are used, depending on the size of the rupture. Cranial partial ruptures can be reattached with one anchor; complete ruptures are repaired with two to four anchors, depending on size. The anchors were positioned from caudal to cranial in accordance with the nearly trapezoid footprint [4]. If a complete rupture is present that affects the upper 50% of the tendon, or if the tendon is completely ruptured, then a double-row reconstruction can be carried out. Biomechanical study has demonstrated this to be better than a single-row repair [5]. For a double-row repair, two anchors are placed medial and two anchors are placed lateral.

Using an awl, preliminary drilling is carried out via the anterosuperior portal at an angle of 45° to the bone surface for a "deadman's angle" [4]. Depending on the anchor type and the hardness of the bone, it may also be necessary for a thread to be tapped. Resorbable or nonresorbable screw anchors can be used (Fig. 6.7). The anchor is checked by applying tension to the sutures. The sutures are then led out anterolaterally, and the first suture is placed using grasping forceps.

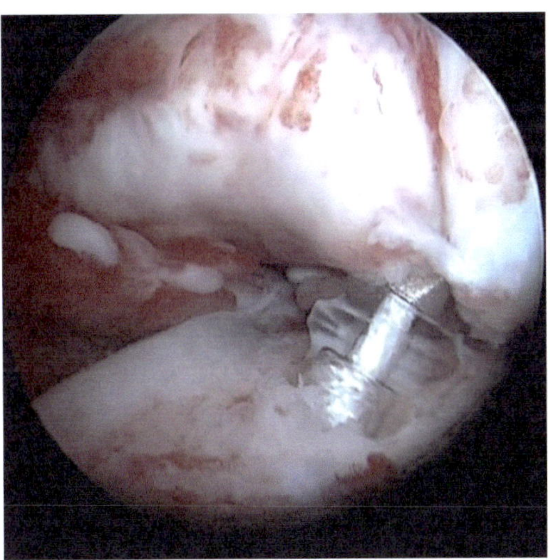

Figure 6.7 Positioning of the screw anchor via the anterosuperior portal at an angle of 45° to the bone surface (dorsal view)

The tendon is penetrated, and the suture is led out in the anterosuperior direction with the help of a shuttle instrument with tension being applied to the tendon with the tension sutures. To reattach the tendon, a modified Mason–Allen stitch was used (Fig. 6.8) or alternatively a single- or double-mattress suture can be used. To avoid suture entanglement, the pairs of sutures were drawn out through the cannulas and kept under tension. The sutures were tied in slight abduction and 20° of external rotation without applying excess tension to the tendon. After placement of a sliding knot, three opposed half-hitches and blocking of the knots using a knot pusher was carried out via the anterosuperior portal.

The sutures were cut using arthroscopic scissors. Figure 6.9 shows the reattached subscapularis tendon. For a complete

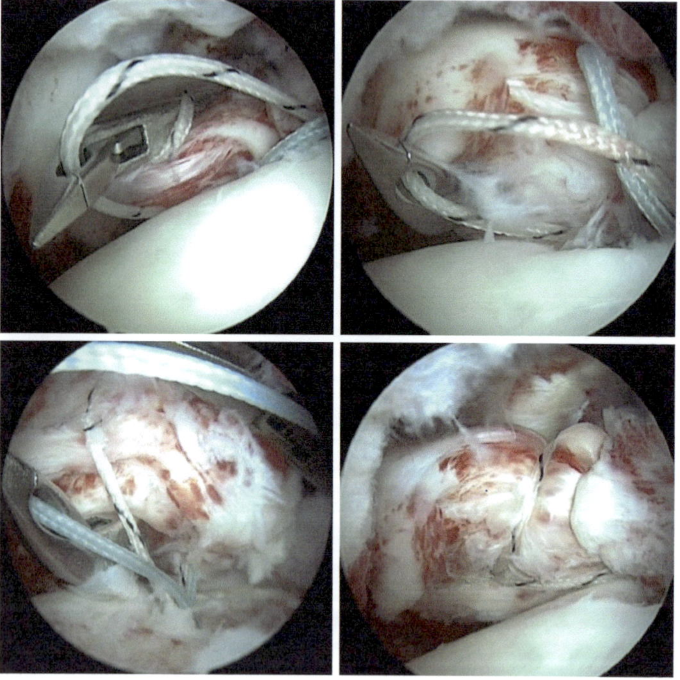

FIGURE 6.8 Penetration and reattachment of the subscapularis tendon

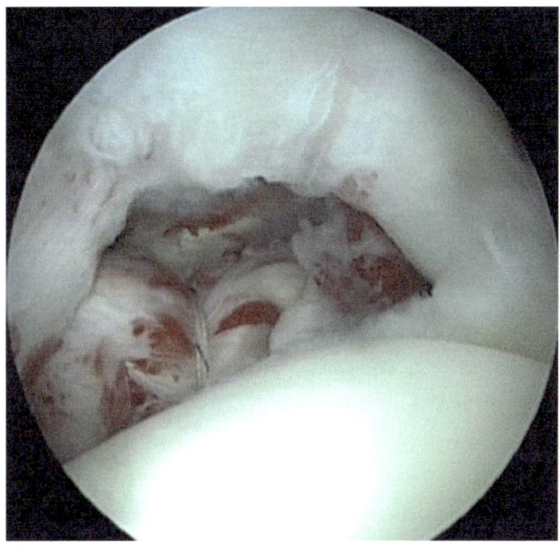

FIGURE 6.9 Reattached tendon (view from dorsal)

rupture in which several anchors are required, the same procedure can be repeated, or alternatively knotless fixation can be used (e.g., SpeedBridge™; Arthrex Inc.). The arthroscopy portals were closed with interrupted sutures and a sterile dressing was applied.

Postoperative Treatment

The patient was placed in a shoulder abduction orthotic device with 15° abduction for 6 weeks. For the first 6 weeks he was allowed no active biceps exercises because of biceps tenotomy. The same is true for patients with a biceps tenodesis. For the first 3 weeks postoperative passive abduction is allowed to 90° and adduction to 0°, passive flexion is allowed to 90°, passive extension is allowed to 0°, passive internal rotation is allowed to 0°, and external rotation is allowed to 0°. He was allowed active assisted external rotation up to 0°. At 4weeks postoperative he was allowed active assisted motion with the same limits of range of motion. Starting at postoperative week 7 he was allowed full actively assisted movement and starting at postoperative week 9 he was allowed full active movement. Strengthening was begun 3 months postoperative using resistance bands and light weights.

Outcome

The patient was discharged from the hospital 2 days after the operation wearing a shoulder abduction orthotic device with 15° abduction for 6 weeks. At intermediate follow-up, functional scores improved and the patient's satisfaction was excellent. Three months after the operation the range of motion of the shoulder was unrestricted except for a 10° external rotation deficit. The patient started a strengthening program for the shoulder and 5 months after the operation he went back to work without any limitation in the right shoulder.

Literature Review

As an internal rotator and static and dynamic stabilizer, the subscapularis is the only anterior component of the transverse "force couple" [6, 7] of the shoulder. If the tendon is torn, the stabilizing force couple is ruptured, leading not only to weakness in internal rotation but also to anterosuperior decentration of the head of the humerus. Subscapularis tendon ruptures occur much more rarely than supraspinatus and infraspinatus tendon ruptures [8]. The majority of subscapularis tendon ruptures result from degenerative changes and affect the upper parts or upper half of the tendon. The diagnosis of a subscapularis tendon tears is based on history and physical examination and confirmed with imaging studies. Repair of the subscapularis tendon can restore the original biomechanical function of the glenohumeral joint. Open procedures with an approach through the deltopectoral interval or an anterior deltoid split have been used for many years for repair of the tendon, but arthroscopic techniques are now increasingly being used [9, 10].

Lafosse et al. [11] reviewed outcomes in 17 patients following arthroscopic subscapularis repair and 29 months postoperatively the average Constant score improved from 58 to 96. Bartl et al. [9] evaluated 21 patients at an average of 27 months after arthroscopic repair of an isolated subscapularis tear and the average Constant score increased from 50 preoperative to 82. Nevertheless, five patients had weakness on the belly press test and the liftoff test. These patients also had atrophy of the upper subscapularis muscle on MRI. In a systematic review, Mall et al. [12] compared the results of three arthroscopic and six open subscapularis repair studies. Both techniques resulted in decreased pain, improved function, and 95% healing rate. Neither technique has been proven to provide better results than the other.

Clinical Pearls/Pitfalls

- With an arthroscopic procedure, careful positioning of the patient is an absolute necessity. With beach chair positioning, excessive elevation of the patient's head can lead to cerebral ischemia, while with lateral decubitus positioning neurological injury to the brachial plexus or musculocutaneous nerve can occur with poor positioning of the arm in balanced suspension.
- Attention needs to be given to correct placement of the portals. A needle should be used to check the entrance level and potential working radius. Twist in cannulas can be screwed in to maintain water pressure.
- The SSC footprint must be inspected during internal rotation. The long biceps tendon and the pulley system must be inspected precisely. An unstable long biceps tendon can endanger the result of the SCC reconstruction due to medial subluxation or luxation. The "comma sign" must not be wrongly interpreted as an intact tendon insertion.

- When there are concomitant additional rotator cuff lesions in the supraspinatus and infraspinatus tendons, reconstruction of the SSC tendon must be carried out first, since visualization of the anterior part of the joint declines due to increasing swelling as the duration of the arthroscopy lengthens.
- Anchors that are placed too shallowly may tear out of the bone. The stability of the anchors must be checked before reinsertion of the tendon, by applying tension to the sutures. If necessary, a switch must be made to a larger anchor. Confident mastery of arthroscopic suturing and knotting techniques is required.

References

1. Fox JANM, Noerdlinger MA, Romeo AA. Arthroscopic subscapularis repair. Tech Shoulder Elbow Surg. 2003;4:154–68.
2. Lo IK, Burkhart SS. The comma sign: an arthroscopic guide to the torn subscapularis tendon. Arthroscopy. 2003;19:334–7.
3. Bauer GJ, Kniesel B. Arthroscopic reconstruction of the rotor cuff. Unfallchirurg. 2006;109:619–27.
4. Richards DP, Burkhart SS, Lo IK. Subscapularis tears: arthroscopic repair techniques. Orthop Clin North Am. 2003;34:485–98.
5. Wellmann M, Wiebringhaus P, Lodde I, et al. Biomechanical evaluation of a single-row versus double-row repair for complete subscapularis tears. Knee Surg Sports Traumatol Arthrosc. 2009;17:1477–84.
6. Burkhart SS. Arthroscopic treatment of massive rotator cuff tears. Clinical results and biomechanical rationale. Clin Orthop Relat Res. 1991;267:45–56.
7. Turkel SJ, Panio MW, Marshall JL, et al. Stabilizing mechanisms preventing anterior dislocation of the glenohumeral joint. J Bone Joint Am. 1981;63:1208–17.
8. Gerber C, Hersche O, Farron A. Isolated rupture of the subscapularis tendon. J Bone Joint Surg Am. 1996;78:1015–23.
9. Bartl C, Salzmann GM, Seppel G, et al. Subscapularis function and structural integrity after arthroscopic repair of isolated subscapularis tears. Am J Sports Med. 2011;39(6):1255–62.

10. Burkhart SS, Brady PC. Arthroscopic subscapularis repair: surgical tips and pearls A to Z. Arthroscopy. 2006;22:1014–27.
11. Lafosse L, Jost B, Reiland Y, Audebert S, et al. Structural integrity and clinical outcomes after arthroscopic repair of isolated subscapularis tears. J Bone Joint Surg Am. 2007;89:1184–93.
12. Mall NA, Chahal J, Heard WM, et al. Outcomes of arthroscopic and open surgical repair of isolated subscapularis tendon tears. Arthroscopy. 2012;28:1306–14.

Chapter 7
Arthroscopic Treatment of Combined Shoulder Instability and Rotator Cuff Tear

Aharon Z. Gladstein and John D.A. Kelly IV

Case Presentation

A 64-year-old, right-hand-dominant male presented for follow-up after traumatic left shoulder dislocation. He underwent closed reduction in the emergency department. On his first clinic visit, he was unable to abduct the left shoulder. His past medical history revealed hypertension, type 2 diabetes mellitus, and Hodgkin's disease. On physical examination of the normal right shoulder forward elevation was 170°, external rotation with the arm at the side was 60°, external rotation at 90° of shoulder abduction was 90°, and internal

A.Z. Gladstein, M.D.
Department of Orthopedics, Texas Children's Hospital,
Baylor College of Medicine, Houston, TX, USA

J.D.A. Kelly IV, M.D. (✉)
Center for Throwing Disorders and Shoulder Preservation,
University of Pennsylvania, Perelman School of Medicine,
Philadelphia, PA, USA
e-mail: john.kelly@uphs.upenn.edu

© Springer International Publishing AG 2018
P.J. McMahon (ed.), *Rotator Cuff Injuries*,
DOI 10.1007/978-3-319-63668-9_7

rotation at 90° of shoulder abduction was 30°. There was no muscle wasting noted. No tenderness was elicited about the acromioclavicular joint, biceps tendon, coracoid process, or greater tuberosity. Strength of the abduction and external and internal rotation was normal at 5/5. The left shoulder forward elevation was 90°. External rotation with the arm at the side was 45°. At 90° of shoulder abduction there was 70° of external rotation and 20° of internal rotation. Tenderness was elicited about the greater tuberosity. There was no coracoid or acromioclavicular joint tenderness. Weakness in abduction and external rotation was noted. Sensation was intact in all distributions.

Figure 7.1 shows the shoulder in a reduced position. Glenohumeral degenerative changes were noted. The patient was referred for MRI to evaluate for a rotator cuff tear. Figure 7.2a–c shows a retracted rotator cuff tear with evidence of a Hill-Sachs lesion. Partial tear of the subscapularis was noted.

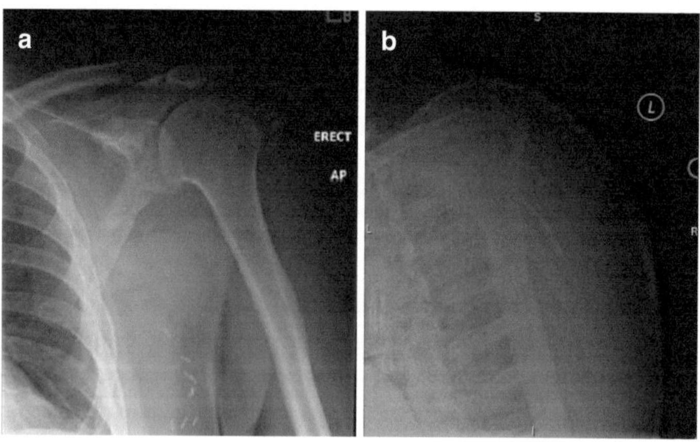

FIGURE 7.1 (**a, b**) Post-reduction AP and Y-lateral x-rays after initial dislocation demonstrating reduction of the joint. Note glenohumeral degenerative changes

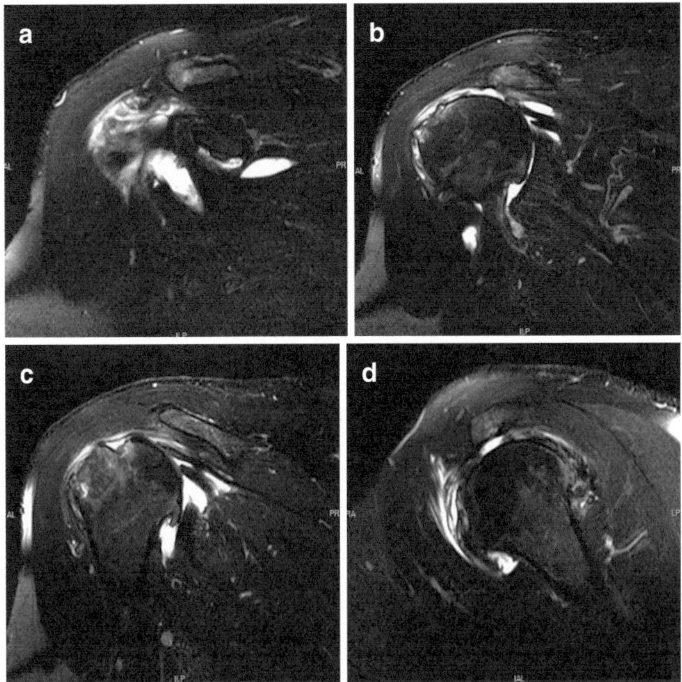

FIGURE 7.2 T2-weighted MRI images. (**a**) Coronal section showing intact subscapularis with tendinosis. (**b, c**) Coronal sections demonstrating large, retracted rotator cuff tear with Hill-Sachs impaction fracture. (**d**) Sagittal section demonstrating massive rotator cuff tear

Diagnosis/Assessment

Treatment of combined instability and rotator cuff tear is usually operative, and accomplished arthroscopically. The aims of surgical treatment are the restoration of the dynamic coronal and axial force couples of the shoulder, as well as the static stabilizers of the shoulder joint [1]. Repair of the rotator cuff is usually sufficient to restore glenohumeral stability and shoulder function [2]. Arthroscopic techniques for labral repair and rotator cuff repair have been well described.

Management

The patient was placed in the right lateral decubitus position with a beanbag. The operative arm was held with a suspension apparatus. The scope was entered traumatically and immediately seen were significant glenohumeral degenerative changes without full-thickness chondral defect. There was a small tear of the subscapularis tendon that was not retracted, so the coracoid was exposed and its connections with the subscapularis tendon were released. No repair was attempted as repair of the subscapularis was felt to lead to loss of external rotation, tightening of the glenohumeral joint, and worsening of degenerative changes. No Bankart lesion was noted. Following this, the posterior capsule was released followed by the anterior inferior capsule in order to reduce proximal humeral migration and lessen tension on the rotator cuff repair. Attention was taken to the rotator cuff which had a large, retracted tear of the supraspinatus and infraspinatus tendons. The infraspinatus had more mobility so this was repaired as a "reverse L"-type tear. Despite appreciable supraspinatus atrophy 2 margin convergence sutures approximated the posterior cuff to the coracohumeral ligament. Following this, an anchor with fiber tape in the remaining anterior and posterior limbs affected a near-complete repair. An arthroscopic photograph of the repair is shown in Fig. 7.3. The patient was placed in a sling with range of motion initiated 6 weeks postoperative.

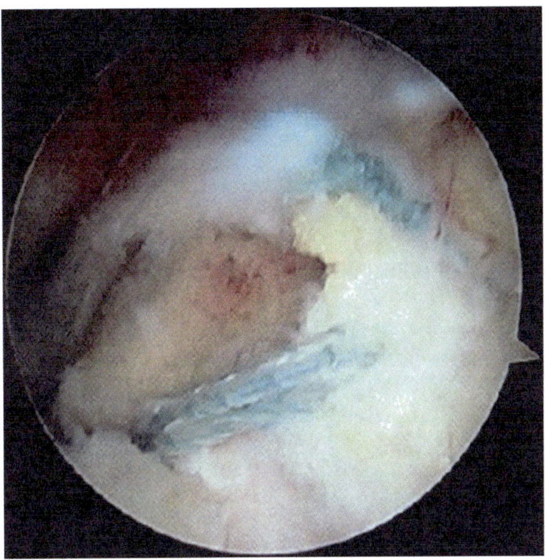

FIGURE 7.3 Arthroscopic photo demonstrating repair of the rotator cuff to the greater tuberosity

Outcome

At 6-month follow-up, the patient had no complaints of left shoulder pain. Shoulder external rotation was 4+/5 in adduction and abduction range of motion was full. However, 1 year post op, the patient fell and sustained a recurrent dislocation. Figure 7.4 shows pre- and post-reduction X-rays of the glenohumeral joint. He again demonstrated weakness in shoulder abduction. He also had internal rotation weakness and tenderness over the coracoid. He consented for revision rotator cuff repair and shoulder stabilization.

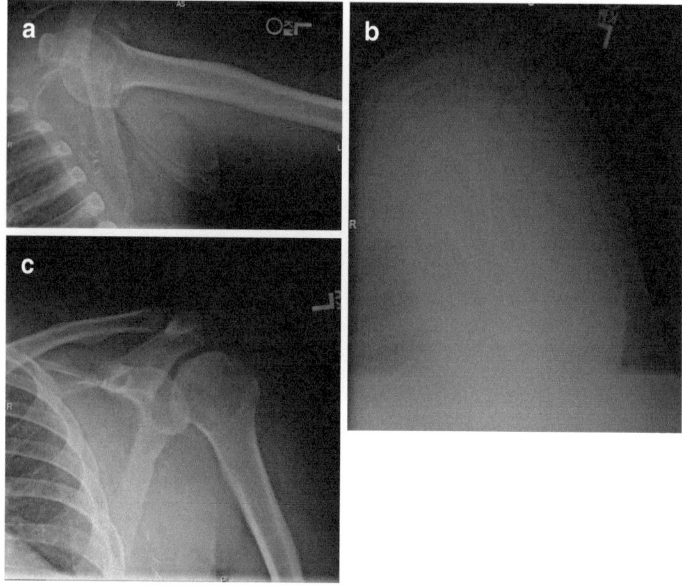

FIGURE 7.4 (**a, b**) AP and lateral x-ray views of the left shoulder show anterior glenohumeral dislocation. (**c**) Post-reduction AP shows reduction of the glenohumeral joint with degenerative changes again noted

Upon arthroscopic evaluation, again noted were degenerative changes in the glenohumeral joint. No Bankart lesion was seen. The subscapularis tendon was torn from the lesser tuberosity with "comma tissue" (combined retracted SGHL and CHL tissue evident). As we were concerned that the prior surgery had failed to prevent recurrent instability because of worsening of the subscapularis tear over time we repaired the subscapularis. Of note, there was no capsulolabral injury present. The subscapularis tendon was then freed through exposure of the coracoid. The subscapularis footprint on the lesser tuberosity was identified. A suture was passed through the subscapularis tendon using a suture-passing device at the junction of the tendon and comma tissue. A 4.75 mm anchor was then placed in the footprint of the lesser tuberosity with the instruments being as close as possible to the patient's face to allow the appropriate angle for drilling and fixation.

Attention was then directed toward repair of the retracted supra- and infraspinatus tendon tears. Revision repair was carried out after mobilization of the soft tissues and placement of margin convergence sutures. Sutures were placed in the infraspinatus/supraspinatus and secured to the coracohumeral ligament. The converged margin of tissue was fixed to the greater tuberosity with suture anchors. Figure 7.5 shows the subscapularis tear and repair, as well as the repair of the infraspinatus.

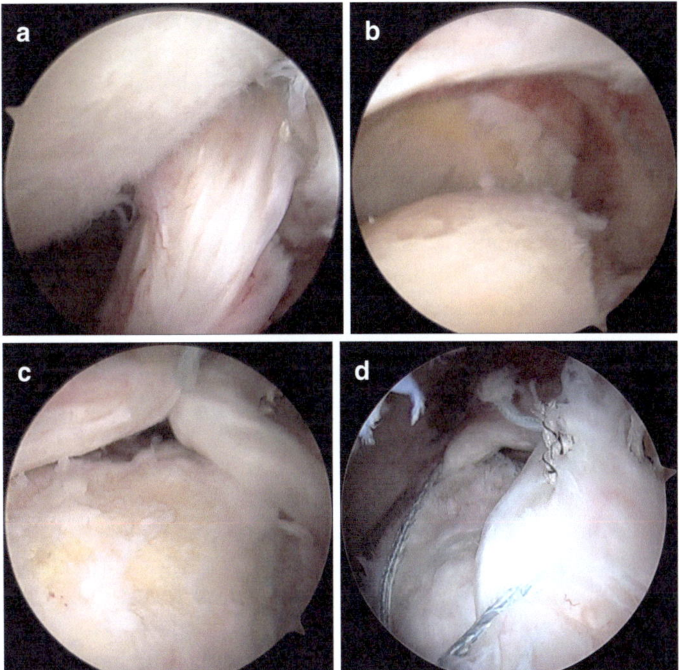

Figure 7.5 Arthroscopic photos from revision rotator cuff repair with mobilization and repair of the subscapularis. (a) Repair of subscapularis to lesser tuberosity. (b) Retracted rotator cuff tear. (c) Margin convergence sutures placed. (d) Approximation of rotator cuff with fiber tape through the anchor

Case Presentation

A 38-year-old, right-hand-dominant male presented with right shoulder pain after a fall 1 month earlier. Since the fall, he has had pain at night and with overhead activity. Pain was localized to the subdeltoid region. His past medical history revealed type 2 diabetes mellitus. On physical examination of the left shoulder he had forward elevation to 170°, external rotation with the arm at the side of 60°, and external rotation at 90° of shoulder abduction was 90° internal rotation and was 30°. There was no muscle wasting. No tenderness was elicited about the acromioclavicular joint, biceps tendon, coracoid process, or greater tuberosity. Strength was normal at 5/5 strength in abduction, external rotation, and internal rotation. The right shoulder had forward elevation to 170°. External rotation with the arm at the side and at 90° of shoulder external rotation was 90° and internal rotation was 30°. There was some muscle wasting noted of the supraspinatus and infraspinatus. Tenderness was elicited about the coracoid process and greater tuberosity. Weakness in abduction and external and internal rotations was noted.

X-rays were taken and are shown in Fig. 7.6. They revealed calcification within the rotator cuff as well as sclerosis and cystic changes about the greater tuberosity. No significant glenohumeral degenerative changes were noted. A large rotator cuff tear was suspected, and an MRI was ordered. Representative images are shown in Fig. 7.7. MRI showed a high-grade undersurface tear of the posterior supraspinatus tendon involving greater than 50% tendon thickness and measuring 10 mm anteroposterior with underlying moderate tendinopathy, and no fatty muscle atrophy. There was a low-grade partial-thickness undersurface tearing of the anterior infraspinatus tendon with moderate underlying tendinosis without atrophy. The teres minor muscle was normal without atrophy. Moderate subscapularis tendinosis with interstitial tearing distally was also noted, without muscle atrophy. Also noted was tendinosis and medial subluxation of the proximal long head of the biceps tendon into the substance of the subscapularis tendon. There was also extensive tearing of the superior and posterior glenoid labrum. Finally, full-thickness cartilage loss along the posterior superior glenoid with associated subchondral bone marrow edema was seen.

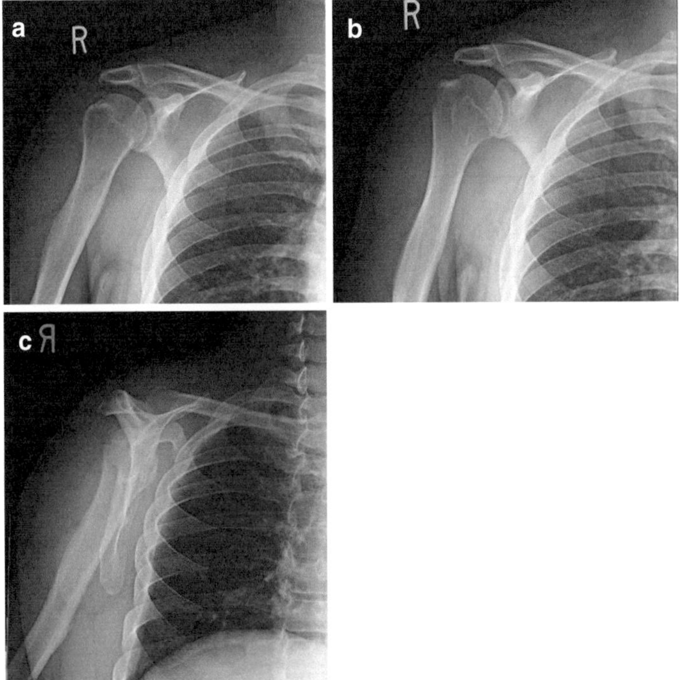

FIGURE 7.6 (**a–c**) AP in internal and external rotation and scapular Y x-ray views of the shoulder demonstrating calcification in the rotator cuff as well as productive changes in the greater tuberosity

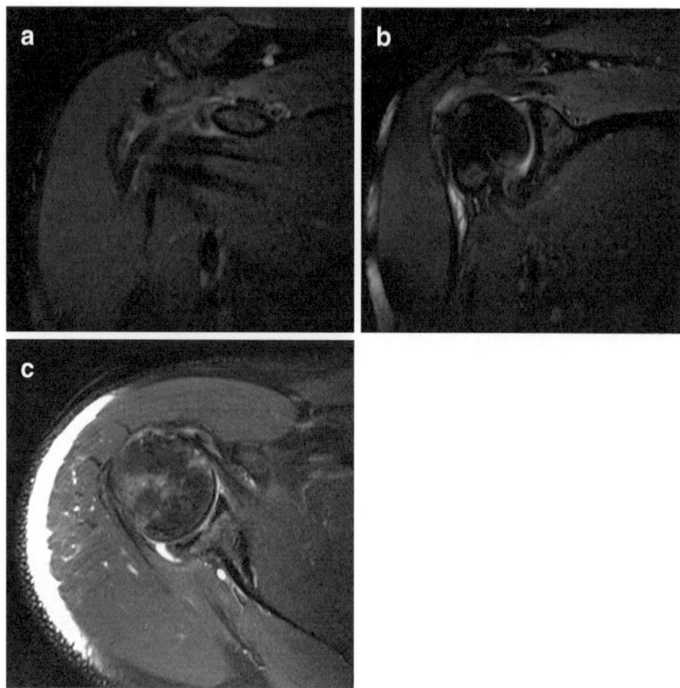

Figure 7.7 T2-weighted MRI images. (**a**) Coronal section showing medial displacement of the biceps tendon. (**b**) Coronal section showing articular sided supraspinatus tear with tendinosis. (**c**) Sagittal section demonstrating increased signal at the subscapularis insertion. Note the medial displacement of the biceps tendon

Diagnosis/Assessment

Because this patient had profound shoulder dysfunction in the absence of overt glenohumeral instability or massive superior rotator cuff tear we thought that the subscapularis tear had led to weakness of shoulder elevation. Repair of the subscapularis and supraspinatus tendons was done to restore motion and stability. The posterior chondral injury suggested posterior instability that caused shear of the articular cartilage due to failure of the posterior cuff to counteract the posterior force exerted by the subscapularis.

Management

The patient was placed in the left lateral decubitus position with a beanbag. The operative arm was held with a suspension apparatus. The 30° arthroscope was introduced into the glenohumeral joint from a standard posterior portal. Inspection of the anterior structures showed subscapularis tendon tearing and medial subluxation of the biceps. A full-thickness supraspinatus tendon tear was seen as well. An anterolateral portal was established. A full-thickness chondral lesion was seen on the posterior glenoid while viewing from anterior. Arthroscopic photos are shown in Fig. 7.8.

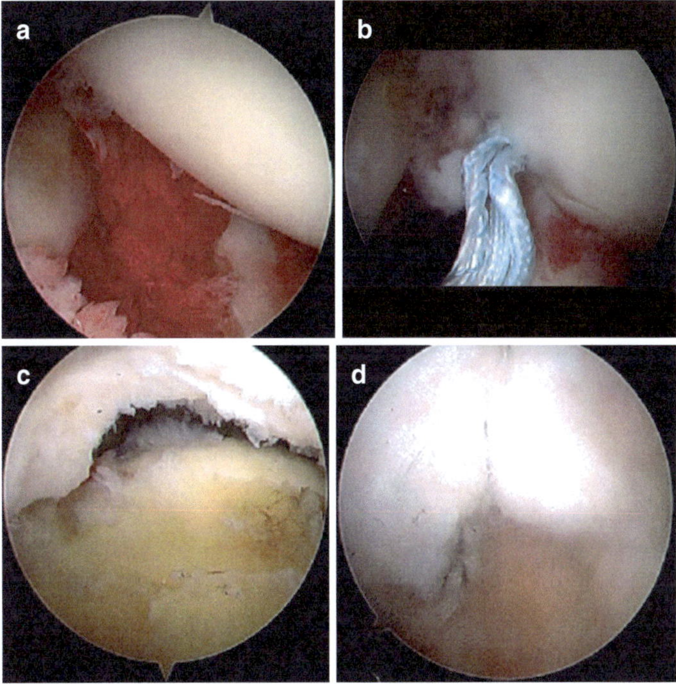

FIGURE 7.8 Arthroscopy photos. (**a**) Synovitis and subluxation of the biceps tendon. (**b**) Subscapularis repair with knotless anchor. (**c**) Supraspinatus tear with bed prepared. (**d**) Convergence stitch placed in supraspinatus. (**e**) Supraspinatus repaired with knotless anchor. (**f**) Full-thickness glenoid articular cartilage defect. (**g**) Microfracture of glenoid articular cartilage defect

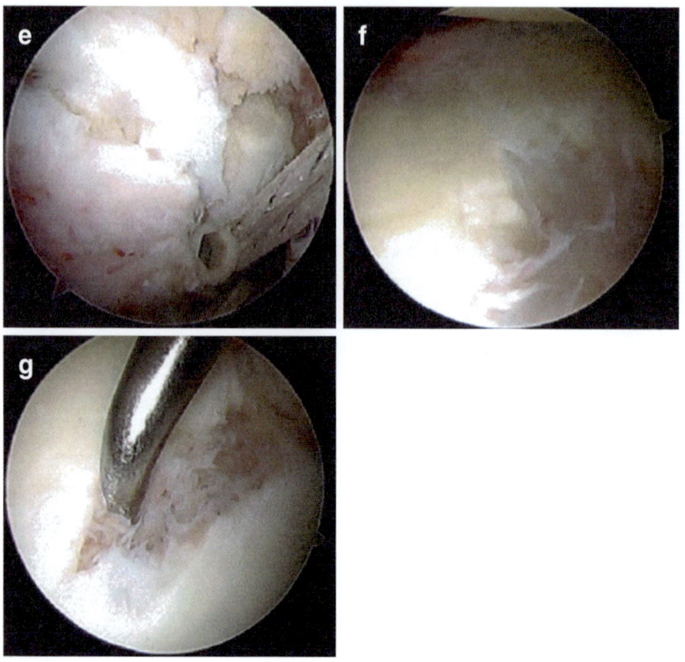

Figure 7.8 (continued)

The chondral lesion was treated with microfracture awl, through the posterior portal.

The subscapularis tendon was then freed from the coracoid using a thermal ablation device. Using a 70-degree scope, the subscapularis footprint on the lesser tuberosity was identified. A suture was passed through the subscapularis tendon using a suture-passing device. A 4.75 mm anchor was then placed in the footprint of the lesser tuberosity keeping the instruments brought as close as possible to the patient's face to allow the appropriate angle for drilling and fixation.

Attention was turned to the subacromial space where an anterolateral debridement and bursectomy were performed revealing the supraspinatus lesion, roughly 2–3 cm in width. Margin convergence sutures were placed in the anterior tear, brought to the posterior, and tied arthroscopically. A suture was then passed in a horizontal mattress configuration in the remaining tear. The insertion site was then prepared with a burr. The suture was used to bring the anterior portion to the lateral cortex, where it was secured with a suture anchor. The patient was placed in a sling with range of motion initiated 6 weeks postoperative.

Outcome

The patient began range-of-motion exercises 6 weeks postoperative and strengthening 3 months postoperative. He regained full range of motion and strength was normal at 5/5 4 months postoperative when he returned to work.

Literature Review

Rotator cuff tears have been noted in the setting of shoulder instability, particularly in older patients [3]. Anterior glenohumeral instability in young athletes has also been associated with tears of the rotator cuff [4, 5]. Efforts to understand rotator cuff pathomechanics have shown relationships between various anatomic lesions and glenohumeral instability [6]. Craig [7] popularized the idea that failure of an attenuated posterior rotator cuff occurs in older patients, with relative sparing of the anterior capsule and labrum. The failure of the infraspinatus to restrain anterior humeral head translation may lead to anterior instability. This posterior mechanism of anterior dislocation is in contrast to the more common mechanism seen in younger patients, in which anterior capsular and labral structures fail, with the rotator cuff uninjured.

The shoulder joint is stabilized by both static (e.g., the labrum and joint capsule) and dynamic (e.g., the shoulder muscles) restraints in both the mid-range and end range of glenohumeral motion. With little inherent bony constraint, these restraints function through the concavity-compression mechanism to compress the humeral head into the glenoid so that translation is minimized throughout the range of motion. In a quantitative analysis, increased resistance to glenohumeral translation was found with the application of a compressive force [8] and there was also decreased resistance to translation after glenoid labrum excision. Differences in the depth of the glenoid labrum were found to account for variation in the force needed to dislocate the joint in different directions. The rotator cuff is an important stabilizer at both the mid- and end ranges of motion [9]. Lastly, in a biomechanical study, simulated rotator cuff lesions allowed for humeral head dislocation with less extensive capsular lesions then with an intact rotator cuff [10] again demonstrating the synergy between static and dynamic stabilizers.

Rotator Cuff Tears and Glenohumeral Instability

Neviaser et al. [11] reported 31 patients who had inability to abduct the arm after shoulder dislocation that were over the age of 35 and all of the patients had rotator cuff tears. Most patients had delay of treatment due to misdiagnosis with presumption of isolated axillary nerve injury but the authors found that only 7.8% of patients who underwent electromyograms had axillary nerve injury. In a subsequent study [9] a similar low, 10.8% incidence of axillary nerve injury in patients who failed to recover shoulder function after dislocation was reported and all had rotator cuff rupture. The average time between injury and diagnosis was 7.2 months. All of the patients were over 40 years of age and were treated with rotator cuff repair. Gumina et al. observed that the incidence of rotator cuff tear after shoulder dislocation increased with age [12]. The supraspinatus tendon is almost always involved [2, 9]. Itoi et al. [2] reported 16 rotator cuff tears after glenohumeral dislocation and 11 were treated with repair of the rotator cuff without repair of capsulolabral injuries. They concluded that repair of the rotator cuff tear is likely sufficient for stabilization of the dislocated shoulder with concurrent capsulolabral repair.

Recurrent Instability

Neviaser et al. [13] reported a subset of patients who had almost immediate recurrent anterior glenohumeral instability after closed reduction. In contrast to patients who maintained reduction, who nearly all had supraspinatus and/or infraspinatus tendon tears, these patients had subscapularis tendon avulsion from the lesser tuberosity with the absence of Bankart lesions. Repair of the subscapularis tendon was sufficient to restore glenohumeral stability. They concluded that recurrent glenohumeral instability in patients over 40 are due to subscapularis tendon injury.

Terrible Triad of the Shoulder

Shoulder dislocation, combined with massive rotator cuff tear and neurologic injury, has been termed the "terrible triad of the shoulder" [14]. Those with this rare entity [15, 16] typically present with the same physical examination finding of inability to raise the arm as those with a rotator cuff tear alone. Numbness in the axillary nerve distribution can aid the clinician with the diagnosis. However, the absence of sensory disturbance does not preclude axillary neuropathy [16]. It is generally understood that patients with this combination of injuries fare more poorly than those without nerve injury. Simonich and Wright [16] reported six patients with the terrible triad and they did not explore the axillary nerve at the time of cuff repair. They advocate early repair of the rotator cuff in those with a terrible triad to minimize muscle atrophy while the nerve recovers [16]. One study indicated that the terrible triad may be as uncommon as previously thought as Pevny et al. reported rotator cuff tears in all of their patients over the age of 40 with axillary nerve palsy after shoulder dislocation [17].

The relationship between rotator cuff insufficiency and shoulder dysfunction is further understood with the concept of force couples of the shoulder. In order for the deltoid to elevate the arm, its moment must be balanced by the moment of the inferior rotator cuff [18]. This is termed the coronal plane force couple. This coronal plane force couple is essential to maintain a fulcrum for glenohumeral joint motion [1]. The transverse plane force couple is comprised of the subscapularis anteriorly and the infraspinatus and teres minor tendons posteriorly. Imbalance of either of these force couples can lead to rotator cuff dysfunction since the stable glenohumeral fulcrum is compromised. Conversely, function may be well preserved in patients with rotator cuff tears with maintenance of the coronal and transverse plane force couples.

Clinical Pearls/Pitfalls

Glenohumeral Instability with Onset over Age 40

- Suspect rotator cuff tear in all shoulder dislocation in those over age 40. Rotator cuff tears are much more common than axillary nerve injury in those over age 40.
- Labral injury may not be present on imaging or arthroscopy.
- Repair of the rotator cuff is usually sufficient to restore glenohumeral stability without repair of capsulolabral injuries.
- Failure to address subscapularis insufficiency may result in recurrent instability.
- Patients over age 40 with axillary nerve injury after dislocation will also commonly have rotator cuff tear.
- Consider early rotator cuff repair in those over age 40 with axillary nerve injury after dislocation whether or not there is an axillary nerve injury.
- Loss of coronal and/or transverse plane force couples can lead to profound glenohumeral dysfunction.
- Clinical presentation may suggest a large rotator cuff tear due to nerve injury or cuff strain even though a tear is not present.
- If a severe rotator cuff tear is not evident on MRI, carefully scrutinize the subscapularis tendon for an occult tear.
- Surgery should include repair of the subscapularis tendon for restoration of the transverse force couple of the shoulder.

References

1. Lo IK, Burkhart SS. Current concepts in arthroscopic rotator cuff repair. Am J Sports Med. 2003;31(2):308–24.
2. Itoi E, Tabata S. Rotator cuff tears in anterior dislocation of the shoulder. Int Orthop. 1992;16(3):240–4.
3. Porcellini G, Caranzano F, Campi F, Pellegrini A, Paladini P. Glenohumeral instability and rotator cuff tear. Sports Med Arthrosc. 2011;19(4):395–400.
4. Savoie FH 3rd, Field LD, Atchinson S. Anterior superior instability with rotator cuff tearing: SLAC lesion. Orthop Clin North Am. 2001;32(3):457–61. ix
5. Goldberg JA, Chan KY, Best JP, Bruce WJ, Walsh W, Parry W. Surgical management of large rotator cuff tears combined with instability in elite rugby football players. Br J Sports Med. 2003;37(2):179–81. discussion 81
6. Gombera MM, Sekiya JK. Rotator cuff tear and glenohumeral instability: a systematic review. Clin Orthop Relat Res. 2014;472(8):2448–56.
7. Craig EV. The posterior mechanism of acute anterior shoulder dislocations. Clin Orthop Relat Res. 1984;190:212–6.
8. Lippitt SB, Vanderhooft JE, Harris SL, Sidles JA, Harryman DT 2nd, Matsen FA 3rd. Glenohumeral stability from concavity-compression: a quantitative analysis. J Shoulder Elb Surg. 1993;2(1):27–35.
9. Neviaser RJ, Neviaser TJ, Neviaser JS. Anterior dislocation of the shoulder and rotator cuff rupture. Clin Orthop Relat Res. 1993;291:103–6.
10. Pouliart N, Gagey O. Concomitant rotator cuff and capsuloligamentous lesions of the shoulder: a cadaver study. Arthroscopy. 2006;22(7):728–35.
11. Neviaser RJ, Neviaser TJ, Neviaser JS. Concurrent rupture of the rotator cuff and anterior dislocation of the shoulder in the older patient. J Bone Joint Surg Am. 1988;70(9):1308–11.
12. Gumina S, Postacchini F. Anterior dislocation of the shoulder in elderly patients. J Bone Joint Surg. 1997;79(4):540–3.
13. Neviaser RJ, Neviaser TJ. Recurrent instability of the shoulder after age 40. J Shoulder Elb Surg. 1995;4(6):416–8.
14. Groh GI, Rockwood CA Jr. The terrible triad: anterior dislocation of the shoulder associated with rupture of the rotator cuff and injury to the brachial plexus. J Shoulder Elb Surg. 1995;4(1 Pt 1):51–3.

15. Gonzalez D, Lopez R. Concurrent rotator-cuff tear and brachial plexus palsy associated with anterior dislocation of the shoulder. A report of two cases. J Bone Joint Surg Am. 1991 Apr;73(4):620–1.
16. Simonich SD, Wright TW. Terrible triad of the shoulder. J Shoulder Elb Surg. 2003;12(6):566–8.
17. Pevny T, Hunter RE, Freeman JR. Primary traumatic anterior shoulder dislocation in patients 40 years of age and older. Arthroscopy. 1998;14(3):289–94.
18. Inman VT, Saunders JB, Abbott LC. Observations of the function of the shoulder joint. 1944. Clin Orthop Relat Res. 1996;(330):3–12.

Chapter 8
Arthroscopic Repair of Severe Rotator Cuff Tears

Brett Sanders and Edwin E. Spencer

Case Presentation

A 78-year-old female with a history of breast cancer presented with a 6-month history of severe anterolateral arm pain that was worse with overhead activity. She had a history of minor trauma with acute worsening in shoulder strength and function over the prior 6 weeks. On physical examination, she had active forward flexion of 150° and internal rotation to L3. Abduction strength was 4/5 and internal rotation strength was 5/5 and she had disproportionate external rotation weakness of 2/5 with a 30° external rotation lag with the arm at the side. Radiographs revealed the shoulder to be normal except for moderate AC joint osteoarthritis. She had failed nonoperative treatment of physical therapy and a steroid injection. Magnetic resonance imaging (MRI) revealed

B. Sanders, M.D. (✉)
Department of Sports Medicine, Center for Sports Medicine and Orthopedics, Chattanooga, TN, USA
e-mail: sandbrett@gmail.com

E.E. Spencer, M.D.
Shoulder and Elbow Service, Knoxville Orthopaedic Clinic, Knoxville, TN, USA
e-mail: spencershoulder13@gmail.com

© Springer International Publishing AG 2018
P.J. McMahon (ed.), *Rotator Cuff Injuries*,
DOI 10.1007/978-3-319-63668-9_8

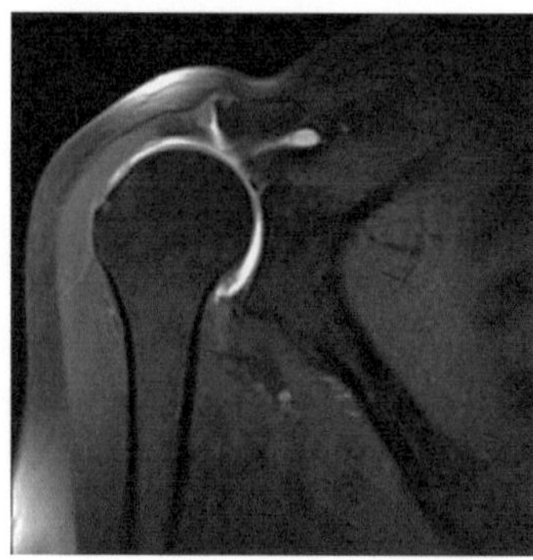

FIGURE 8.1 Preoperative MRI demonstrating massive rotator cuff tear with retraction to the glenoid

retracted tears of the supraspinatus and infraspinatus tendons with no atrophy and minimal fatty infiltration of the muscles (Fig. 8.1).

Diagnosis/Assessment

This patient has a symptomatic severe, full-thickness tear involving two tendons of the rotator cuff with disproportionate loss of external rotation strength. She had already failed nonoperative treatments and was referred for consideration of operative treatment. The decision was made to attempt repair of the rotator cuff because the humeral head was centered on the glenoid; there were normal rotator cuff muscle with no glenohumeral arthritis, and despite the severe tendon retraction, the history indicated that she was likely to have had an acute-on-chronic tear. We thought that anatomic repair of the tendons would likely yield better function and specifically better external rotation strength than a functional muscle transfer, reverse shoulder arthroplasty, or reverse arthroplasty with latissimus dorsi tendon transfer. She understood that if a rotator cuff repair was not possible, a partial repair, patch augmentation, or debridement would be done, as well as treatment of the biceps tendon for pain relief.

Management

Anesthesia was induced and the patient was placed in the beach chair position with an interscalene regional block. Diagnostic arthroscopy was performed which demonstrated tears of the supraspinatus and infraspinatus tendons, with severe retraction of the infraspinatus (Fig. 8.2). Double-traction sutures were placed in the supraspinatus and infraspinatus tendons. A rotator interval slide in continuity was performed by releasing circumferentially around the corocoid intra- and extra-articularly, but retaining the lateral rotator interval tissue in continuity with the subscapularis tendon.

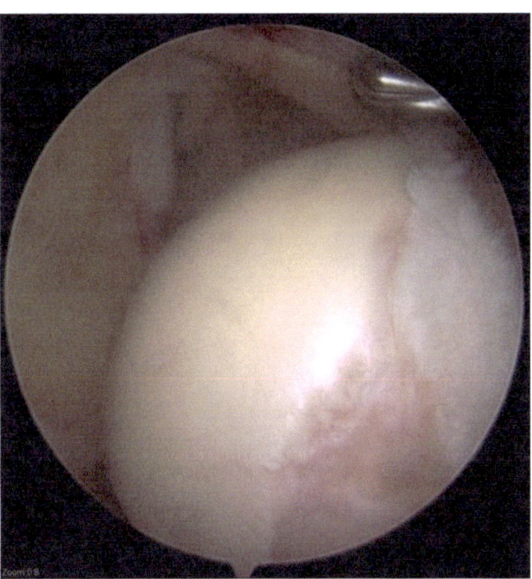

FIGURE 8.2 Posterior arthroscopic view of severely retracted supra and infraspinatus tear

Intra- and extra-articular releases were also performed about the supraspinatus and infraspinatus tendons which allowed the rotator cuff to be brought out to length onto the greater tuberosity. A reverse "L"-shaped tear pattern was present, with softer bone present in the greater tuberosity at the infraspinatus tendon insertion.

Two suture anchors were placed posteriorly with a tunnel between them to repair the infraspinatus tendon (Fig. 8.3). A transosseous equivalent-type repair with two lateral row anchors was then completed posteriorly, while the supraspinatus tendon was repaired with arthroscopic transosseous tunnels anteriorly. High-strength sutures in transosseous tunnels were utilized, which created simultaneous medial and lateral row fixation, obviating the need for lateral row anchors and sparing bone in this location. The medial tunnel was 2.9 mm in diameter, while the lateral tunnel was 1.9 mm in diameter (Fig. 8.4).

The patient was placed in a sling for 6 weeks postoperatively. She had an uneventful recovery until she fell on her outstretched arm 4 months postoperatively and presented with

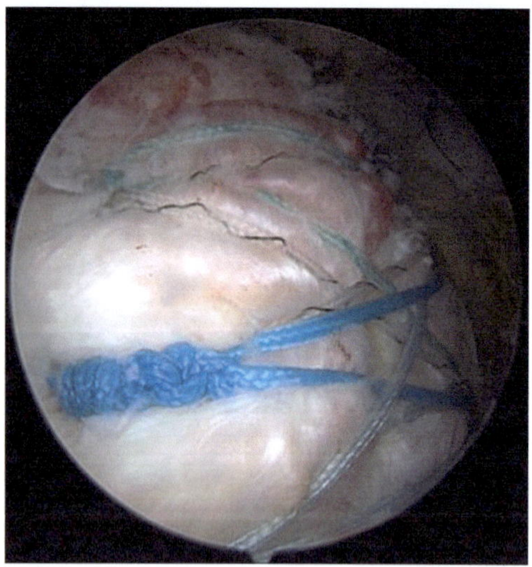

FIGURE 8.3 Posterior view of infraspinatus repair using a transosseous equivalent technique with two anchors medially and two laterally

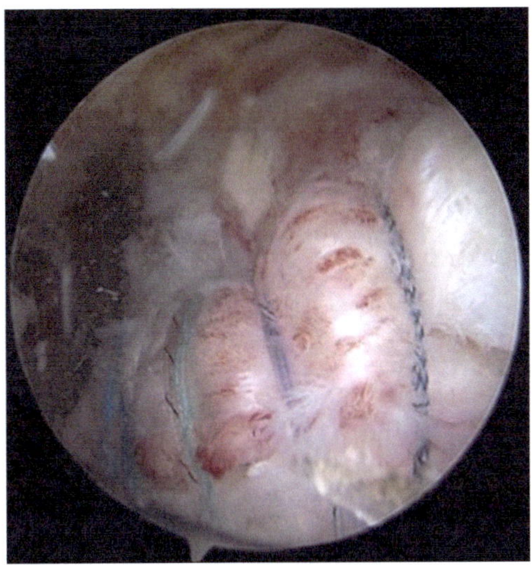

FIGURE 8.4 Arthroscopic transosseous tunnels are utilized to repair the supraspinatus and rotator interval anteriorly

worsening pain and function. A repeat MRI showed failure at the anchor-based infraspinatus repair, with the transosseous repair of the supraspinatus predominantly intact (Fig. 8.5). The decision was made to proceed with revision rotator cuff repair.

At surgery, arthroscopy confirmed a tendon remnant medially, but the majority of the lateral tendon remained on the tuberosity (Fig. 8.6). A 12–14 mm anchor void was created by removal of the loose anchor, creating concern of placing an anchor or stacked anchors in this void and obtaining fixation (Fig. 8.7). The anterior transosseous tunnels had healed to the rotator cuff. The previous tunnels had healed with bone and offered good bone which was available for revision anchor placement (Figs. 8.8 and 8.9). The previous tunnels were replaced with anchors, and transosseously placed sutures were placed in the previous anchor holes, inverting the prior construct. Figure 8.10 shows the guide arm of the suture tunneler in the anchor void. The tendon remnant was repaired with the inverted hybrid construct with anchor placed in the previous tunnels and tunnels placed in the previous anchor

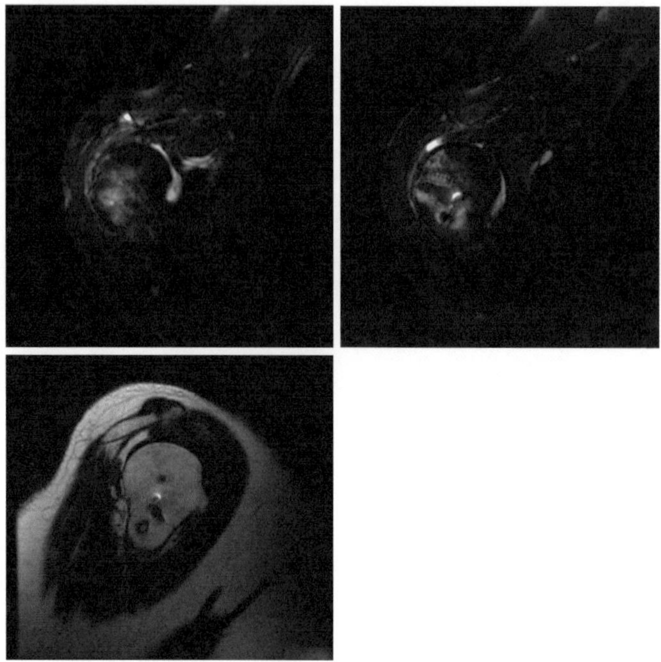

Figure 8.5 Coronal T2 MRI image showing intact supraspinatus repaired transosseously. Sagittal and coronal views show type 2 re-tear of the infraspinatus

hole positions. This allowed the rotator cuff to heal to the remaining bone with ample access to marrow elements. A "side-to-side" repair effect was also done at the tunneled sites, essentially mimicking a biological patch (Fig. 8.11).

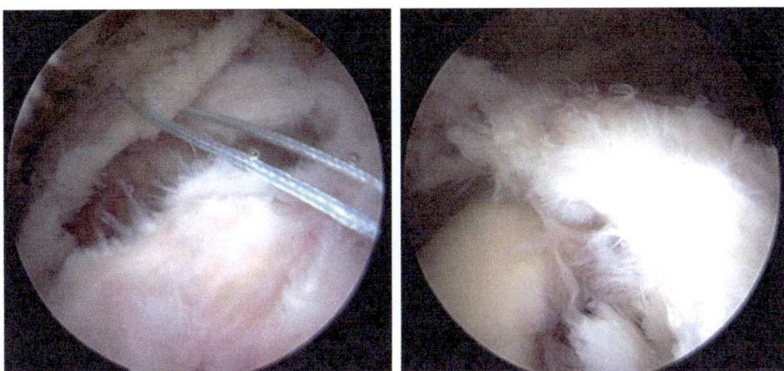

FIGURE 8.6 Arthroscopic views confirming a reparable tendon remnant with a type 2 failure of the previous repair. The anatomic footprint of the infraspinatus remains on the tuberosity

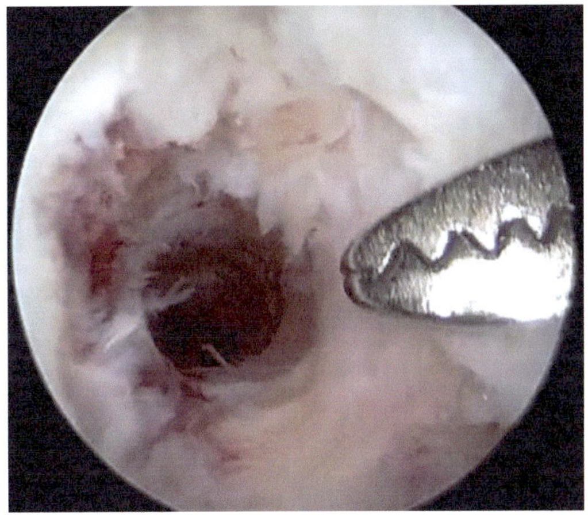

FIGURE 8.7 Large 12–14 mm anchor void is shown in the footprint of the rotator cuff

Outcome

At 6-month follow-up, the patient was pleased with the pain relief, range of motion, and strength of the shoulder, and she had an ASES score of 75.

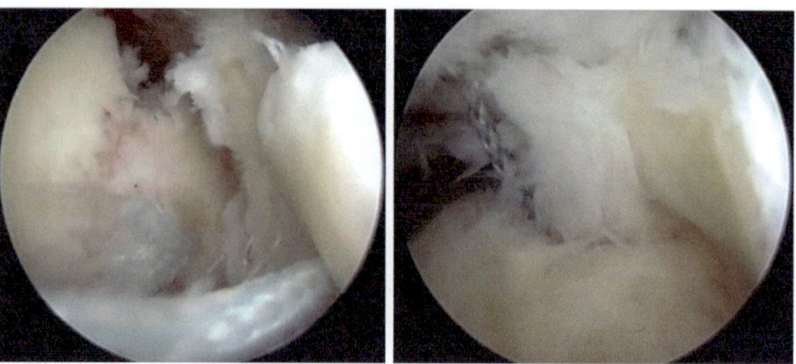

FIGURE 8.8 A small posteriorly based transosseous tunnel with a suture healed in the bone is seen adjacent to the large void created by the loose anchor. The anterior tunnel shows healing of the rotator cuff into the defect

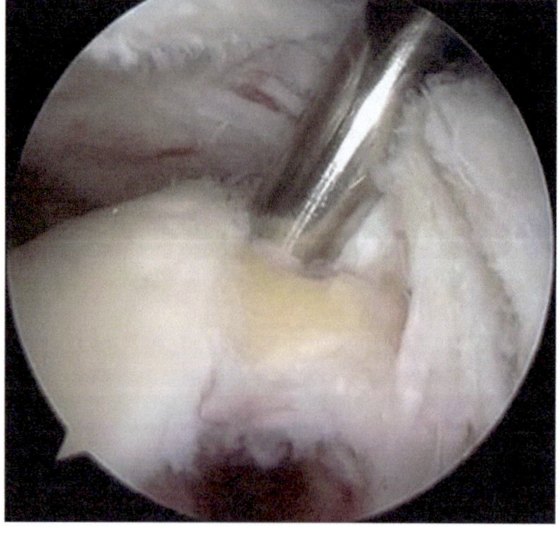

FIGURE 8.9 The previously placed tunnels are revised to anchors with excellent purchase of the bone

Literature Review

Open transosseous repair of tendons offers a cost-effective [1–9], biologically desirable [10, 11], biomechanically sound

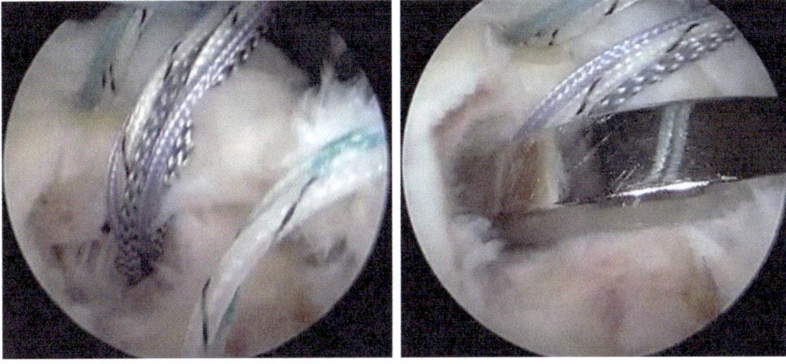

FIGURE 8.10 Sutures are placed in the bone void, while anchors are used to revise the previous transosseous tunnels. The tunneling guide is shown in position

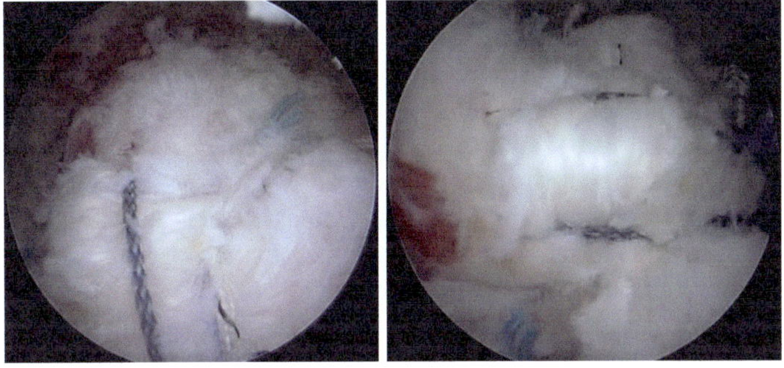

FIGURE 8.11 Lateral and posterior views of final revision repair

[12–16], and clinically effective [17–27] fixation method for healing of human tendons to bone. As a result, it has been considered the gold standard of rotator cuff repair for decades [27–31]. Anchor-based single- or double-row repairs became popular in the 1990s and early 2000s because of technical advances of arthroscopic treatments. Although healing of early single-row anchor constructs was relatively poor [30, 32], more recent double-row and transosseous repairs have had satisfactory outcomes [33]. There is no substantial difference in outcomes or re-tear rates between anchor-based and transosseous techniques [27]. Regardless of the technique, re-tear rates of the rotator cuff are about

25% overall and are even higher after repair of severe rotator cuff tears. Surprisingly, functional outcomes may fail to correlate with repair integrity [34, 35].

Arthroscopic methods of transosseous cuff repair have been described which have similar clinical results and decreased cost to anchor-based repairs [17–19, 23, 36]. Anchor-based and transosseous techniques have various benefits, but are not mutually exclusive, and thus can be used synergistically to treat severe rotator cuff tears [36]. This is advantageous when there is tendon or bone loss, revision scenarios, need for multiple fixation points, and poor local biology, and when the surgeon wants to use allograft or synthetic tissue augments and other biologically active substances.

Basic science has supported several principles for rotator cuff repair: high initial fixation strength, adequate resistance to cyclic loading, and anatomic footprint reconstruction with crossing sutures meant to provide compression and decrease shear forces at the tendon-bone interface [37]. Anchor-based constructs can satisfy many of these requirements including stiff and strong initial fixation, as well as ease of insertion and inherent bone augmentation in areas of soft bone at risk for anchor pullout. Transosseous equivalent (TOE) methods can mimic the cerclage effect about the footprint created by transosseous repair [38]. Because one anchor per fixation point is necessary, multiple anchors must be used, increasing cost and hardware in the greater tuberosity, as well as creating abrupt stress and strain transitions across delicate and poorly vascularized tissue which remains the weakest link in the repair. Some mechanical and biological concerns regarding anchor fixation are tissue strangulation [39], stress concentration [40], and modulus mismatch at the anchor-suture-tendon interface. Since the healing capability of the rotator cuff is poor and consists predominantly of controlled reparative, scar-based healing rather than regenerative healing with a new tendon insertion [41], these factors can produce "failure in continuity" seen as failure at the medial anchor. Previous authors have described this failure mode to be associated with, if not unique to, anchor constructs [42, 43]. When there is cuff failure it can be a type 1 failure defined as a torn cuff with no tendon left on the tuberosity, or type 2 failure where the tendon is torn at the medial anchors, leaving the tendon attached to the greater tuberosity. With a type 2 failure the shortened remaining tendon makes revision more difficult and increases tension in the repair. Techniques such as patch augmentation, bridging of tendon gaps, superior capsular reconstruction, bone loss management around anchor voids, and tension reduction strategies increase cost and technical difficulty. The exact interplay of biological factors such as vascularity and mechanical factors such as tension, stiffness, and ultimate failure strength necessary for healing remains unknown but matching local tissue mechanics rather than trying to exceed them may be more beneficial to biological healing. In summary, we consider both biological and mechanical factors for each patient in their rotator cuff repair.

Transosseous techniques have several relevant differences compared to anchor-based repairs. Small-diameter suture tunnels are easier to manage in revision settings, and don't preclude the placement of anchors or repeat tunnels in the same position. Transosseous tunnels offer benefits similar to double-row fixation with only a single tunnel, as there may be less re-tear in double-row repair patterns [44]. The failure mode of transosseous repairs generally spare tendon substance with a type 1 failure [25]. In addition, multiple repeat fixation points may be utilized, and various numbers and configurations of sutures per fixation point can be selected by the surgeon, creating a myriad of different repair constructs for complex cases. Additional high-strength sutures are generally more cost effective than additional anchors. In transosseous repair, there is no hardware blocking egress of bone marrow into the repair site that may improve the local biology [10, 11]. Since the strength of the repair is proportional to the number of sutures crossing the repair site [13], high-strength biomechanical constructs can be achieved. Some concerns regarding transosseous tunnels are deformation of the bone or the suture cutting through the bone, especially in chronic tears where the bone is soft. Cortical buttons, screw augmentation, suture tapes, or anchor hybrids may alleviate this concern [17, 36]. The ramifications of the suture cutting through the bone include fixation loss, but this is preferable to third body wear that may occur with failure of suture anchors. Regardless of the repair technique, the sutures pulling through the tendon are likely the biggest reason for failure of rotator cuff repairs with current techniques of repair of severe rotator cuff tears.

Clinical Pearls/Pitfalls

- Arthroscopic transosseous tunnels are bone and tendon sparing in repair of severe rotator cuff tears and avoid problems with loose or broken hardware.
- Anchors and tunnels can be used synergistically in repair of a severe rotator cuff tear, and revised in a complementary fashion.
- Hybrid techniques of anchors and tunnels allow the surgeon to use the advantages of each method to greatest effect while maintaining revision options in the future.
- Transosseous tunneling can provide multiple, repeat fixation points for sutures to share load with minimal costs.
- For soft bone into which an awl can be driven by hand, we will often use anchor support. If the awl requires a mallet, tunnels are usually sufficient. Mattress sutures rarely if ever cut through bone across a large bone bridge, but this must be tempered with concern over tissue tearing at the medial fixation of the repaired cuff.
- Large bone voids can be treated with transosseous tunnels, allowing the tendon to heal. Additional cortical support can be obtained with cortical buttons, screws, or anchors placed laterally and inferiorly. High-surface-area tapes can be used as well in tunnels to prevent or reduce the chances of sutures cutting through tendon or bone.

References

1. Yu S, Zuckerman J. 5 points on orthopedics in US healthcare. Am J Orthop. 2015;44:12.
2. Payne A, et al. Orthopaedic implant waste: analysis and quantification. Am J Orthop. 2015;44(12):554–60.
3. Black EM, Higgins LD, Warner JJP. Value based shoulder surgery: practicing outcomes driven, cost conscious care. J Shoulder Elb Surg. 2013;22:1000–9. http://dx.doi.org/10.1016/j.jse.2013.02.008
4. Srikumaran U, et al. Arthroscopic transosseous rotator cuff repair is cost effective compared to anchored technique. Poster presentation at San Diego Shoulder Meeting, 2013.
5. Churchill RS, Ghorai JK. Total cost and operating room time comparison of rotator cuff repair techniques at low, intermediate, and high volume centers: mini-open versus all-arthroscopic. J Shoulder Elb Surg. 2010;19:716–21. http://dx.doi.org/10.1016/j.jse.2009.10.011
6. Genuario JW, Donegan RP, Hamman D, Bell JE, Boublik M, Schlegel T, et al. The cost-effectiveness of single-row compared with double-row arthroscopic rotator cuff repair. J Bone Joint Surg Am. 2012;94:1369–77. http://dx.doi.org/10.2106/JBJS.J.01876
7. Adla DN, Rowsell M, Pandey R. Cost-effectiveness of open versus arthroscopic rotator cuff repair. J Shoulder Elb Surg. 2010;19:258–61. http://dx.doi.org/10.1016/j.jse.2009.05.004
8. Vitale MA, Vitale MG, Zivin JG, et al. Rotator cuff repair: an analysis of utility scores and cost-effectiveness. J Shoulder Elb Surg. 2007;16(2):181–7.
9. Narvy S, Ahluwalia A, Vangsness CT. Analysis of direct cost of outpatient arthroscopic rotator cuff repair. Am J Orthop. 2016;45(1):E7–E11.
10. Jo CH, Shin JS, Park IW, Kim H, Lee SY. Multiple channeling improves the structural integrity of rotator cuff repair. Am J Sports Med. 2013;41(11):2650–7. doi:10.1177/0363546513499138. Epub 2013 Aug 13
11. Milano G, Saccomanno MF, Careri S, Taccardo G, Vitis RD, Fabbriciani C. Efficacy of marrow stimulating technique in rotator cuff repair: a prospective randomized study. Abstract presented at AANA San Francisco, April 2011.

12. Behrens GA. Initial fixation strength of transosseous equivalent suture bridge repair is comparable with transosseous repair. Am J Sports Med. 2012;40:133.
13. Johst PW, Khair MM, Chen DX, Wright TM, Kelly AM, Rodeo SA. Suture number determines strength of rotator cuff repair. J Bone Joint Surg Am. 2012;94(14):e100. doi:10.2106/JB- JS.K.00117.
14. Bicos J, Mazzoca A, Hallab N, Santangelo S, Bach B. The multi-suture technique for rotator cuff repair: a biomechanical evaluation. Orthopaedics. 2007;30(11):910–9.
15. Kummer FJ, Hahn M, Day M, Muslin RJ, Jazrawi LM. Laboratory comparison of a new arthroscopic transosseous rotator cuff repair technique to a double row transosseous equivalent repair using anchors. Bull Hosp Joint Dis. 2013;71(2):128–31.
16. Bisson LJ, Manohar LM. A biomechanical comparison of transosseous suture anchor and suture bridge rotator cuff repairs in cadavers. Am J Sports Med. 2009;37(10):1991–5.
17. Garrigues GE, Lazarus MD. Arthroscopic bone tunnel augmentation for rotator cuff repair. Orthopaedics. 2012;35(5):392–7.
18. Cicak N, Klobucar H, Bicanic G, Trsek D. Arthroscopic transosseous suture anchor technique for rotator cuff repairs. Arthroscopy. 2006;22(5):565.e1–6.
19. Kim KC, Rhee KJ, Shin HD, Kim YM. Arthroscopic transosseous rotator cuff repair. Orthopaeidcs. 2008;31(4):327–30.
20. Garofalo R, Castagna A, Borroni M, Krishnan S. Arthroscopic transosseous (anchorless) rotator cuff repair. Knee Surg Sports Traumatol Arthrosc. 2012;20:1031–5. doi:10.1007/500167-001-1725.4.
21. Fox MP, Auffarth A, Tauber M, Hartmann A, Resch H. A novel transosseous button technique for rotator cuff repair. Arthroscopy. 2008;24(9):1074–7. doi:10.1016/j.arthro.2008.02.014. Epub 2008 Apr 21
22. Burkhart SS, Nassar J, Schenck RC Jr, Wirth MA. Clinical and anatomic considerations in the use of a new anterior inferior submaxillary nerve portal. Arthrsocopy. 1996;12(5):634–7.
23. Kuroda S. Advantages of arthroscopic transosseous suture repair of the rotator cuff without the use of anchors. Clin Orthop Relat Res. 2013;471(11):3514–22. doi:10.1007/s11999-013-3146-7.
24. Nho S, et al. Systematic review of arthroscopic rotator cuff repair and mini-open rotator cuff repair. J Bone Joint Surg Am. 2007;89(Suppl 3):127–36. doi:10.2106/JBJS.G.00583.

25. Black EM, Linn A, Skrikumaran U, Jain N, Freehill M. Arthroscopic transosseous rotator cuff repair: technical note, outcomes, and complications. Orthopaedics. 2015;38(5):e352–8.
26. Srikumaran U, Hannan C, Kilcoyne K, Petersen S, Mcfarland E, Zikria B. Arthroscopic anchored versus transosseous cuff repair: a comparison of clinical outcomes and structural integrity. AAOS presentation, March 2016, Orlando, Florida. Abstract #356.
27. Flanagin BA, Garofalo R, Lo EY, Feher L, Castagna A, Qin H, Krishnan SG. Midterm clinical outcomes following arthroscopic transosseous rotator cuff repair. Int J Shoulder Surg. 2016 Jan-Mar;10(1):3–9.
28. McLaughlin HL. Lesions of the musculotendinous cuff of the shoulder: the exposure and treatment of tears with retraction. J Bone Joint Surg Am. 1944;26:31–51.
29. Ramsey ML, Getz CL, Parsons BO. What's new in shoulder and elbow surgery. J Bone Joint Surg Am. 2009;91(5):1283–93.
30. Bishop J, Klepps S, Lo IK, Bird J, Gladstone JN, Flatow EL. Cuff integrity after arthroscopic versus open rotator cuff repair: a prospective study. J Shoulder Elb Surg. 2006;15(3):290–9.
31. McCallister WV, Parson IM, Titleman RM, Matsen FA III. Open rotator cuff repair without acromioplasty. J Bone Joint Surg Am. 2005;87(6):1278–83.
32. Galatz LM, Ball CM, Teefey SA, Middletown WD, Yamaguchi K. The outcome and repair integrity of completely arthroscopically repaired large and massive rotator cuff tears. J Bone Joint Surg Am. 2004;86-A(2):219–24.
33. Imam MA, Abdelkafy A. Outcomes following arthroscopic transosseous equivalent suture bridge double row rotator cuff repair: a prospective study and short-term results. SICOT J. 2016;2:7. doi:10.1051/sicotj/2015041. PMID: 27163096
34. Russell RD, et al. Structural integrity after rotator cuff repair does not correlate with patient function and pain: a meta-analysis. J Bone Joint Surg Am. 2014;96(4):265–71. doi:10.2106/JBJS.M.00265.
35. Moosmayer S, et al. Tendon repair compared with physiotherapy in the treatment of rotator cuff tears. A randomized controlled study in 103 cases with a five-year follow up. J Bone Joint Surg Am. 2014;96:1504–14.
36. Sanders B. Novel reusable transosseous tunnel based soft tissue repair techniques about the shoulder: a rational, value-based approach. MOJ Orthop Rheumatol. 2016;5(1):00164. doi:10.15406/mojor.2016.05.00164.

37. Lee TQ. Current biomechanical concepts for rotator cuff repair. Clin Orthop Surg. 2013;5(2):89–97. doi:10.4055/cios.2013.5.2.89. PMCID: PMC3664677

38. Franceschi F, Papalia R, Franceschetti E, Palumbo A, Del Buono A, Paciotti M, Maffulli N, Denaro V. Double-row repair lowers the retear risk after accelerated rehabilitation. Am J Sports Med. 2016;44(4):948–56. doi:10.1177/0363546515623031. Epub 2016 Jan 21. PMID: 26797698

39. Christoforetti JJ, Krupp RJ, Singleton SB, Kissenberth MJ, Cook C, Hawkins RJ. Arthroscopic suture bridge transosseus equivalent fixation of rotator cuff tendon preserves intratendinous blood flow at the time of initial fixation. J Shoulder Elbow Surg. 2012;21:523–30.

40. Sano H, Yamashita T, Wakabayashi I, Itoi E. Stress distribution in the supraspinatus tendon after tendon repair: suture anchors versus transosseous suture fixation. Am J Sports Med. 2007;35(4):542–6. Epub 2007 Jan 11

41. JA MC, Derwin KA, Bey MJ, Polster JM, Schils JP, Ricchetti ET, Iannotti JP. Failure with continuity in rotator cuff repair "healing". Am J Sports Med. 2013;41(1):134–41. doi:10.1177/0363546512459477. Epub 2012 Sep 27

42. Cho NS, Yi JW, Lee BG, Rhee YG. Retear patterns after arthroscopic rotator cuff repair: single-row versus suture bridge technique. Am J Sports Med. 2010;38(4):664–71. doi:10.1177/0363546509350081. Epub 2009 Dec 29

43. Trantalis JN, Boorman RS, Pletsch K, Lo IK. Medial rotator cuff failure after arthroscopic double-row rotator cuff repair. Arthroscopy. 2008;24(6):727–31. doi:10.1016/j.arthro.2008.03.009.

44. Panella A, Amati C, Moretti L, Damato P, Notarnicola A, Moretti B. Single-row and transosseous sutures for supraspinatus tendon tears: a retrospective comparative clinical and strength outcome at 2-year follow-up. Arch Orthop Trauma Surg. 2016;136:1507–11.

Chapter 9
Arthroscopic Debridement for Massive Rotator Cuff Tears

Steven Cohen and Kirsten Poehling-Monaghan

Case Presentation

We present the case of a patient undergoing arthroscopic debridement along with capsular release and subacromial decompression for a massive, immobile, and atrophied rotator cuff tear in her nondominant shoulder. This was a 73-year-old right-hand-dominant female presenting with pain in her left shoulder for approximately 1 year. She described a deep, aching pain over the superolateral shoulder, occurring intermittently and worsened with overhead or forward activities. Recently, it had become difficult to drive and the pain awakened her at night. The pain was relieved only by rest and occasionally with a heating pad over the posterior periscapular muscles. She denied any radiating pain or paresthesias, and had no mechanical symptoms such as catching or clicking.

S. Cohen, M.D.
Rothman Institute of Orthopeadics,
925 Chestnut St., Philadelphia, PA 19107, USA
e-mail: steven.cohen@rothmaninstitute.com

K. Poehling-Monaghan, M.D. (✉)
Precision Orthopedics and Sports Medicine, Silver Springs, MD, USA
e-mail: drkpmonaghan@gmail.com

© Springer International Publishing AG 2018
P.J. McMahon (ed.), *Rotator Cuff Injuries*,
DOI 10.1007/978-3-319-63668-9_9

She had previously undergone several courses of physical therapy, three subacromial cortisone injections, and a course of prescription anti-inflammatories without improvement in her symptoms. Two weeks prior her primary care provider gave her a prescription for hydrocodone, which she had been taking, but it often made her sleepy. She noticed a decrease in her range of motion secondary to weakness, though when prompted to quantify she stated that this was only 10% of her disability, with pain comprising the remaining 90%. She felt as though the pain not only limited her recreational activities (which include gardening and volunteer work) but had also begun to affect her activities of daily living.

The patient was 5′3″ tall and 165 lbs, with a BMI of 29. Range of motion of the cervical spine was painless and slightly decreased in extension, with a negative Spurling maneuver. She was neurologically intact throughout her bilateral upper extremities with symmetric and intact sensation and reflexes. Range of motion for bilateral upper extremities is documented in Table 9.1.

When testing rotator cuff strength, the patient had significant weakness with resisted abduction at 90° (i.e., supraspinatus testing), with a positive drop-arm sign. She had 3/5 strength in resisted external rotation, and normal resisted internal rotation equal to the contralateral side. She was able to perform a belly-press and liftoff test, indicating a competent subscapularis muscle. Her deltoid and biceps strength were normal and equal to the contralateral side.

TABLE 9.1 Pre-op range of motion

	Left	**Right**
Elevation/ABD supine	100 (active) 160 (passive)	150 (active) 160 (passive)
Elevation/ABD upright	80 (active) 130 (passive)	130 (active) 150 (passive)
External rotation	50 (active) 60 (passive)	60 (active) 75 (passive)
Internal rotation	L1	L1

There was mild tenderness over the biceps tendon in the groove, with similar tenderness in the contralateral shoulder. Biceps testing (Speed and Yergason) was negative for pain or weakness. She had no tenderness over the acromioclavicular (AC) joint, and no significant pain with cross-body abduction. She had positive impingement signs (both Neer and Hawkins).

Radiographs included upright AP of the shoulder in internal and external rotation as well as axillary and scapular-Y views. These revealed that the humeral head was centered on the glenoid so there was no evidence of significant humeral head elevation, and preserved glenohumeral joint space. She had a type II acromion with minimal AC joint arthrosis.

A 1.5 T non-contrast MRI of the shoulder taken 2 months prior to our initial office evaluation was read by the radiologist as a full-thickness tear of the supraspinatus involving approximately 70% of the tendon footprint. There was significant tendinopathy throughout the remaining tendon as well as partial-thickness bursal-sided tearing (approximately 30%) of the infraspinatus tendon. The supraspinatus tendon was retracted to the glenoid. On T1-weighted sagittal views, there was approximately 40% atrophy of the supraspinatus muscle. The infraspinatus muscle was normal in appearance. There was a minimal amount of fluid within the AC joint. Degenerative fraying of the labrum was noted both anteriorly and posteriorly without a frank tear. The biceps tendon was located within the groove and was normal in appearance. The subscapularis was intact. A small amount of humeral head chondrosis was noted but the majority of the joint space appeared well preserved.

Diagnosis/Assessment

Based on imaging, the patient was diagnosed with a full-thickness rotator cuff tear with significant retraction. A number of surgical options were presented and the risks and benefits of each were explained. Ultimately, the surgeon's recommendation was shoulder arthroscopy to address any chondrolabral pathology that may be encountered, capsular release if indicated, subacromial decompression, and attempted rotator cuff repair. Based on the degree of tendinopathy and atrophy seen on the MRI, the patient was cautioned that the quality and integrity of the remaining tendon may not be amenable to repair. If this were the case, then an arthroscopic debridement would be performed. The patient was made aware that with a debridement we would seek to diminish the pain, without significant improvements in strength and motion.

Management

In the weeks before surgery, the patient was weaned from her hydrocodone. No nerve block was used and once in the operating room, the patient was placed in the beach-chair position and underwent general anesthesia without paralysis. Examination of the shoulder under anesthesia showed minimal change in passive range of motion from her clinical encounter. The operative extremity was prepped and draped and preoperative antibiotics were given (Table 9.2).

A standard posterior-viewing portal was established after the joint was insufflated with 50 cc of normal saline utilizing an 18-guage spinal needle through the same path. A diagnostic arthroscopy was performed (Fig. 9.1).

TABLE 9.2 Pearls: pre-op

Patient selection	Imaging	Discussion
Elderly (>65)	X-ray: elevation of humeral head, GH arthritis	Partial repair vs. debridement only
Lower demand	MRI: amount of retraction, subscap tears, fatty atrophy	Pain relief realistic but gains in motion are *not*
Pain > ROM loss		

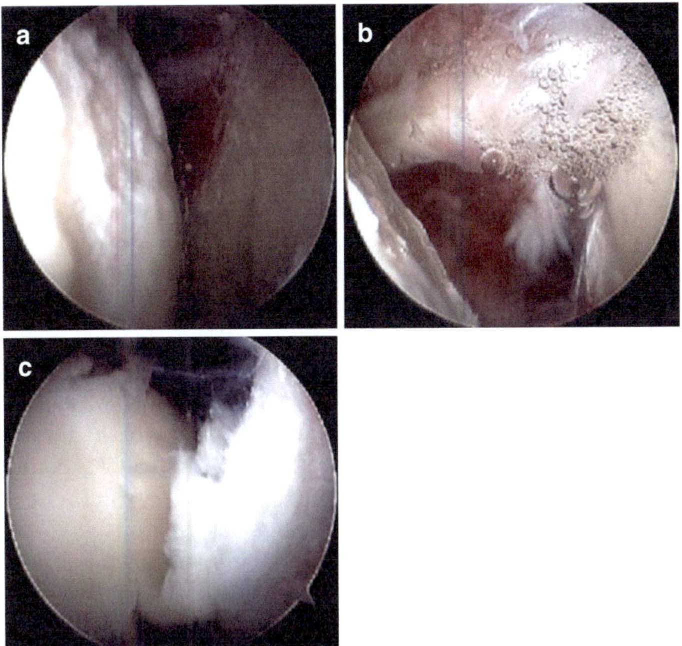

FIGURE 9.1 The intra-articular portion of the diagnostic arthroscopy shows Grade III degenerative changes at the glenohumeral articulation (**a**). The biceps anchor is probed and a type I SLAP tear is noted (**b**). The rotator cuff tear is seen (**c**) with significant retraction

There was noted to be Grade III chondrosis of approximately 20% of the humeral head articular surface. A type I SLAP tear was encountered, with both the intra-articular and proximal-groove portion of the biceps tendon appearing normal. The rotator cuff was visibly torn with retraction to the level of the glenohumeral articulation. The axillary pouch was free of loose bodies. The subscapularis was covered in a thickened synovium but was intact. The middle and superior glenohumeral ligaments were contracted.

Under direct visualization, an anterior working portal was created between the biceps and subscapularis. A 5.5 mm cannula was introduced. A 4.0 mm shaver was used to lightly debride the degenerative anterior labrum and type I SLAP tear, as well as a small chondral flap on the humeral head. The anterior capsule was released using a combination of arthroscopic electrocautery and the shaver. Finally, a 0-PDS suture was introduced as a traction stitch through the rotator cuff using an 18-gauge spinal needle (Fig. 9.2).

The arthroscope was then removed and the portal was redirected through the same posterior skin incision to enter the subacromial space. After sweeping the space with the blunt trocar of the scope, a large amount of scar and inflamed bursa remained. An anterolateral accessory portal was created under direct visualization and a 4.0 mm shaver was used to perform a thorough subacromial and subdeltoid bursectomy. The anterior and lateral boundaries of the acromion were established using arthroscopic cautery, and the coracoacromial ligament was gently debrided but left intact. Care was taken not to elevate the deltoid from the lateral acromial border. Any bleeding encountered, particularly anteromedial adjacent to the coracoacromial ligament and medially past the myotendinous junction, was controlled using arthroscopic electrocautery. Such an extensive bursectomy was necessary for two important reasons: first, extensive debridement of the subacromial bursa, particularly medially

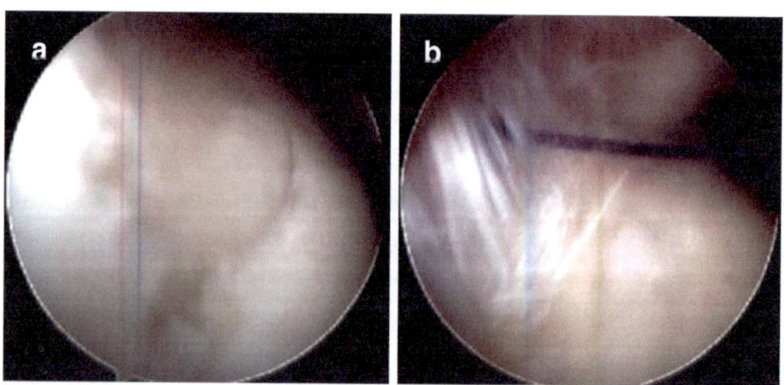

FIGURE 9.2 The chondral lesion on the humeral head was debrided (**a**), and the rotator cuff tear was tagged using a percutaneously placed 0-PDS suture (**b**) for adequate visualization from the subacromial space

(with care to electrocauterize inevitable bleeders), mobilizes the cuff tissue significantly, which is vital for best chances for repair. Second, decompression of the subdeltoid space results in improved visualization of the rotator cuff footprint on the greater tuberosity, which is necessary to determine the degree of retraction. In addition, patients with shoulder stiffness are likely to gain motion from releasing any adhesions in this space.

Once the subacromial and subdeltoid bursae were cleared, the shaver was switched to a 5.5 mm sheathed barrel burr, and the subacromial spurs were removed without removing any of the normal acromion or resecting the CA ligament. This is different than the subacromial decompression we normally perform with rotator cuff repair when working from anterior to posterior; the bony decompression is considered finished once the anterior acromion is flush with the spine of the scapula posteriorly (Table 9.3).

With improved visualization and increased working space, attention was turned back to the rotator cuff. The traction PDS suture was retrieved out the lateral portal, and light traction was applied. The suture, which penetrated the tendon approximately 5.0 mm from the free edge, pulled through the tissue. Using the 4.0 mm shaver and light suction, the edges of

TABLE 9.3 Pearls: intra-op

Intra-articular	Subacromial
Perform thorough assessment of GH chondral changes	Thorough bursectomy is key both to visualization and mobilization of cuff
Document status of biceps and subscap, addressing biceps if needed	Preserve the CA ligament
Perform capsular release for more significant limits in motion	Adequate debridement of the cuff to *viable tissue*
Scar/bursa can mask a cuff tear from the subacromial space: tag with PDS from inside the joint if in question	Care not to debride too far posterior into viable cuff or too far anterior into biceps

the rotator cuff were debrided and large amount of bursa and scar was removed. The remaining tissue was extremely friable, and a large defect was quickly identified. Using the arthroscopic grasper, we attempted to mobilize the remaining tissue which also pulled apart easily. Despite efforts to mobilize the tendon and attempt marginal convergence, the tendon was not able to be restored to the tuberosity and we therefore decided to proceed with arthroscopic debridement of the rotator cuff. Using a 4.0 mm shaver, the edges of the cuff that came freely to the shaver with moderate suction were debrided (Fig. 9.3). Care was taken not to extend into

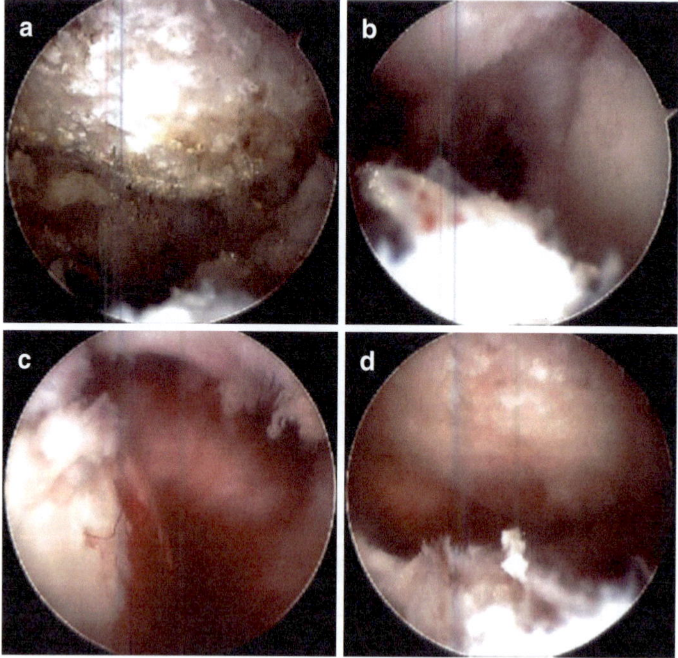

FIGURE 9.3 An adequate bursectomy and subacromial decompression are performed to ensure adequate visualization and aid in potential mobilization of the cuff (**a**). After debridement of nonviable cuff tissue and bursa, the remaining rotator cuff is noted to be significantly retracted and difficult to mobilize (**b**). At that point, a formal debridement was performed (**c**, **d**)

TABLE 9.4 Pearls: post-op

Begin early ROM to prevent stiffness

Focus on periscapular muscle strengthening

No lifting restrictions: let pain be their guide

Follow closely with biannual or annual X-rays to assess acromiohumeral distance

the remaining intact cuff posteriorly, or to violate the biceps tendon which was partially exposed anteriorly. The cuff remnant on the tuberosity was also debrided, but no tuberoplasty was performed due to the lack of significant bony prominence. Were we to have encountered a more significant overgrowth of the tuberosity or roughened edges and spurring, the prominence would have been shaved down to a smooth surface to prevent future impingement.

Once the debridement was sufficient, the arthroscope was removed and the portals were closed using interrupted #3-0-nylon sutures. The portals and subacromial space were injected with 15 cc of half-percent Marcaine. The wounds were dressed with Xeroform, 4 × 4 gauze and a single abdominal (ABD) pad and covered with foam tape. A simple sling was applied to the left arm. The patient was transferred to the postanesthesia care unit and returned to home later that day after adequate recovery from anesthesia. The patient was given instructions on donning the sling, and gentle pendulum exercises to perform on her own until her follow-up visit.

The patient was seen back at 10 days post-op to remove her sutures and initiate gentle physical therapy to work on regaining motion, stretching, and gradual increase in strength. There were no lifting restrictions (Table 9.4).

Outcome

The patient was lost to follow-up until 1 year from the date of surgery and she said that she had been pain free until recently when there had been a return in pain and increase in disability.

Repeat radiographs showed a narrowed acromiohumeral distance. She was referred for reverse shoulder arthroplasty.

Literature Review

Repair of massive, retracted, and largely atrophied rotator cuff tears is often not possible and even when it is, the needs of the patient are sometimes best served by arthroscopic debridement. Given the potential for unfavorable outcomes with this procedure, adequate patient selection is crucial. We feel that those best served by debridement alone are those complaining primarily of pain over loss of motion, and those with lower demand and functional requirements. While hand dominance does not play a crucial role, debridement in the nondominant shoulder may have better outcome.

Arthroscopic debridement for irreparable rotator cuff tears has favorable outcomes and in the correct patient population outcomes can rival arthroscopic repair. A randomized study of partial repair versus arthroscopic debridement for massive cuff tears with associated grade 3 and 4 fatty atrophy noted equal pain relief and DASH scores in the two groups [1]. Yet another study of massive tears undergoing debridement, partial, or complete repair showed no difference in clinical outcome scores (Constant, DASH, and patient satisfaction) among the three groups [2].

With debridement alone it has long been thought that preserving the coracohumeral arch is important, so no acromioplasty or violation of the CA ligament is done. The worry is "anterior humeral head escape"; instead of rolling to elevate the arm, the humeral head instead slides anterior to the acromion and the arm does not go up. In a series of patients undergoing debridement without acromioplasty, elderly, low-demand individuals showed improved pain and function scores at 4 years, but with a concomitant decrease in acromiohumeral distance [3]. In a similar series, 33 elderly patients underwent arthroscopic rotator cuff debridement along with tuberoplasty and biceps tenotomy (a so-called reverse acromioplasty) with preservation of the acromion and CA ligament. At a mean of 38 months, 94% of patients had significant improvements in Constant scores, though acromiohumeral height was still decreased by an average of 2.58 mm [4].

In some instances, overgrowth of the CA arch is thought to contribute to pain and acromioplasty is performed. Patients undergoing arthroscopic cuff debridement as well as both acromioplasty and tuberoplasty saw significantly improved clinical outcome scores and range of motion provided that their preoperative acromiohumeral interval was not decreased [5]. The questionable contribution of the biceps to both pain and stability of the humeral head has also been questioned, and comparisons of rotator cuff debridement with or without biceps tenotomy in elderly patients showed no difference in outcomes with improved pain and function in both groups [6].

When considering this procedure, the surgeon should be aware that a number of negative prognostic factors have also been identified, including significant limits in preoperative range of motion, preoperative superior migration of the humeral head, concomitant subscapularis tears, and presence of glenohumeral arthritis at the time of debridement [7].

Clinical Pearls/Pitfalls

- The key to the management of a massive rotator cuff tear with debridement is patient selection; those with lower demand who have pain as the greatest concern over loss of motion and strength.
- Perform a thorough bursectomy to visualize and aid in potential mobilization.
- Not taking down CA ligament to minimize the risk of anterior humeral head escape.
- Include concomitant capsular release if there is shoulder stiffness.
- Begin early ROM postoperative.
- Follow postoperative with radiographs to assess for decreased acromiohumeral distance.

References

1. Neri BR, Chan KW, Kwon YW. Management of massive and irreparable rotator cuff tears. J Shoulder Elb Surg. 2009;18(5):808–18.
2. Heuberer PR, Kölblinger R, Buchleitner S, Pauzenberger L, Laky B, Auffarth A, Moroder P, Salem S, Kriegleder B, Anderl W. Arthroscopic management of massive rotator cuff tears: an evaluation of debridement, complete, and partial repair with and without force couple restoration. Knee Surg Sports Traumatol Arthrosc. 2016;24:3828–37.
3. Klinger HM, Spahn G, Baums MH, Steckel H. Arthroscopic debridement of irreparable massive rotator cuff tears—a comparison of debridement alone and combined procedure with biceps tenotomy. Acta Chir Belg. 2005;105(3):297–3013.
4. Verhelst L, Vandekerckhove PJ, Sergeant G, Liekens K, Van Hoonacker P, Berghs B. Reversed arthroscopic subacromial decompression for symptomatic irreparable rotator cuff tears: mid-term follow-up results in 34 shoulders. J Shoulder Elb Surg. 2010;19(4):601–8.
5. Lee BG, Cho NS, Rhee YG. Results of arthroscopic decompression and tuberoplasty for irreparable massive rotator cuff tears. Arthroscopy. 2011;27(10):1341–50.
6. Liem D, Lengers N, Dedy N, Poetzl W, Steinbeck J, Marquardt B. Arthroscopic debridement of massive irreparable rotator cuff tears. Arthroscopy. 2008;24(7):743–8.
7. Klinger HM, Steckel H, Ernstberger T, Baums MH. Arthroscopic debridement of massive rotator cuff tears: negative prognostic factors. Arch Orthop Trauma Surg. 2005;125(4):261–6.

Chapter 10
Open Repair of Severe Rotator Cuff Tears

Robert J. Neviaser and Andrew S. Neviaser

Case Presentation

A 58-year-old right-handed man presents having fallen a week ago injuring his right shoulder. He was seen in an emergency room and the shoulder was reduced successfully after an X-ray showed that he had an anterior dislocation but no associated fractures. He had never dislocated this shoulder before but had noted non-disabling mild pain at night and pain after playing tennis over the past few years. After the shoulder was reduced, he was not able to elevate the arm, but that had improved somewhat over the ensuing few days.

On physical examination, he is 5′10″ tall and weighs 185 lbs. His neck and neurologic exam is normal. His axillary nerve in particular is normal. There is some supraspinatus and infraspinatus atrophy, and the long head of the biceps is intact but tender. He can elevate the arm actively but cautiously to 80°,

R.J. Neviaser, M.D. (✉) • A.S. Neviaser, M.D.
Department of Orthopaedic Surgery, The George Washington University School of Medicine, GWU-MFA,
5th Floor, 2300 M St., NW, Washington, DC 20037, USA
e-mail: rneviaser@mfa.gwu.edu

© Springer International Publishing AG 2018
P.J. McMahon (ed.), *Rotator Cuff Injuries*,
DOI 10.1007/978-3-319-63668-9_10

externally rotate in abduction to 70°, externally rotate at the side to 30°, and internally rotate to L3 compared to 170°, 85°, 45°, and T11 with the other shoulder. His liftoff and abdominal press tests are negative, but his impingement sign, palm-down abduction, and biceps resistance tests are positive. His strength in external rotation and elevation is 4/5.

He brings his injury and post-reduction films with him. They confirm the anterior dislocation and satisfactory reduction. Because his injury was a primary dislocation and he was over the age of 40, it is suspected that he has a traumatic rotator cuff rupture or tear [1].

Diagnosis/Assessment

An MRI is ordered which shows an extensive tear (Fig. 10.1a, b) with some fatty infiltration on the T1 sagittal oblique images (Fig. 10.1c). This confirms the diagnosis. The discussion with the patient includes the state of his rotator cuff, the fact that it is not going to heal spontaneously, and that if surgical repair is undertaken before the 3-week mark, his chances of a successful outcome are better than they are if the surgery is delayed much beyond that [2].

Management

The surgery can be done under general anesthesia with or without an associated interscalene block or under an interscalene block with sedation. The patient is positioned in a sitting position with the head secured on a headrest and the entire shoulder and right side of the chest—anterior and posterior—exposed. An arthroscope is introduced into the glenohumeral joint through a posterior portal, and an anterior portal established from inside-out. A shaver is passed though the anterior portal, and the joint debrided as needed. The long head of the biceps and the joint side of the cuff tear are inspected. The scope is redirected to the subacromial space and a lateral portal is made through which the shaver

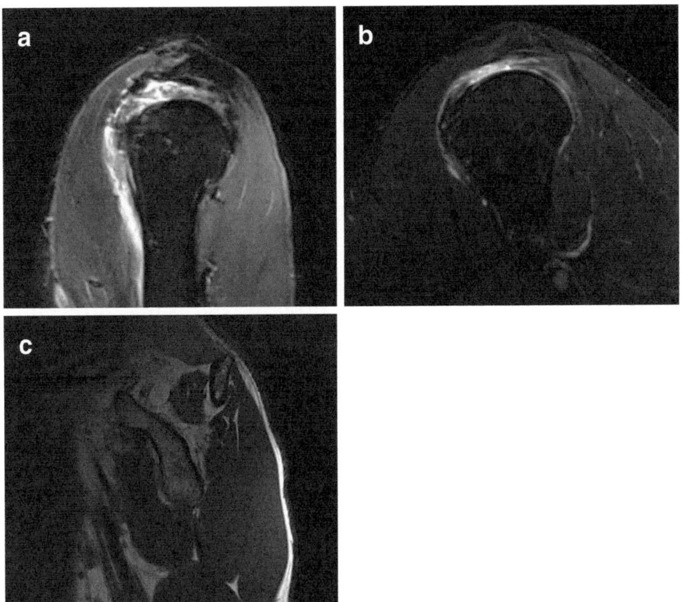

Figure 10.1 (**a**) Coronal T2-weighted MRI image revealing large rotator cuff tear. (**b**) Sagittal oblique image showing AP extent of tear. (**c**) TI-weighted image documenting moderate fatty infiltration of the supraspinatus

is reintroduced to debride enough of the bursa to allow clear visualization of the cuff tear, the coracoacromial ligament, and the anterior inferior acromion. This step can be facilitated by using an electrocautery wand.

Before doing an acromioplasty, a grasper is placed through the lateral portal as well as a small elevator to free the tendons up. Traction via the grasper allows us assessment of the mobility of the tendons, which determines if they can be repaired. If the tendons are not mobile and we do think a repair can be done, a subacromial decompression is not done so as to minimize the complication of anterior-superior escape. Using the electrocautery wand, the coracoacromial ligament is released. If we think a repair is possible we further tailor the amount of release by how confident we are about the strength and security of the repair. If a good repair can be achieved, then a complete ligament release is done; but if there is any concern about the security of a repair, then the lateral one-third only is released in order to avoid the complication of anterior-superior escape. The periosteum of the undersurface of the acromion is removed with the wand and a burr is used to perform an acromioplasty to give the repaired cuff room to glide under the acromion. One can also place nonabsorbable traction sutures through the torn cuff with a suture punch to provide traction to the tendons throughout the mobilization process but only after any decompression is performed; otherwise these sutures may be cut during the decompression.

An incision is made slightly medial to the anterolateral corner of the acromion and extended through and in line with the fibers of the deltoid. An elevator is used to free the subdeltoid space around the entire glenohumeral joint. If traction sutures have not already been placed, serial traction sutures are placed in the cuff. After placing each, further mobilization is done with an elevator, bringing the torn edges farther and farther toward the anatomic neck and tuberosity. Using these steps, eventually the apex of the tear is reached, which completes the control of the cuff. If additional mobility is needed, the intervals between the supraspinatus and subscapularis as well as those between the infraspinatus and teres minor can be split longitudinally to allow the supraspinatus and infraspinatus additional mobility. The subscapularis and most of the teres minor are often intact. Release of the coracohumeral ligament from the coracoid base is also helpful. If necessary, a small elevator can be placed between the undersurface of the cuff and the superior labrum to free the tendons even more. A biceps tenodesis is done by suturing the tendon of the long head to the transverse humeral ligament with three, figure-of-eight, nonabsorbable sutures, and the intra-articular portion is excised and saved for possible use later.

If mobilization has allowed the cuff edges to be brought to the anatomic neck at the greater tuberosity, this area is then lightly roughened with a curette; a deep trough is not

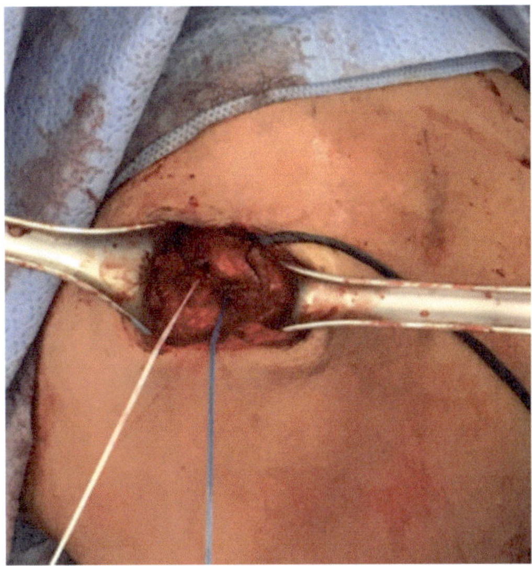

Figure 10.2 Suture anchors placed in a roughened area at the anatomic neck

necessary. The torn edges of the tendons are minimally trimmed, and suture anchors, loaded with #1 nonabsorbable sutures, are placed into the anatomic neck (Fig. 10.2). The sutures are passed through the cuff tendons from inside-out spaced approximately 8–10 mm apart (Fig. 10.3). The number of anchors is determined by how many are needed to bring the cuff to its desired insertion. The suture limbs are then arranged in twos or threes to cross and be secured in a transosseous pattern and secured below the greater tuberosity with pushlock anchors (Fig. 10.4).

Because this patient had a history of shoulder pain before the current injury, this tear may represent an acute on chronic, preexisting tear. In some instances, direct repair may not be possible. There are alternative techniques available which can be used. Fortunately, they are rarely needed. These include partial repair, interpositional grafts, and local or distant tendon transfers. Partial repair involves inserting the tendon edges into a site on the humeral head that is medial

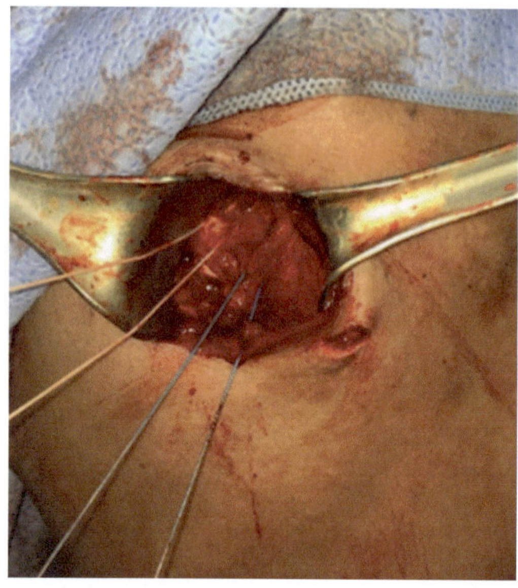

FIGURE 10.3 Sutures passed from the deep surface of the cuff tendons to exit on the bursal side

to the greater tuberosity. This can be successful if the insertion site itself is lateral to the apex of curvature, or very top, of the humeral head.

Interpositional Grafts

The absolute requirement for grafting is that the residual, intact portion of the rotator cuff tendons is mobile and that the muscles do not have extensive fatty infiltration. A graft is only a means of extending the length of the functioning muscle unit so that it can perform its natural function. If the native muscle does not work, the graft itself cannot replace the muscle's function. Thus, the residual cuff should exhibit a springy feel when traction is applied to it. These interpositional graft techniques are not the same as and do not serve the same purpose as the so-called patch graft.

For smaller residual defects, the previously excised intra-articular tendinous portion of the long head of the biceps is filleted (Fig. 10.5) and placed into the defect [3]. It is contoured

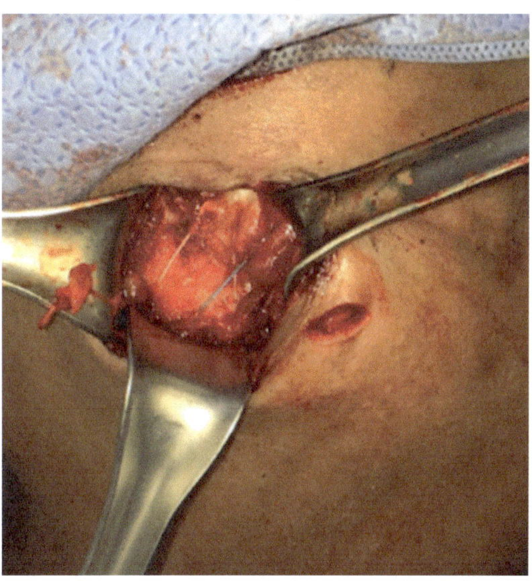

FIGURE 10.4 Cuff reduced to tuberosity and secured with a transosseous equivalent configuration secured below the tuberosity using pushlocks

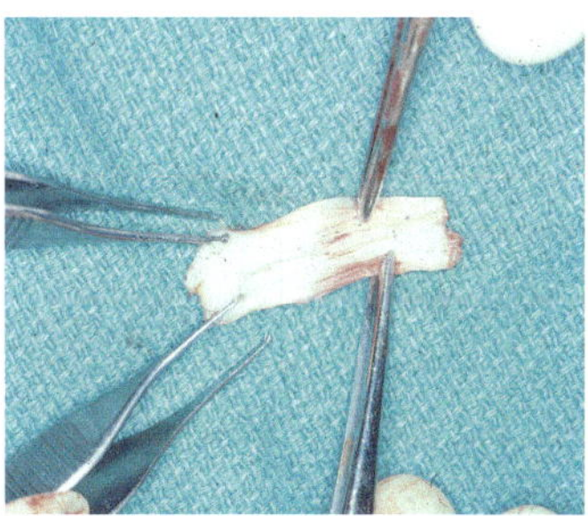

FIGURE 10.5 Intra-articular portion of the long head of the biceps is filleted to be used as an intercalated graft (from Neviaser RJ. Tears of the rotator cuff. Orthopedic Clin North Am. 1980;11(2):295–306)

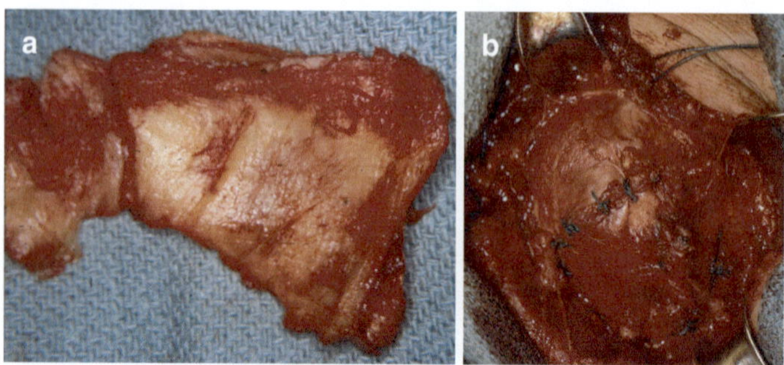

FIGURE 10.6 (**a**) Reconstituted freeze-dried cadaver rotator cuff. (**b**) Freeze-dried cadaver rotator cuff contoured to fit the defect of the remaining, mobile rotator cuff (from Neviaser JS, Neviaser RJ, Neviaser TJ. The repair of chronic massive ruptures of the rotator cuff by use of a freeze-dried rotator cuff. J Bone Joint Surg. 1978;60-A:681–4)

to accommodate the configuration of the defect and sutured to the residual cuff tendons. Its lateral edge is then sutured to the roughened area of the anatomic neck at the greater tuberosity as described above for a direct repair.

With larger defects, a freeze-dried cadaver rotator cuff is used [4]. It requires reconstitution in sterile saline for 30 min or until pliable in the operating room (Fig. 10.6a). It is contoured to fit the residual defect, sutured first to the residual native cuff and then to the roughened area at the anatomic neck adjacent to the greater tuberosity (Fig. 10.6b). For both of these techniques, the tension on the graft should be such that they are smooth and not lax or floppy, replicating the resting tension of an intact cuff with the arm at the side.

Tendon Transfers

Local tendons available for transfer include the subscapularis alone [5] and the teres minor in combination with the subscapularis [6]. To mobilize them, each is separated from the underlying capsule medial to the musculotendinous junction and then dissected laterally sharply peeling the tendon off of the capsule. It is important to leave the capsule intact to prevent instability. It is also critical to protect the axillary nerve, which lies at the inferior margin of the subscapularis anteriorly and the inferior margin of the teres minor posteriorly. The subscapularis is mobilized first and rotated superiorly to see if it can close the residual defect in the cuff that could not be closed directly (Fig. 10.7a). If it does, then the teres is left in place. If additional coverage is needed, then the teres minor is mobilized as well. The muscle tendon units are mobilized bluntly and rotated superiorly to meet on top of the humeral head (Fig. 10.7b). They are sutured to each other to form a new broad tendon and then inserted into the roughened area at the anatomic neck where it joins the greater tuberosity. The inferior edge of each tendon is then sutured to the superior edge of the undisturbed anterior (for the subscapularis) and posterior (for the teres minor) capsule (Fig. 10.7c).

The most common distal tendon transfer is the latissimus dorsi [7]. This technique is covered in another chapter.

For all of the procedures done through the mini open incision, the deltoid split is closed with two inverted #1 nonabsorbable sutures, and the skin with a subcuticular 3-0 nonabsorbable suture.

In an unusual case, additional exposure may be necessary to perform any of these alternative techniques, or even a direct repair. One can use the anterior superior surgical approach [8, 9]. An incision is made from the posterior edge of the acromioclavicular joint vertically to a point just lateral to the coracoid tip. The deltoid is split in line with its fibers but not beyond the coracoid. The deltoid origin is dissected subperiosteally, and not detached from the superior surface of the lateral clavicle and anterior acromion, as far laterally as the anterior lateral corner. The outer 7–8 mm of the clavicle can be excised to allow the scapula to be rotated posteriorly for exposure of the posterior rotator cuff (Fig. 10.8). At closure, the deltoid is simply replaced on top of the acromion and lateral clavicle and the split repaired side to side with two

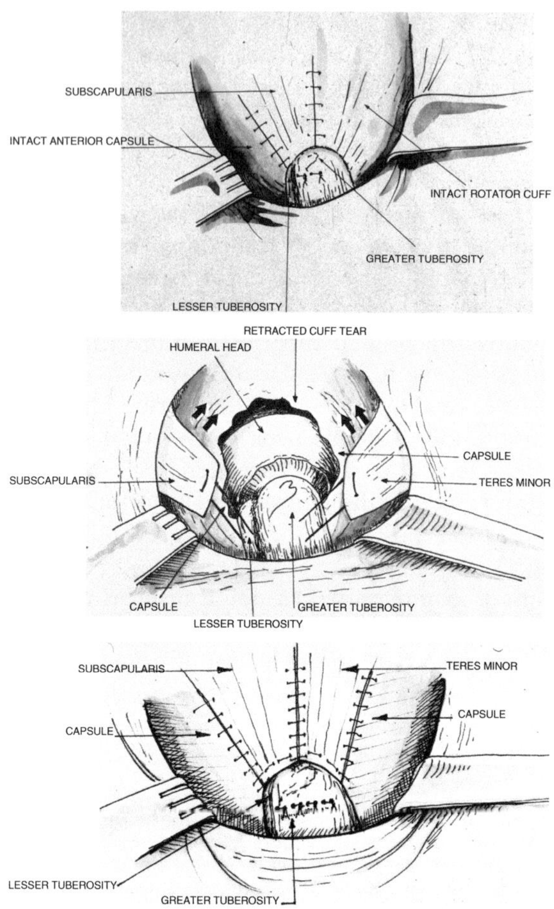

FIGURE 10.7 (**a**) Subscapularis musculotendinous unit mobilized, freed from the intact underlying capsule, rotating superiorly. (**b**) Subscapularis tendon sutured to the remaining rotator cuff, the undisturbed intact anterior capsule, and the greater tuberosity. (**c**) Subscapularis and teres minor tendons rotated superiorly to meet, sutured together to form a broad tendon, sutured to the greater tuberosity and their respective undisturbed capsules (from Neviaser RJ, Neviaser AS. Open repair of massive rotator cuff tears: tissue mobilization techniques. In: Zuckerman JD, editor. Advanced reconstruction shoulder. Rosemont, IL: American Academy of Orthopaedic Surgeons; 2007. p. 175–82)

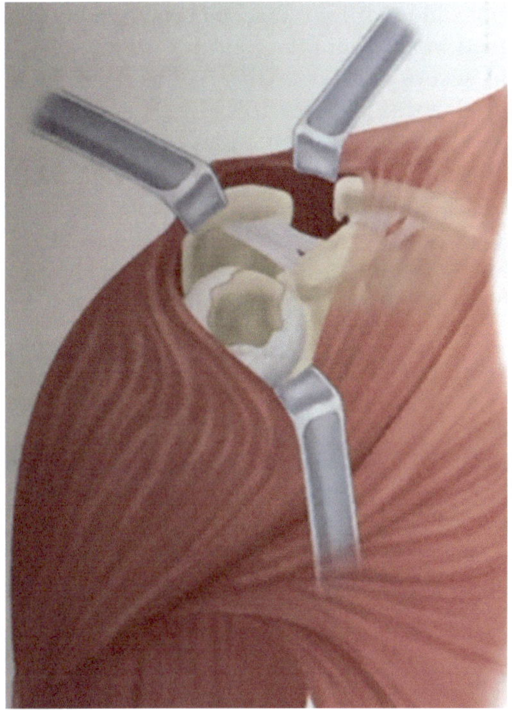

FIGURE 10.8 Anterior-superior approach to the shoulder utilizing subperiosteal dissection of the deltoid origin from the superior acromion and lateral clavicle, avoiding detaching the deltoid origin from these structures (from Neviaser AS, Neviaser RJ. Open treatment of large and massive rotator cuff tears. In: Lee DH, Neviaser RJ, editors. Shoulder and elbow surgery. New York: Elsevier; 2011, p. 63–86)

#1 nonabsorbable inverted sutures. The skin is closed with a subcuticular 3-0 suture and steri-strips.

Postoperatively, the extremity is immobilized at the side in an immobilizer sling. Abduction bracing is not used. Within the first few days, the patient is shown how to mobilize the elbow, wrist, fingers, and thumb without moving the shoulder. He is seen weekly, the sutures being removed at 10 days, and placed supine on the examining table. The surgeon passively moves the arm into approximately 90° of forward elevation and to a maximum of 15° of external rotation at the side. This is continued weekly until the fourth to sixth weeks (depending on the security of the repair). At this point, the patient is allowed to do these two exercises himself and is sent to physical therapy with specific instructions to do exercises to regain motion but not to strengthen, and use weights, rubber bands, or resistive machines. At 12 weeks, while motion exercises are continued, progressive strengthening is added. Maximum improvement in motion and function is reached by 1 year, although normal use of the arm is allowed at 4–6 months.

Outcome

This patient had an uneventful early postoperative recovery. Following the just described protocol, he returned to swimming by 14 weeks and tennis at 20 weeks. By 1 year, he had active motion of forward elevation to 165°, external rotation in abduction to 85°, external rotation at the side to 45°, and internal rotation to T11 compared to 170°, 85°, 45°, and T11 of the contralateral shoulder. His strength in external rotation and elevation was 5/5.

Literature Review

With an acute injury, whether a result of a dislocation or not, it has been shown that repair within the first 3 weeks produces a superior outcome to waiting a longer period [2]. If the patient does not show marked improvement in motion in the first couple of weeks, then repair should be strongly considered. A careful history is important as in many instances the patient may have experienced prior shoulder symptoms or even been treated for them, indicating the possibility of a preexisting tear, resulting in an acute-on-chronic injury. In such circumstances, one should be prepared for the possibility that a direct repair may not be possible. In those cases reconstructive techniques as described above [3–7] can be employed with reasonable chances of success.

Patients who cannot raise the arm after an injury need to be followed every 5–7 days in order to assess the progress of their recovery of motion. An important issue is to realize that the inability to elevate the arm after an acute primary dislocation in a patient over the age of 40 is more likely to be due to an acute rotator cuff rupture than an axillary nerve injury. In our series, all cases had a tear of the cuff, while only 7.8% of cases had an associated axillary nerve injury [1]. Even in the presence of the combined injuries—rotator cuff and axillary nerve—repair of the cuff should be considered as there can eventually be enough recovery of the nerve to allow functional use of the arm if the cuff has also recovered.

Interpositional grafting [3, 4] is not the same as patch grafting. Rather its intent is to extend the reach of a functional musculotendinous unit in an attempt to restore its length at a normal resting tension but not to augment the substance or thickness of the native tendon itself. It is analogous to a flexor tendon graft in the hand.

The course of rehabilitation after the surgery should be carefully monitored by the treating surgeon. Strengthening or resistive exercised should be avoided until at least 3 months postoperatively. We have found that introduction of such exercises before that time is a significant risk for failure of the repair [10].

Clinical Pearls/Pitfalls

- With first-time dislocation in a patient over age 40, suspect a rotator cuff tear rather than an axillary nerve injury.
- Follow such patients closely and if little or no improve-ment in function is noted in the first 2 weeks obtain an MRI.
- Significant fatty infiltration on the T1-weighted sagittal oblique images should alert one for the possibility that this is an acute-on-chronic tear and reconstructive techniques may be necessary.
- Whether to do a subacromial decompression and if chosen, then its extent is determined by the security of the repair.

- Tendon mobilization is key to successful repair.
- Introduction of strengthening or weights in the postoperative period before 3 months creates a risk for failure of repair via re-rupture.

References

1. Neviaser RJ, Neviaser TJ, Neviaser JS. Concurrent rupture of the rotator cuff and anterior dislocation of the shoulder in the older patient. J Bone Joint Surg. 1988;70-A:1308–11.
2. Bassett RW, Cofield RH. Acute tears of the rotator cuff. The timing of surgical repair. Clin Orthop Relat Res. 1983;175:18–24.
3. Neviaser JS. Ruptures of the rotator cuff of the shoulder. New concepts in the diagnosis and treatment of chronic ruptures. Arch Surg. 1971;102:483–5.
4. Neviaser JS, Neviaser RJ, Neviaser TJ. The repair of chronic massive ruptures of the rotator cuff by use of a freeze-dried rotator cuff. J Bone Joint Surg. 1978;60-A:681–4.
5. Cofield RH. Subscapular muscle transposition for repair of chronic rotator cuff tears. Surg Gynecol Obstet. 1982;154:667–72.
6. Neviaser RJ, Neviaser TJ. Transfer of the subscapularis and teres minor for massive defects of the rotator cuff. In: Bayley J, Kessel L, editors. Shoulder surgery. Heidelberg: Springer Verlag; 1982. p. 60–9.
7. Birmingham PM, Neviaser R. Outcome of latissimus dorsi transfer as a salvage procedure for failed rotator cuff repair with loss of elevation. J Shoulder Elbow Surg. 2008;17:871–4.
8. Neviaser RJ, Neviaser TJ. Major ruptures of the rotator cuff. In: Watson M, editor. Practical shoulder surgery. New York: Grune and Stratton; 1985. p. 171–224.
9. Neviaser AS, Neviaser RJ. Open repair of rotator cuff tears. In: Lee DH, Neviaser RJ, editors. Shoulder and elbow surgery. Philadelphia: Elsevier; 2011. p. 63–86.
10. Neviaser RJ, Neviaser TJ. Reoperation for failed rotator cuff repair: analysis of 50 cases. J Shoulder Elbow Surg. 1992;1(6):283–6.

Chapter 11
Latissimus Dorsi Transfer for Severe Rotator Cuff Tears

Robert J. Thorsness and Gregory P. Nicholson

Case Presentation

The patient is a 45-year-old male with a history of hypertension who presented after he injured his right shoulder while trying to throw a bag of garbage and felt a ripping sensation in his shoulder. Prior to presentation, he had intermittent anterolateral shoulder pain that was mild and worse with overhead activity. The trauma dramatically worsened his pain, and he also noticed significant weakness in the shoulder. He denies a prior history of surgery or trauma to the ipsilateral shoulder, and had yet to trial physical therapy.

Physical exam demonstrated a well-developed, well-nourished male, 5 feet 8 inches tall weighing 245 pounds. The cervical spine was mildly limited in its range of motion with

R.J. Thorsness, M.D. (✉)
Department of Orthopaedic Surgery, Rush University Medical Center, 1611 W Harrison St., Suite 200, Chicago, IL 60654, USA
e-mail: Robert_j_thorsness@rush.edu

G. P. Nicholson, M.D.
Department of Orthopaedic Surgery, Rush University Medical Center, 1611 West Harrison St, Chicago, IL 60612, USA

© Springer International Publishing AG 2018
P.J. McMahon (ed.), *Rotator Cuff Injuries*,
DOI 10.1007/978-3-319-63668-9_11

flexion to 25°, extension to 20°, and rotation to 30° right and left, with a negative Spurling's sign. On the healthy, contralateral left shoulder he demonstrated active forward elevation to 170°, and active external rotation to 60°, and demonstrated 5/5 external rotation strength, and 5/5 belly press strength. On the affected, right shoulder he demonstrated passive forward elevation to 160°, and passive external rotation 60°, but was unable to actively forward elevate. He had a remarkably positive external rotation lag sign and positive Hornblower's sign, with 3/5 external rotation strength. He had a negative belly press test and 5/5 internal rotation strength. His AC joint was nontender, as well as the remainder of the shoulder girdle including the biceps tendon within the bicipital groove. He possessed a normal, symmetric bicipital contour.

True AP, scapular Y, and axillary lateral radiographs were obtained which demonstrated moderate superior migration of the humeral head without evidence of glenohumeral arthritis (Fig. 11.1). There was no evidence of early rotator

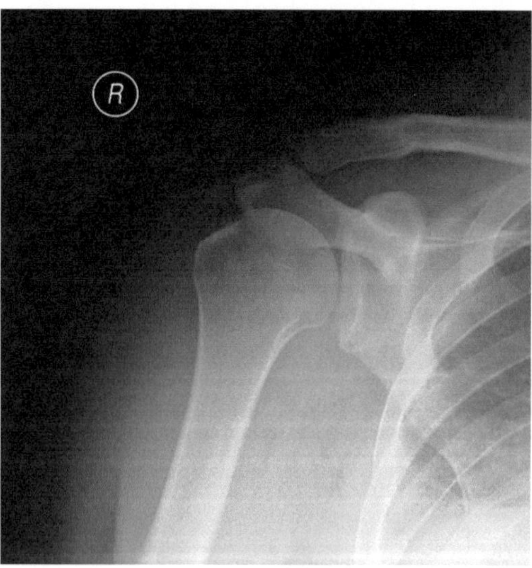

FIGURE 11.1 True AP x-ray view of the right shoulder in this patient demonstrating moderate superior migration of the humeral head and narrowing of the acromiohumeral interval. There are no arthritic changes present

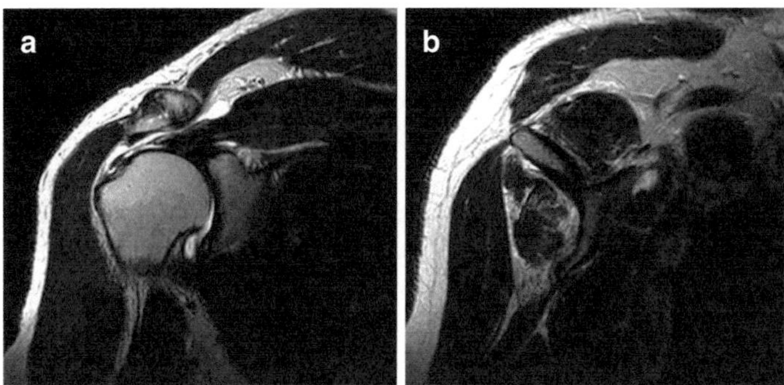

FIGURE 11.2 Magnetic resonance imaging demonstrating a full-thickness, retracted posterosuperior rotator cuff tear on coronal T2 image (**a**), with grade 1 atrophy of the supraspinatus, grade 2 atrophy of the infraspinatus, grade 4 atrophy of the teres minor with a normal subscapularis (**b**)

cuff arthropathy present. An MRI from an outside hospital was reviewed which demonstrated a large, moderately retracted posterosuperior tear of the rotator cuff involving the supraspinatus, infraspinatus, and teres minor. On sagittal T1 images, there was Goutallier grade 1 atrophy of the supraspinatus, grade 2 atrophy of the infraspinatus, and unexpectedly severe grade 4 atrophy of the teres minor with a normal, intact subscapularis (Fig. 11.2).

Diagnosis/Assessment

This patient is presenting with an acute exacerbation of a posterosuperior rotator cuff tear after a minor trauma. The patient's history, physical exam, and imaging all corroborate this diagnosis. The tear likely propagated anteriorly during the acute exacerbation leaving the supraspinatus with less severe atrophy compared to the infraspinatus and teres minor. While tears and atrophy of the teres minor are rare on presentation, this warranted an electromyographic study (EMG) to evaluate for a neurologic etiology such as a C5 radiculopathy. The EMG was obtained and demonstrated normal testing of the C5 distribution, as well as no evidence of suprascapular nerve or axillary nerve deficit.

While repair of the supraspinatus would likely improve his forward elevation, the chronicity of the posterior component of the tear involving the infraspinatus and teres minor would likely lead these to be less amenable to repair, and less predictable with regard to improving his profound external rotation weakness. For young, active patients with large, irreparable posterosuperior rotator cuff tears with an intact, functional subscapularis, a latissimus dorsi transfer to the greater tuberosity remains a viable, though unpredictable, option for restoring external rotation.

Management

The decision was made to pursue an open rotator cuff repair and latissimus dorsi transfer.

The patient was positioned in a sloppy lateral decubitus position after an interscalene regional block was performed. The first incision was carried out in Langer's lines just medial to the lateral border of the acromion. Skin flaps were raised, and the raphe between the anterior and middle thirds of the deltoid was incised and released off the acromion with the coracoacromial ligament. The deltoid was split 2.5 cm laterally and a stay suture placed to prevent propagation of the split. An acromioplasty was then performed as well as a thorough subacromial bursectomy in standard fashion. The supraspinatus and infraspinatus tendons were able to be identified and were tagged with heavy-braided #2 suture. The greater tuberosity footprint was then prepared to a bleeding base to optimize the biologic environment for healing. A transosseous rotator cuff repair was then performed through four drill holes double-loaded with heavy-braided #2 suture.

The bed was then tilted away to optimize the positioning for the latissimus transfer. A hockey-stick incision was then made along the lateral border of the latissimus dorsi and then parallel to the humerus. The latissimus was then identified, mobilized from the adjacent teres major, and released off the humerus. A heavy-braided #2 Dyneema suture was then run in Krackow fashion through the tendon, and a separate differing color #2 Dyneema suture was placed in similar fashion on the adjacent edge of the tendon, creating four limbs. The latissimus was then bluntly mobilized down to its neurovascular pedicle and off the fascia. Through the original incision, the latissimus sutures were retrieved deep to the deltoid and superficial to the repaired infraspinatus. The tendon was mobilized to the level of the posterior greater tuberosity footprint. This was then repaired to the level of the posterior greater tuberosity with a similar transosseous technique through drill holes.

The wounds were irrigated, and the deltoid split closed with heavy-braided #2 suture incorporating the coracoacromial ligament into the repair. The subcutaneous tissue and skin were closed in standard fashion. The patient was placed into a sling with a derotation wedge to maintain the arm in mild abduction but also approximately 10° external rotation. He was then extubated and transferred to the postanesthesia care unit in stable condition. There were no intraoperative complications.

Outcome

The patient was started with a guided physical therapy regimen beginning 1 week after surgery. He was maintained in a sling for 6 weeks to protect the repair. Phase 1 of therapy consisted of pendulums, passive external rotation limited to 30°, and passive forward elevation to 90° for weeks 1–6. Avoiding internal rotation behind the back or across the midline for the first 4 weeks is emphasized. At week 6, phase 2 of therapy began with active assisted range of motion as tolerated, pulleys, and isometric strengthening of the deltoid and periscapular musculature. Feedback to the patient is provided while doing isometric ER and IR to begin to try to

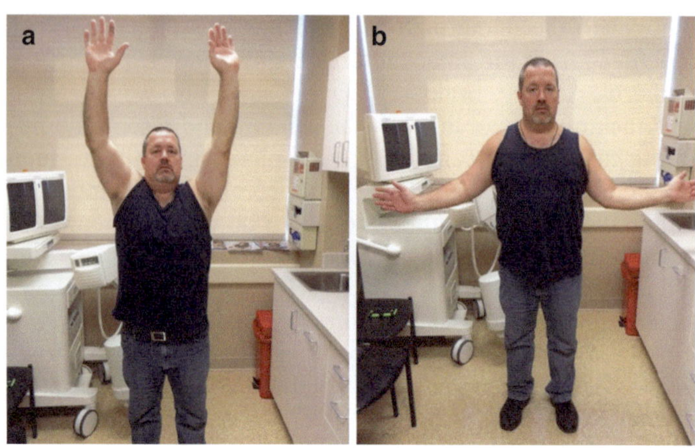

FIGURE 11.3 The patient postoperatively demonstrated excellent range of motion in both forward elevation (**a**) and external rotation (**b**) without pain

"train" the latissimus to become an external rotators. Phase 3 began at 3 months postoperatively, to include active range of motion as tolerated and rotator cuff strengthening.

At most recent follow-up 8 months postoperatively, the patient demonstrated active forward elevation to 160°, and active external rotation to 45°, with 5/5 strength in forward elevation and 5/5 strength in external rotation (Fig. 11.3). He demonstrated a negative Hornblower's sign and external rotation lag sign. The reconstruction completely eliminated his essentially pseudoparalytic state and restored external rotation power.

Literature Review

Massive posterosuperior rotator cuff tears in young patients present a difficult clinical problem. Repair of these tears in these patients is associated with poor outcomes, likely given irreversible changes to muscular function [1–3]. As an alternative to massive rotator cuff repair in this setting, some surgeons have elected for a latissimus dorsi tendon transfer to supplement for loss of function of the posterosuperior rotator cuff [4–9], with a goal of restoring active forward elevation and external rotation.

While reverse total shoulder arthroplasty remains a viable treatment of massive irreparable rotator cuff tears in elderly, lower demand patients, this is often not an ideal treatment strategy for younger, more active patients given the risk of component loosening and subsequent revision [10–12]. Latissimus dorsi tendon transfer does remain a reasonable option for these younger patients, but unfortunately the clinical outcomes are mixed [5–7, 13–20]. The ideal candidate is a young, active patient with an irreparable posterosuperior rotator cuff tear, with an intact and functional subscapularis, without glenohumeral arthritis.

While latissimus transfer will often lead to significant improvements in pain and function, it is imperative for surgeons to manage expectations with these patients as a return to normal or near-normal function is unlikely. Patient should be counseled that they can expect approximately 35° increase in forward elevation, 10° increase in external rotation, and a 70% increase in abduction strength following the procedure [20]. However, it is imperative to instruct patients that latissimus transfer does not preclude cuff tear arthropathy in young patients, and they should expect continued progression of glenohumeral arthritis with age. There are a variety of factors that may influence outcome including age, sex, surgical technique, and concomitant transfer of the teres major, but most studies are heterogeneous and likely underpowered to detect the influence of these factors on outcome [20]. Further, the litcraturc lacks appropriate studies to evaluate comparative outcomes in similar patients undergoing partial rotator cuff repair, patch augmentation, or reverse total shoulder arthroplasty, further highlighting the need for high-quality studies of this procedure.

When indicating patients for a latissimus transfer, it is imperative to understand the factors that are associated with poor outcome. Surgeons should expect poor functional results following latissimus transfer in patients undergoing revision surgery, in patients with a torn or deficient subscapularis, or those with advanced teres minor atrophy [20]. The integrity of the subscapularis is paramount, as the subscapularis is necessary to maintain a balanced, centered humeral head following a latissimus transfer during forward elevation and external rotation.

Clinical Pearls and Pitfalls

- The ideal candidate for a latissimus transfer is a young, active patient with an irreparable posterosuperior rotator cuff tear, with a functional subscapularis in the absence of glenohumeral arthritis, and poor external rotational ability and compromised motors of the posterior rotator cuff.
- If the patient is lower demand, or elderly, then a reverse total shoulder will provide a more predictable functional outcome.
- Latissimus transfer does not preclude cuff tear arthropathy, and patients must be instructed that they should expect progression of arthritic changes over time that may necessitate a reverse total shoulder arthroplasty in the future.

References

1. Denard PJ, Ladermann A, Jiwani AZ, Burkhart SS. Functional outcome after arthroscopic repair of massive rotator cuff tears in individuals with pseudoparalysis. Arthroscopy. 2012;28(9):1214–9.
2. Millett PJ, Warth RJ. Posterosuperior rotator cuff tears: classification, pattern recognition, and treatment. J Am Acad Orthop Surg. 2014;22(8):521–34.
3. Omid R, Lee B. Tendon transfers for irreparable rotator cuff tears. J Am Acad Orthop Surg. 2013;21(8):492–501.
4. Gerber C, Vinh TS, Hertel R, Hess CW. Latissimus dorsi transfer for the treatment of massive tears of the rotator cuff. A preliminary report. Clin Orthop Relat Res. 1988;232:51–61.

5. Gerber C. Latissimus dorsi transfer for the treatment of irreparable tears of the rotator cuff. Clin Orthop Relat Res. 1992;275:152–60.
6. Gerber C, Maquieira G, Espinosa N. Latissimus dorsi transfer for the treatment of irreparable rotator cuff tears. J Bone Joint Surg Am. 2006;88(1):113–20.
7. Gerber C, Rahm SA, Catanzaro S, Farshad M, Moor BK. Latissimus dorsi tendon transfer for treatment of irreparable posterosuperior rotator cuff tears: long-term results at a minimum follow-up of ten years. J Bone Joint Surg Am. 2013;95(21):1920–6.
8. Debeer P, De Smet L. Outcome of latissimus dorsi transfer for irreparable rotator cuff tears. Acta Orthop Belg. 2010;76(4):449–55.
9. Birmingham PM, Neviaser RJ. Outcome of latissimus dorsi transfer as a salvage procedure for failed rotator cuff repair with loss of elevation. J Shoulder Elb Surg. 2008;17(6):871–4.
10. Cuff D, Pupello D, Virani N, Levy J, Frankle M. Reverse shoulder arthroplasty for the treatment of rotator cuff deficiency. J Bone Joint Surg Am. 2008;90(6):1244–51.
11. Wall B, Nove-Josserand L, O'Connor DP, Edwards TB, Walch G. Reverse total shoulder arthroplasty: a review of results according to etiology. J Bone Joint Surg Am. 2007;89(7):1476–85.
12. Matsen FA 3rd, Boileau P, Walch G, Gerber C, Bicknell RT. The reverse total shoulder arthroplasty. J Bone Joint Surg Am. 2007;89(3):660–7.
13. Aoki M, Okamura K, Fukushima S, Takahashi T, Ogino T. Transfer of latissimus dorsi for irreparable rotator-cuff tears. J Bone Joint Surg Br. 1996;78(5):761–6.
14. Codsi MJ, Hennigan S, Herzog R, et al. Latissimus dorsi tendon transfer for irreparable posterosuperior rotator cuff tears. Surgical technique. J Bone Joint Surg Am. 2007;89(Suppl 2 Pt.1):1–9.
15. Costouros JG, Espinosa N, Schmid MR, Gerber C. Teres minor integrity predicts outcome of latissimus dorsi tendon transfer for irreparable rotator cuff tears. J Shoulder Elb Surg. 2007;16(6):727–34.
16. Degreef I, Debeer P, Van Herck B, Van Den Eeden E, Peers K, De Smet L. Treatment of irreparable rotator cuff tears by latissimus dorsi muscle transfer. Acta Orthop Belg. 2005;71(6):667–71.
17. Iannotti JP, Hennigan S, Herzog R, et al. Latissimus dorsi tendon transfer for irreparable posterosuperior rotator cuff tears. Factors affecting outcome. J Bone Joint Surg Am. 2006;88(2):342–8.

18. Irlenbusch U, Bracht M, Gansen HK, Lorenz U, Thiel J. Latissimus dorsi transfer for irreparable rotator cuff tears: a longitudinal study. J Shoulder Elb Surg. 2008;17(4):527–34.
19. Miniaci A, MacLeod M. Transfer of the latissimus dorsi muscle after failed repair of a massive tear of the rotator cuff. A two to five-year review. J Bone Joint Surg Am. 1999;81(8):1120–7.
20. Namdari S, Voleti P, Baldwin K, Glaser D, Huffman GR. Latissimus dorsi tendon transfer for irreparable rotator cuff tears: a systematic review. J Bone Joint Surg Am. 2012;94(10):891–8.

Chapter 12
Pectoralis Major Transfer

Jens Stehle

Case Presentation

The 57-year-old patient presented with pain (visual analog scale, VAS 8–9) and reduced strength of internal rotation of the left shoulder. He reported trauma of the shoulder consistent with a subscapularis tear 8 months before, but the treatment was conservative and the diagnosis of a traumatic tear of the subscapularis was not confirmed yet. He was a worker in a psychiatric institution, and his general health status was reduced and his weight was 55 kg.

An MRI of the left shoulder was conducted and revealed a complete tear of the subscapularis with retraction of the tendon behind the glenoid and severe atrophy of the subscapularis muscle belly (grade 3–4). Additionally, a luxated long head of the biceps was seen.

J. Stehle, M.D.
Department of Shoulder Surgery, Bodensee-Sportklinik,
Moettelistraße 5, Friedrichshafen 88045, Germany
e-mail: jensstehle@gmx.de

© Springer International Publishing AG 2018
P.J. McMahon (ed.), *Rotator Cuff Injuries*,
DOI 10.1007/978-3-319-63668-9_12

Diagnosis/Assessment

The patient's history, physical, and imaging findings are consistent with the diagnosis of symptomatic full-thickness subscapularis tendon tear. Based on the clinical findings and the MRI, an arthroscopy was indicated to evaluate if the subscapularis tendon could be repaired. Pectoralis major transfer is indicated for a painful, irreparable subscapularis tear. Ideal patients are active and younger than 60 years with an intact or a reparable supraspinatus. Patients must have a functioning deltoid muscle and minimal glenohumeral joint arthritic changes. Pectoralis transfers may also be considered in cases of failure of subscapularis healing after shoulder arthroplasty or open shoulder stabilization. In these scenarios, decreased pain can be expected; however, the results are less predictable and the functional results are also inferior in the setting of recurrent glenohumeral subluxation and instability [1]. A pectoralis major transfer has been described for the treatment of anterior-superior escape in the setting of rotator cuff arthropathy and/or failed rotator cuff repair [2]. Although the reverse shoulder arthroplasty has become the standard treatment in this clinical scenario, a pectoralis major transfer may still be considered in younger patients or in patients in whom a reverse shoulder arthroplasty is not indicated. The results of a transfer in this setting are not as promising; however pain relief and some functional improvement can be expected. The pectoralis major transfer is not able to correct a forward flection pseudoparalysis. In these cases, a reverse shoulder arthroplasty will provide better functional results [1].

Management

An arthroscopy of the left shoulder revealed a completely torn and retracted subscapularis tendon with poor tissue quality and no chance to repair, even if the surgery would have been converted to an open procedure. Therefore, only a tenodesis of the long head of the biceps with an acromioplasty was performed to reduce the pain. The postoperative X-rays showed only a slightly superior humeral head and only a slight ventral subluxation of the humeral head on the glenoid in the axial plane (Figs. 12.1 and 12.2). However, the patient showed up with almost the same deficits as before the surgery and pain (VAS 8) even after an intensive rehabilitation program. The different treatment options were discussed with the patient. The patient chose the recommended pectoralis major transfer.

The pectoralis major transfer was performed with the subcoracoid technique described by Resch et al. [3] with a partial subcoracoid transfer of the pectoralis major. In

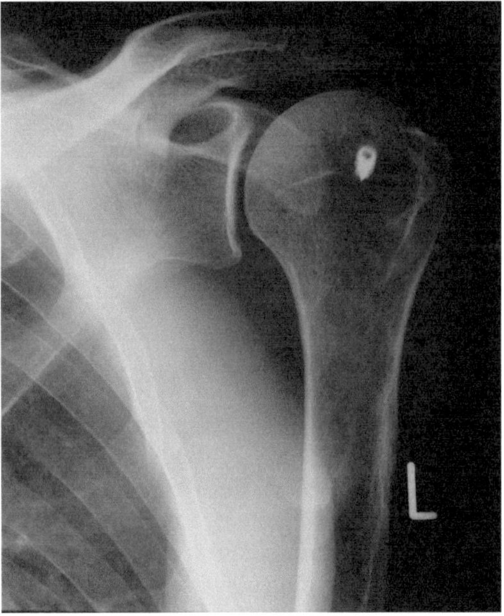

FIGURE 12.1 True AP X-rays of the left shoulder showed only a slight superior humeral head migration after the tenodesis of the long head of the biceps with chronic rupture of the subscapularis

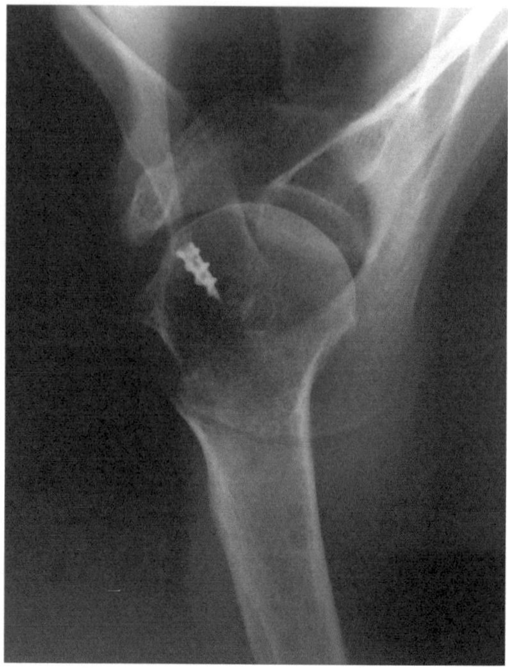

Figure 12.2 Axial plane X-ray showed only minimal ventral subluxation of the humeral head on the glenoid

brief, the patient was positioned in the beach-chair position. A standard deltopectoral incision was used. The deltoid was retracted laterally with the cephalic vein. Subdeltoid, subacromial, and subcoracoid adhesions were released. Another attempt was made to mobilize the retracted subscapularis tendon but it could not be repaired. The lesser tuberosity was exposed. The insertion of the pectoralis major tendon on the humerus was identified lateral to the intertubercular sulcus. The superior one-half to two-thirds of the tendon was tagged with stay sutures and taken for the transfer and detached from the humerus. Medial blunt dissection along the fibers up to 8 cm medially to achieve the necessary elongation was performed. The space medial to the conjoined tendon and lateral to the pectoralis minor was bluntly developed. A path was bluntly cleared for passage with the two index fingers from both sides. The musculocutaneous nerve was identified visually and digitally with its entrance to the muscle. If a small proximal nerve branch is encountered that would be under tension from the transfer, an attempt can be undertaken to release this nerve branch digitally with minimal force, causing minimal pathology [1]. In most cases the interval between the nerve and the conjoined tendons is big enough to pass the muscle through. If this seems possible with no tension of the nerve, the preferred subcoracoid transfer can be used. (If the nerve might be under excessive tension after the transfer with pending neurapraxia, one must consider the supracoracoid transfer described by Wirth and Rockwood [4] as an alternative.) The sutures of the tendon were grasped behind the conjoined tendons but in front of the nerve with a curved forceps and transferred to the lesser tuberosity. Lastly, the transferred tendon was attached by use of transosseous sutures or bone anchors. Between 2 and 4 nonabsorbable sutures are placed in a modified Mason-Allen technique to securely fix the thin tendon of the distal pectoralis major muscle. A deep and a superficial drain was used to reduce the risk of postoperative hematoma. The patient's arm was placed in a sling. Postoperative care was similar to that after a massive anterosuperior rotator cuff repair. The operated shoulder was immobilized for 6 weeks. Passive exercises were allowed early to encourage tendon gliding and prevent adhesions. However, external rotation was limited to 0° for 6 weeks after surgery to protect the tendon transfer. Active-assisted and strengthening exercises were started 6 weeks after the surgery. Internal rotation against resistance was restricted until 12 weeks after surgery. After this, patients will notice functional gains throughout the first year. Fortunately, the subscapularis and pectoralis major are in phase, and transfers do not require retraining protocols [3, 5].

Outcome

The patient showed up 6 weeks and 3 months after surgery. He reported no complications and the pain was significantly reduced (VAS 2–3). However, he showed up again 2 years after the pectoralis tendon transfer with increasing pain (VAS 8–9) and reduced function of the left shoulder. Active forward flection was reduced to 80°. Atrophy of the upper part of the pectoralis major was clearly seen. Also, the trapezius, deltoideus, supraspinatus, and infraspinatus showed visible atrophy. In the meantime, he had surgeries of internal organs with life-threatening complications. During this time, he neglected his shoulder problems. His general health status was further reduced and his weight was 50 kg. MRI of the left shoulder showed that the transferred pectoralis tendon and muscle were very thin with subcoracoid impingement, superior head migration, and ventral subluxation of the humeral head on the glenoid. Because of his reduced general health status conservative treatment with physiotherapy was performed, but the pain and the function did not improve over time. Therefore, after his general health improved and his weight was 53 kg, the arguments for and against surgery were discussed, and since his life expectancy was considered low, he had a low activity level, and his quality of life was low, a reverse total shoulder arthroplasty was performed three years after the pectoralis tendon transfer when he was 62 years old. During operation the transferred pectoralis major tendon was observed to be very thin but intact. However, the signs of subcoracoid impingement, superior head migration, and ventral subluxation of the humerus were clearly seen. The operation was carried out without any complication and the transferred tendon again attached to the lesser tuberosity. The operated shoulder was immobilized for 6 weeks in an abduction pillow. Passive exercises were allowed and supported with a shoulder motion device for 6 weeks for abduction. However, external rotation was limited to 0° for 6 weeks after surgery to protect the pectoralis major tendon and prevent luxations. Active-assisted exercises were allowed after the 6-week point. The patient showed up 6 weeks and 3 months after surgery. He reported no complications and the

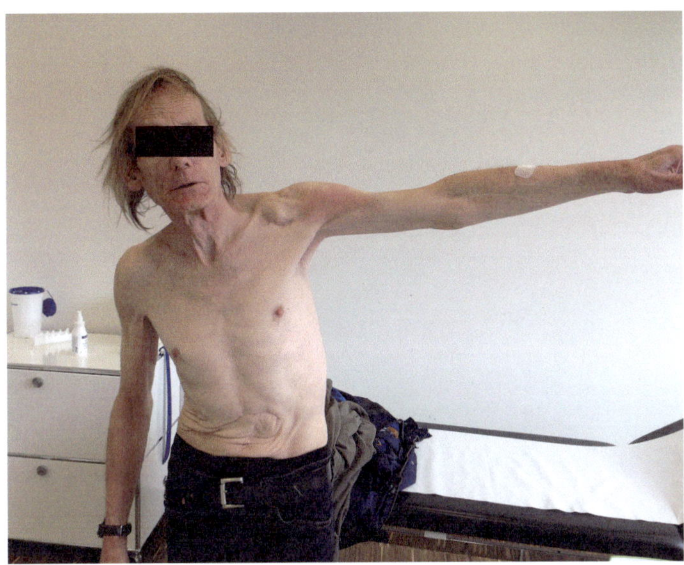

FIGURE 12.3 Clinical findings 2 years after reverse shoulder arthroplasty: Active forward flection and abduction are reduced to 90°. Note the multiple scars on the belly after multiple surgeries and the reduced general condition of the patient

pain was again significantly reduced (VAS 3). Two years after the reverse total shoulder arthroplasty he reported increased pain (VAS 7) and decreasing function of the left shoulder. Active forward flection and abduction were reduced to 90° (Fig. 12.3). He is able to comb his hair (Fig. 12.4) with strong external rotation but could only reach the lateral hip (Fig. 12.5), because his active internal rotation was markedly reduced. Atrophy of the upper part of the pectoralis major could be clearly seen (Fig. 12.6). On the ventral aspect of the shoulder the arthroplasty can be outlined because the patient is so slim. Also, the trapezius, deltoideus, supraspinatus, and infraspinatus showed visible atrophy (Fig. 12.7). The neurological findings were normal. He had also a rash of the ventrolateral shoulder, but the lab values showed a normal CRP. The X-rays 2 years after surgery show a reverse arthroplasty with no signs of loosening or notching (Fig. 12.8). In the meantime, he again had surgeries of internal organs with

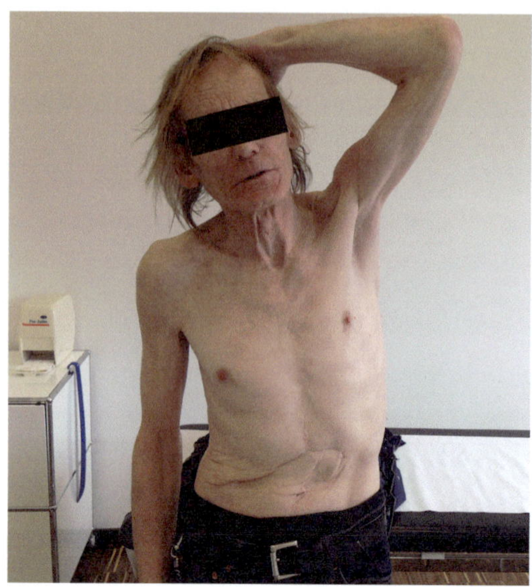

FIGURE 12.4 Satisfactory external rotation in abduction 2 years after reverse shoulder arthroplasty

life-threatening complications and his weight was again 50 kg. He was asked to follow up closely every 3 months to check on his status.

This example shows that the pectoralis major transfer is not always successful in terms of permanent pain relief, even though the indication was right, based on the current literature. This patient had always only a partial and temporary pain relief after surgery. A reverse shoulder arthroplasty is sometimes the last alternative when pain and function deteriorate over time, but after multiple operations and weakened internal rotators the results are sometimes frustrating.

Literature Review

The majority of rotator cuff tears involve the posterosuperior cuff and can often be treated with repair of the tendons, even months and years after rupture. However, tears of the

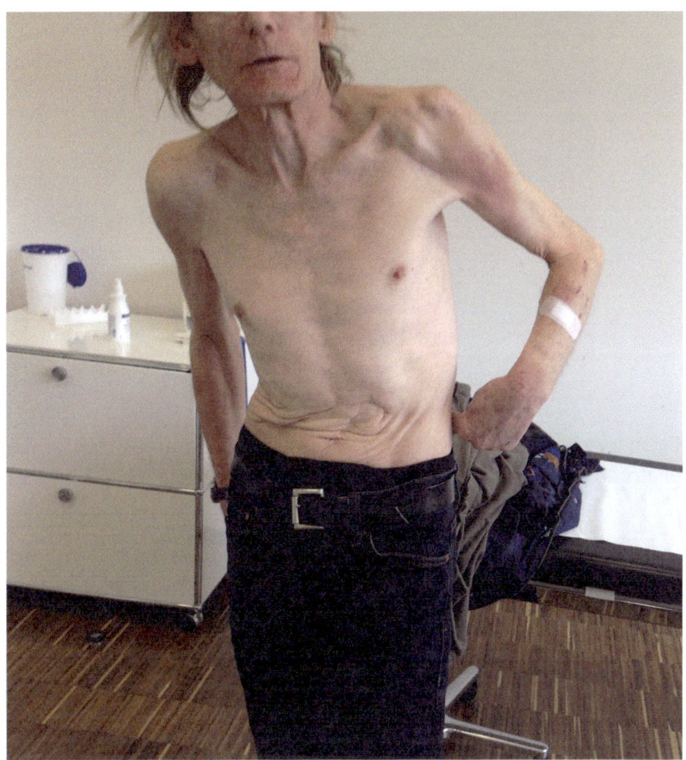

FIGURE 12.5 Reduced active and passive internal rotation 2 years after reverse shoulder arthroplasty. The arthroplasty can be seen through the skin with significant atrophy of the upper part of the pectoralis major after the transfer

subscapularis tend to retract fast, and show rapid fatty degeneration of the muscle belly, leading to irreparable situations, especially when the diagnosis is delayed [3, 4, 6].

The subscapularis is an important factor for the muscular force couple of the glenohumeral joint. An insufficiency of the subscapularis caused by a tendon tear or neurologic disorder leaves the humeral head unbalanced, producing functional disabilities [7, 8]. Additionally, chronic and recurrent anterior subluxation and instability with associated pain are characteristics of subscapularis insufficiency [2, 9].

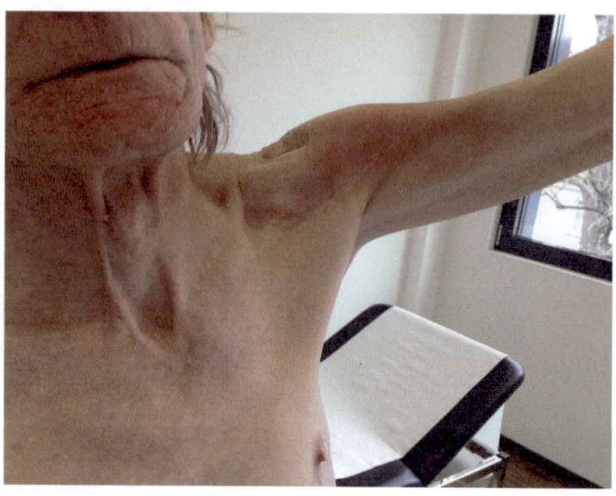

FIGURE 12.6 The atrophy with a visible gap of the upper part of the pectoralis major can be clearly seen in abduction

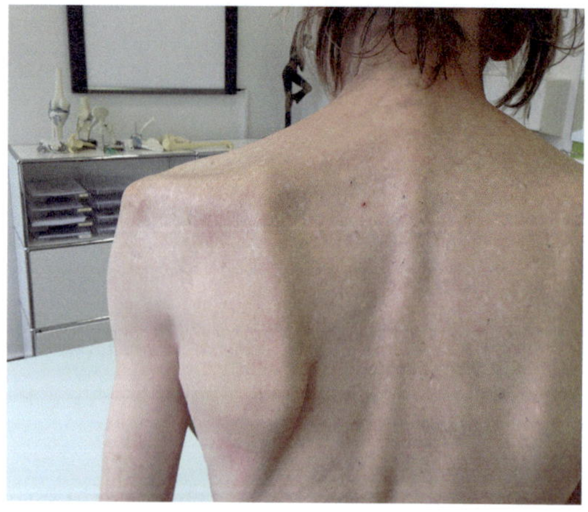

FIGURE 12.7 Atrophy of the trapezius, deltoideus, supraspinatus, and infraspinatus from the posterior view

Arthroplasty is a treatment option, depending on the patient's level of glenohumeral arthritis, age, and activity level, in combination with or without a pectoralis major transfer. Hemiarthroplasty has been attempted with moderate and unreliable pain relief and functional results [10–13].

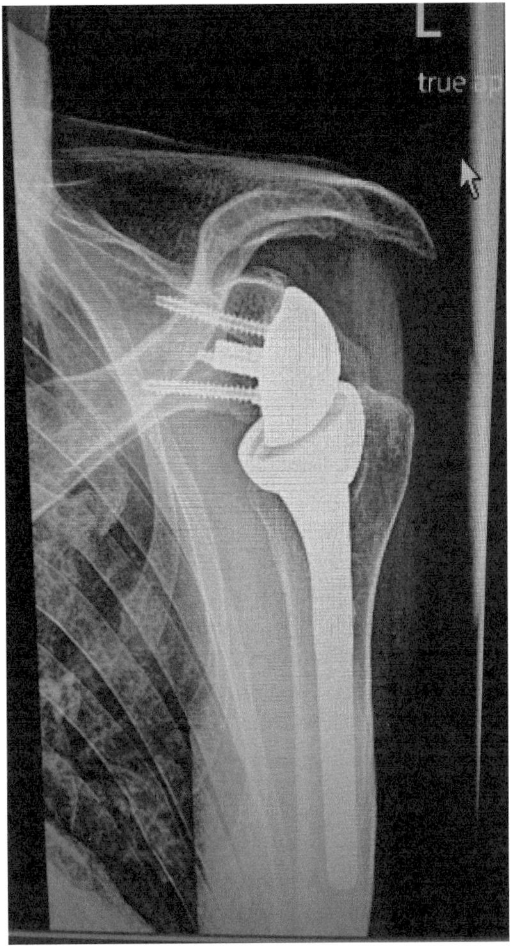

FIGURE 12.8 The X-ray's true AP from 2 years after surgery shows a reverse arthroplasty with no signs of loosening or notching

Recently, reverse total shoulder arthroplasty has become the standard for older and low-demand patients with good clinical results [8]. Depending on the patient's needs and circumstances other options include arthroscopic debridement with biceps tenotomy or tenodesis to reduce the pain [14].

Although arthroplasty may be the standard in old and low-demand patients, the management of high-demand, active, and/or young patients with an irreparable subscapularis tear is still an important challenge. In these cases, tendon transfers are a feasible option, commonly using the pectoralis major, if the patient has a well-preserved glenohumeral joint [1, 4, 6, 15–19].

The pectoralis major can be transferred using its whole tendon, or it can be split to rebalance the force couple on the humeral head [2–4]. The tendon is then rerouted underneath or left superficially to the conjoined tendon. If rerouted underneath to the conjoined tendon, the pectoralis is thought to additionally reduce subcoracoid impingement through a soft-tissue interposition effect that helps in pain relief. These techniques can be used for subscapularis tears in isolation, for subscapularis tears with anterior supraspinatus tears, or in combination with posterior cuff repair for posterosuperior tears. In addition, they have been used for subscapularis insufficiency after failure of subscapularis repair after open shoulder stabilization or shoulder hemiarthroplasty [20–22]. However, subscapularis insufficiency after hemiarthroplasty presents a significant therapeutic challenge, often because of recurrent instability, with unsatisfactory results [20].

Anatomy

Muscle

The muscle of the pectoralis major originates from the anterior surface of the medial clavicle, sternum, cartilage of ribs 2 through 7, and variably, as a small abdominal belly, aponeurosis of the external oblique muscle. The clavicular muscle belly has a cross-sectional area of about 60% of the total muscle. The clavicular and sternal muscle bellies are separated by an intermuscular septum that can best be seen laterally near the musculotendinous junction [23].

Tendon

The pectoralis major tendinous insertion consists of two distinct layers [4, 23, 24]. The anterior lamina is the terminal portion of the clavicular head, whereas the posterior lamina originates from the sternal head. A variable small third layer, the abdominal lamina, is derived from the aponeurosis of the external oblique muscle medially. The sternal and clavicular lamellae fuse into a single tendon. The sternal lamina is rotated almost 180° about its longitudinal axis before insertion on the humerus. This rotation results in the inferior (sternal) fibers attaching superior and posterior to the clavicular fibers on the humerus when the arm is in an adducted position. The two tendons overlap approximately 2.7 cm, producing a total footprint between 5.7 and 6.3 cm [4, 23, 24].

Nerves

The musculocutaneous nerve is the most important neurovascular structure of concern when a transfer is planned. It enters the undersurface of the coracobrachialis between 5 and 6 cm distal to the coracoid base [23, 24]. In the study of Klepps et al., 18 of 20 specimens had a small proximal branch thought to also innervate the coracobrachialis [24]. This nerve branch was reported to be 4 cm from the coracoid base and, when found, was supposedly small enough to sacrifice without any meaningful functional effect, although this was not investigated clinically [1].

The lateral pectoral nerve originates from the lateral cord of the brachial plexus, passes medial to the pectoralis minor, and enters the clavicular belly superior to the intermuscular septum, about 12 cm medial to its humeral insertion [23, 24].

The medial pectoral nerve originates from the medial cord. In most cases, it travels through the substance of the pectoralis minor before entering the undersurface of the pectoralis major. However, Klepps et al. [24] reported variable paths for the medial pectoral nerve, noting that it sometimes passed lateral to the pectoralis minor. Jennings et al. [23]

further reported that it passed lateral to the pectoralis minor in 4 of 24 cadavers whereas the nerve divided in two specimens, with one branch traveling through and another traveling lateral to the pectoralis minor. The medial pectoral nerve then travels with the lateral thoracic artery and is at some risk of injury during the division of the two muscular units. This nerve was found in the same study to cross the septum at a mean of 9 cm medial to the humeral insertion and entered the sternal head 1.4 cm distal to the septum [23]. Klepps et al. stated that the medial pectoral nerve does not branch to innervate the clavicular head as it travels laterally; blunt dissection along its course allows separation of the clavicular and sternal muscle bellies without the risk of significant denervation [24].

Artery

The subclavian artery provides the blood supply to the pectoralis major, with the thoracoacromial and lateral thoracic branch. The thoracoacromial branch travels medial to the muscular division, whereas the lateral thoracic branch crosses the septum between the two muscle bellies at a mean of 8.5 cm medial to the humeral insertion [23, 24].

Biomechanics of Transfer Techniques

The biomechanics of the supracoracoid and subcoracoid transfers were investigated by Konrad et al. [25]. Six fresh-frozen full upper extremities were mounted into a dynamic shoulder testing apparatus to simulate glenohumeral kinematics when applying force to the different tendons of the shoulder muscles. Four scenarios were tested: intact shoulder, complete subscapularis tear, transfer of the clavicular head superficial to the conjoined tendon, and subcoracoid transfer of the clavicular pectoralis head. The forces applied were determined based on values used in previous studies and finite element modeling. The complete subscapularis tear condition displayed less than 50% of the maximum abduction achieved with the intact condition (40.8° vs. 86.3°). Maximum external rotation (91.8°) and anterior (6.4 mm) and superior (6.1 mm) translation were also increased significantly. Both tendon transfer scenarios resulted in more physiological shoulder motion compared with the tear condition. Specifically, maximum abduction and superior stability were restored in both transfer scenarios. The subcoracoid transfer, however, restored the glenohumeral kinematics closer to those of the intact shoulder than those resulting from the transfer superficial to the conjoined tendon [25].

Different Surgical Techniques for Pectoralis Major Tendon Transfer

The transferred tendon may take different courses. The traditional course is that the tendon can be passed in the plane of its normal course but merely in a more superior direction and can then be attached to the tuberosities of the proximal humerus [4, 26]. In a variation of the traditional course, the tendon (complete or partial) was routed deep, through the interval between the conjoined tendon (superficial) and the musculocutaneous nerve [2, 3, 27]. In another variation the sternal lamina of the pectoralis major was passed deep to the clavicular lamina but superficial to the conjoined tendon [20]. In a cadaveric study, a fourth position was investigated: subcoracoid transfer with the tendon passing deep to the musculocutaneous nerve [24]. This position, however, was found to place tension on the musculocutaneous nerve and is considered to be too risky for clinical practice.

The subcoracoid tendon transfer has the advantage of producing a force vector that better simulates that of the native subscapularis tendon [25]. This inferior and posterior vector of the subscapularis has been well documented and is thought to balance the net superior pull of the deltoid, keeping the humeral head centered in the glenoid fossa [7, 28]. A second advantage of the subcoracoid transfer is that the transferred tendon produces a static soft-tissue interposition (buttress effect) between the humerus and the coracoid process, minimizing anterior humeral translation and decreasing the risk of coracohumeral impingement [23].

One potential downside of the subcoracoid technique is the more extensive surgical dissection, as well as the increased bulk of the pectoralis major transfers may increase the risk of injury of the musculocutaneous nerve and surrounding brachial plexus. Especially when the entire pectoralis major was taken for a subcoracoid transfer, the musculocutaneous nerve was under too much tension, necessitating a release of the proximal branch to relieve the tension in 6 of 20 cadaveric specimens [24]. In addition, there are clinical reports of musculocutaneous nerve injuries; therefore, split-tendon transfers are more frequently advocated [3]. If a partial transfer of the pectoralis is chosen, the most common technique is described by Resch et al. [3] where the superior part of the pectoralis major insertion is taken for the transfer. A different approach was used by Jennings et al. [23] by separating the humeral insertions into the clavicular and sternal laminae of the pectoralis major. The posterior lamina (sternal part, with a more inferior-directed force vector) is chosen for transfer, and the majority of the anterior insertion (clavicular part) was left intact. A study found that a split transfer tensioned the musculocutaneous nerve in 2 of 20 specimens, although this was also relieved with release of the proximal nerve branch [24]. In one reported case, median and ulnar nerve symptoms developed. After the patient underwent revision surgery and rerouting of the transfer from a subcoracoid position to a superficial transfer overlying the conjoined tendon, the neurologic symptoms resolved [29].

Clinical Outcomes

Transfer for Isolated Subscapularis Tears

Pectoralis major tendon transfer for isolated subscapularis tears produced satisfactory improvements in several studies. Resch et al. [3] found the Constant score to increase from

22.6 to 54.4 with patients averaging 65 years of age. Elhassan et al. [20] found also the Constant score to increase from 40.9 to 60.8 in a younger population. Jost et al. [26] reported a final mean relative Constant score of 79% in their series of isolated irreparable subscapularis tears. Also, the subcategories of the scores, e.g., range of motion and strength, were improved by a successful pectoralis transfer. Wirth and Rockwood [4] published a series where 10 of 13 shoulders achieved an elevation between 120° and 170° (mean 143°). For the three transfers that failed, the mean range of motion was significantly lower (110°; range 60°–140°). Resch et al. [3] reported about mean improvements in forward flexion and abduction (from 93° to 129° and from 85° to 113°, respectively). Forward flexion and abduction strength at 90° also improved, as did internal rotation strength. Five patients were able to achieve preinjury levels of shoulder function, and six were able to perform physically rigorous tasks, but not at the same level as before symptoms developed. However, external rotation was limited after successful pectoralis major transfer, decreasing by a mean of 25° [3, 26].

Transfer for Subscapularis in Combination with Multi-Tendon Rotator Cuff Tears

Some studies looked at results after pectoralis major transfer with anterosuperior rotator cuff tears involving both the subscapularis and the supraspinatus, as well as variably the infraspinatus. These patients also regularly benefited from salvage tendon transfer with measured mean Constant score increases from 28.7 to 52.3 [20], 52 to 68 [27], and 38.8 to 63.4 [30]. Jost et al. [26] reported a good mean relative Constant score (79%) when the supraspinatus was repairable compared to a group, where the supraspinatus was not reconstructable (59%). The postoperative Constant score was inversely correlated with preoperative supraspinatus fatty degeneration in the MRI [26]. In support of this observation, Galatz et al. [2] published his series of 14 patients with anterosuperior humeral head subluxation in massive anterosuperior cuff tears treated with pectoralis major transfer of the complete tendon. The American Shoulder and Elbow Surgeons score did improve from 27.2 to 47.7; however, depending on preoperative dysfunction, the outcomes were less uniformly satisfactory. The shoulders with pseudoparesis saw an increase in mean forward flexion from 28.4° to only 60° whereas passive external rotation decreased slightly (from 32° to 28°). Several authors have also reported that instability and anterior subluxation greatly reduced patient satisfaction [5, 20, 26]. Patients without instability, who had small or repairable supraspinatus tears, or whose supraspinatus defect could be simultaneously covered by the transferred pectoralis tendon had better results [26, 27, 30].

Transfer for Subscapularis Insufficiency After Shoulder Arthroplasty

Patients with symptomatic subscapularis insufficiency after anatomic shoulder arthroplasty or hemiarthroplasty had unreliable and often unsatisfactory results. Miller et al. [21] reported of mixed results of surgical outcomes in four patients treated with a pectoralis major tendon transfer. Only two of four patients were satisfied, with ratings of 9 of 10 (good-excellent).

Elhassan et al. [20] looked at eight patients with subscapularis tears after either hemiarthroplasty ($n = 3$) or anatomic total shoulder arthroplasty ($n = 5$). The results in the revision arthroplasty group were unpredictable. Only one of eight patients reported a significant improvement in pain and function. There were no statistically significant improvements in mean Constant scores or pain scores. Six of the eight patients reported no improvement in function or pain, and several required revision surgeries, including treatment for infection, conversion to reverse shoulder arthroplasty, and teres major transfer.

In general, clinical outcomes after pectoralis major transfers in cases of subscapularis insufficiency have been satisfactory for salvage procedures. Reasonable pain relief can be expected, although functional gains are often unpredictable [1, 5].

Although comparisons are difficult because of the heterogeneity of data and operative techniques, the best results are achieved in patients with an isolated subscapularis tear or an anterosuperior tear when the supraspinatus can also be repaired. These patients mostly displayed substantial improvements in the Constant score, as well as increases in mean range of motion to within near-normal range. The worst functional outcomes can be expected in patients who present with anterosuperior escape. This can be explained by the fact that these patients had the worst rotator cuff dysfunction preoperatively [1]. In addition, the pectoralis major transfer does not completely restore the force vector provided by a functional subscapularis. The transferred pectoralis exerts its force along a vector that is still more anterior to the native subscapularis [25].

It can be hypothesized that patients with anterior instability have only little improvement because even with a subcoracoid transfer, the pectoralis major is unable to restore the more posterior and medial directed vector of the subscapularis, which creates concavity compression and shoulder stability [1].

Patients with anatomic total shoulder arthroplasty also had poor results. When directly compared, however, the total shoulder arthroplasty group had higher Constant scores whereas the massive cuff tear patients had lower postoperative pain scores [20].

Improvements in pain were unpredictable across all surgical indications. In a few cases, patients had complete pain relief, whereas other patients only had partial relief. When self-reported pain levels are compared via visual analog scales, it appears that mean pain improvement was generally equivalent across all studies [1].

In conclusion, pectoralis major transfer can be an effective treatment for subscapularis tears that reduces pain and improves function when nonoperative therapies and attempts at anatomic restoration have failed, especially in patients too young or too active for salvage via reverse total shoulder arthroplasty. Moreover, it appears that the best outcomes occur in patients with subscapularis tears in isolation or combined with reparable supraspinatus tears.

Clinical Pearls/Pitfalls

- In potential cases when a pectoralis major transfer is under consideration I always check the alternatives like a reverse shoulder arthroplasty (older and inactive patients when more reliable functional results are favored) or an arthroscopy (to treat the pain or to check the indication) very thoroughly and discuss the alternatives with the patient.
- The subcoracoid tendon transfer is my favored technique and has the advantage of biomechanical superior results and the transferred tendon produces a soft-tissue interposition (buttress effect) between the humerus and the coracoid process.
- In cases when intraoperatively the musculocutaneus nerve seems under tension with the subcoracoid transfer, I consider the supracoracoid transfer as an alternative.
- The split-tendon transfer is my preferred technique to minimize musculocutaneous nerve tension.
- Most patients benefit from a pectoralis major transfer as a salvage procedure. However, the results are less predictable than the standard procedures in shoulder surgery.

References

1. Nelson GN, Namdari S, Galatz L, Keener JD. Pectoralis major tendon transfer for irreparable subscapularis tears. J Shoulder Elb Surg. 2014;23(6):909–18.
2. Galatz LM, Connor PM, Calfee RP, Hsu JC, Yamaguchi K. Pectoralis major transfer for anterior-superior subluxation in massive rotator cuff insufficiency. J Shoulder Elb Surg. 2003;12:1–5.
3. Resch H, Povacz P, Ritter E, Matschi W. Transfer of the pectoralis major muscle for the treatment of irreparable rupture of the subscapularis tendon. J Bone Joint Surg Am. 2000;82:372–82.
4. Wirth MA, Rockwood CA. Operative treatment of irreparable rupture of the subscapularis. J Bone Joint Surg Am. 1997;79:722–31.

5. Omid R, Lee B. Tendon transfers for irreparable rotator cuff tears. J Am Acad Orthop Surg. 2013;21:492–501.
6. Lyons RP, Green A. Subscapularis tendon tears. J Am Acad Orthop Surg. 2005;13:353–63.
7. Burkhart SS. Fluoroscopic comparison of kinematic patterns in massive rotator cuff tears. A suspension bridge model. Clin Orthop Relat Res. 1992;284:144–52.
8. Cuff D, Pupello D, Virani N, Levy J, Frankle M. Reverse shoulder arthroplasty for the treatment of rotator cuff deficiency. J Bone Joint Surg Am. 2008;90:1244–51.
9. Elhassan B, Endres NK, Higgins LD, Warner JJP. Massive irreparable tendon tears of the rotator cuff: salvage options. Instr Course Lect. 2008;57:153–66.
10. Baumgarten KM, Lashgari CJ, Yamaguchi K. Glenoid resurfacing in shoulder arthroplasty: indications and contraindications. Instr Course Lect. 2004;53:3–11.
11. Gadea F, Alami G, Pape G, Boileau P, Favard L. Shoulder hemiarthroplasty: outcomes and long-term survival analysis according to etiology. Orthop Traumatol Surg Res. 2012;98:659–65.
12. Goldberg SS, Bell J-E, Kim HJ, Bak SF, Levine WN, Bigliani LU. Hemiarthroplasty for the rotator cuff-deficient shoulder. J Bone Joint Surg Am. 2008;90:554–9.
13. Williams GR, Rockwood CA. Hemiarthroplasty in rotator cuffdeficient shoulders. J Shoulder Elb Surg. 1996;5:362–7.
14. Edwards TB, Walch G, Nove-Josserand L, Boulahia A, Neyton L, O'Connor DP, et al. Arthroscopic debridement in the treatment of patients with isolated tears of the subscapularis. Arthroscopy. 2006;22:941–6.
15. Dines DM, Moynihan DP, Dines JS, McCann P. Irreparable rotator cuff tears: what to do and when to do it; the surgeon's dilemma. Instr Course Lect. 2007;56:13–22.
16. Gerber C, Maquieira G, Espinosa N. Latissimus dorsi transfer for the treatment of irreparable rotator cuff tears. J Bone Joint Surg Am. 2006;88:113–20.
17. Goutallier D, De Abreu L, Postel JM, Le Guilloux P, Radier C, Zilber S. Is the trapezius transfer a useful treatment option for irreparable tears of the subscapularis? Orthop Traumatol Surg Res. 2011;97:719–25.
18. Tonino PM, Gerber C, Itoi E, Porcellini G, Sonnabend D, Walch G. Complex shoulder disorders: evaluation and treatment. J Am Acad Orthop Surg. 2009;17:125–36.
19. Werner CML, Zingg PO, Lie D, Jacob HAC, Gerber C. The biomechanical role of the subscapularis in latissimus dorsi transfer

for the treatment of irreparable rotator cuff tears. J Shoulder Elb Surg. 2006;15:736–42. doi:10.1016/j.jse.2005.11.002.

20. Elhassan B, Ozbaydar M, Massimini D, Diller D, Higgins L, Warner JJP. Transfer of pectoralis major for the treatment of irreparable tears of subscapularis: does it work? J Bone Joint Surg Br. 2008;90:1059–65.

21. Miller BS, Joseph TA, Noonan TJ, Horan MP, Hawkins RJ. Rupture of the subscapularis tendon after shoulder arthroplasty: diagnosis, treatment, and outcome. J Shoulder Elb Surg. 2005;14:492–6.

22. Miller S. Loss of subscapularis function after total shoulder replacement: a seldom recognized problem. J Shoulder Elb Surg. 2003;12:29–34.

23. Jennings GJ, Keereweer S, Buijze GA, De Beer J, DuToit D. Transfer of segmentally split pectoralis major for the treatment of irreparable rupture of the subscapularis tendon. J Shoulder Elb Surg. 2007;16:837–42.

24. Klepps SJ, Goldfarb C, Flatow E, Galatz LM, Yamaguchi K. Anatomic evaluation of the subcoracoid pectoralis major transfer in human cadavers. J Shoulder Elb Surg. 2001;10:453–9.

25. Konrad GG, Sudkamp NP, Kreuz PC, Jolly JT, McMahon PJ, Debski RE. Pectoralis major tendon transfers above or underneath the conjoint tendon in subscapularis-deficient shoulders. An in vitro biomechanical analysis. J Bone Joint Surg Am. 2007;89:2477–84.

26. Jost B, Puskas GJ, Lustenberger A, Gerber C. Outcome of pectoralis major transfer for the treatment of irreparable subscapularis tears. J Bone Joint Surg Am. 2003;85:1944–51.

27. Gavriilidis I, Kircher J, Magosch P, Lichtenberg S, Habermeyer P. Pectoralis major transfer for the treatment of irreparable anterosuperior rotator cuff tears. Int Orthop. 2010;34:689–94.

28. Burkhart SS, Esch JC, Jolson RS. The rotator crescent and rotator cable: an anatomic description of the shoulder's "suspension bridge". Arthroscopy. 1993;9:611–6.

29. Owens BD, Nelson BJ, Taylor DC. Acute brachial plexus compression after pectoralis major transfer for subscapularis insufficiency. Am J Sports Med. 2008;36:173–5.

30. Lederer S, Auffarth A, Bogner R, Tauber M, Mayer M, Karpik S, et al. Magnetic resonance imaging-controlled results of the pectoralis major tendon transfer for irreparable anterosuperior rotator cuff tears performed with standard and modified fixation techniques. J Shoulder Elb Surg. 2011;20:1155–62.

Chapter 13
Hemiarthroplasty for Cuff Arthropathy

Patrick J. McMahon

Case Presentation

The patient is a 62-year-old active male with a 5-year history of worsening, constant, achy right shoulder pain. There was no specific injury when the pain began. He said that he liked to split wood for his fireplace and wanted to continue to do so. He had persistent moderate, achy constant shoulder pain that was worse with activities and awakened him a night. He was treated with physical therapy and two cortisone injections in the subacromial space that has each resulted in diminished pain for 5–6 weeks before the pain had recurred.

On physical examination, he stood 5 ft 10 in. tall and weighed 185 pounds. He had full range of motion of the right shoulder with pain throughout the arc of motion and the scapula moved normally without a shoulder shrug or winging. There was mild crepitus with motion. He had diffuse mild tenderness of the shoulder and none at the acromioclavicular (AC)

P.J. McMahon, M.D.
Orthopedics and Rehabilitation,
Department of Bioengineering, University of Pittsburgh,
2100 Jane St., Pittsburgh, PA 15203-2076, USA
e-mail: mcmahonp@upmc.edu

© Springer International Publishing AG 2018
P.J. McMahon (ed.), *Rotator Cuff Injuries*,
DOI 10.1007/978-3-319-63668-9_13

and sternoclavicular joints. The right shoulder strength was diminished in abduction and external rotation, rated as 4/5 with pain, and was normal in internal rotation at 5/5. He had no pain at the AC joint with cross-body motion. I did not do impingement or instability testing.

The true lateral (i.e., Grashey), (Fig. 13.1a) axillary lateral, (Fig. 13.1b) supraspinatus outlet (Fig. 13.1c), and acromioclavicular (i.e., Zanca) (Fig. 13.1d) radiographs of the patient's right shoulder revealed that the humeral head was superior and bone-on-bone against the acromion and there was moderate AC joint osteoarthritis. As the patient had failed nonsurgical treatment, and had persistent, constant pain and good shoulder function, he was interested in shoulder

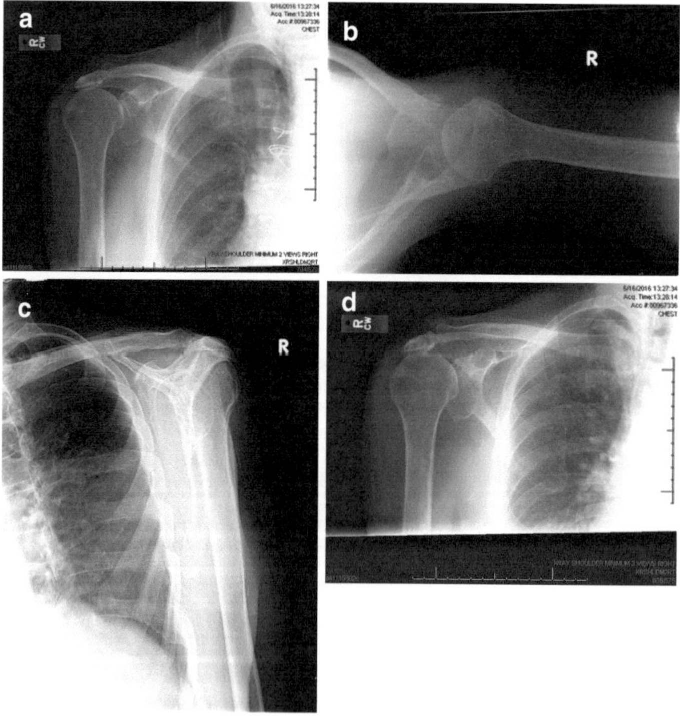

FIGURE 13.1 (**a, b, c, d**) Preoperative radiographs

hemiarthroplasty. We discussed that there was a chance of his having worse function after the surgery and that the goal was to diminish the pain, on average, by about two-thirds.

Diagnosis/Assessment

The patient's history, physical, and imaging findings are consistent with the diagnosis of cuff arthropathy with good shoulder function. Initial treatment was nonoperative including rehabilitation and NSAIDs. A subacromial injection of lidocaine and cortisone that resulted in immediate diminished pain and persisted for several weeks was helpful in ruling out other causes of shoulder pain such as cervical radiculopathy and malingering. He had full range of shoulder motion and did not want to lose internal and external rotation with the arm at the side. When there is AC joint osteoarthritis as with this patient, I have been successful using the absence of tenderness at the AC joint and the absence of pain at the AC joint with cross-body motion in leaving the AC joint alone.

Management

With the patient in the Fowler position (Fig. 13.2) and the arm on a Mayo Stand a deltopectoral incision is made (Fig. 13.3). The deltopectoral interval is split and the shoulder is then extended and internally rotated to expose the rotator cuff tear. A Fukuda retractor is placed into the joint. When the superior subscapularis tendon is torn as is usually the case, the shoulder is then pushed superior to expose the humeral head (Fig. 13.4). If the entire subscapularis tendon is intact it is helpful to incise the superior third of the subscapularis tendon to aid in the exposure, and when I do this, I prefer to incise the subscapularis off the lesser tuberosity with a peel-off method. The long head of the biceps tendon is almost always torn. In the rare instance when it is not, a tenodesis can be done just below the bicipital groove. I use an intramedullary guide and

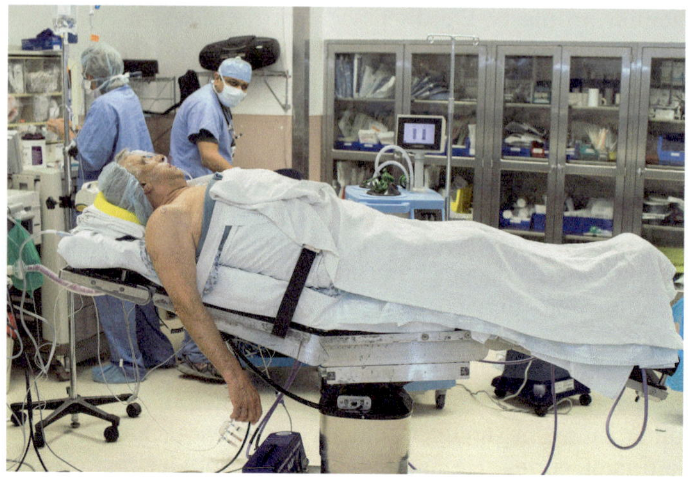

FIGURE 13.2 The patient positioned in the semi-Fowler's position

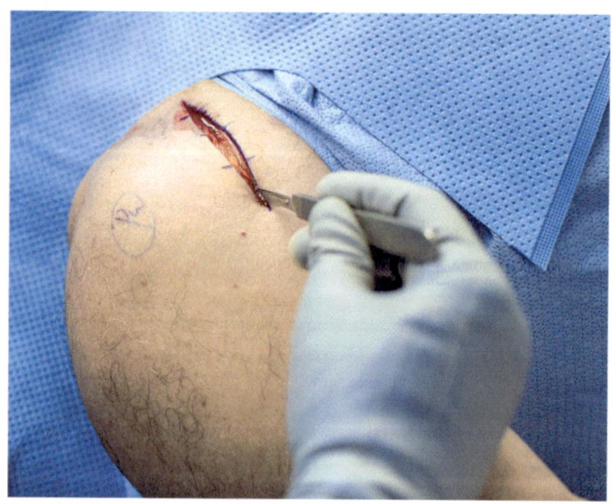

FIGURE 13.3 Surgical incision

a proximal humeral cutting guide to aid in the humeral osteotomy. The intramedullary guide is placed into the lateral
humeral head an average of 9 mm posterior to the bicipital
groove. It is sometimes difficult to find the junction of the
lateral humeral head and the greater tuberosity when the cuff

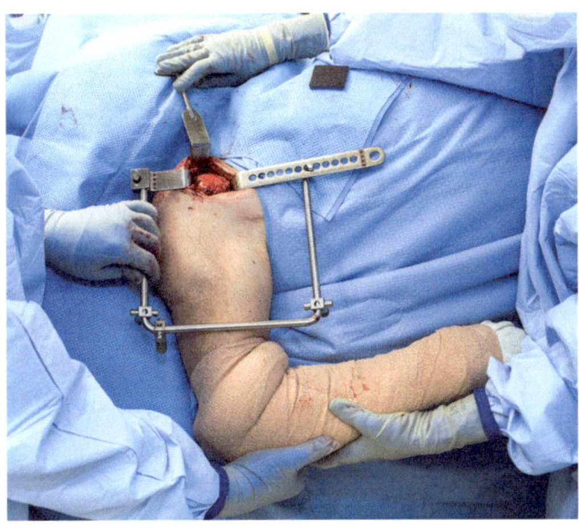

FIGURE 13.4 Exposure of the rotator cuff tear and pushing the humerus superior

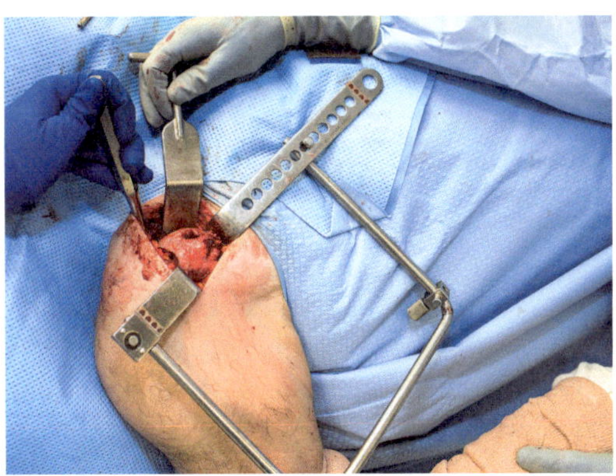

FIGURE 13.5 Exposure of the humeral head for evaluation of humeral retroversion

arthropathy is chronic and proximal humerus has a "bald eagle" appearance. Then a starting point is made so that the intramedullary guide will go straight down the humeral shaft. I position the guide in 30° of retroversion and mark the front of the humerus with a line where the osteotomy will be done (Fig. 13.5). The intramedullary guide is removed. It is helpful

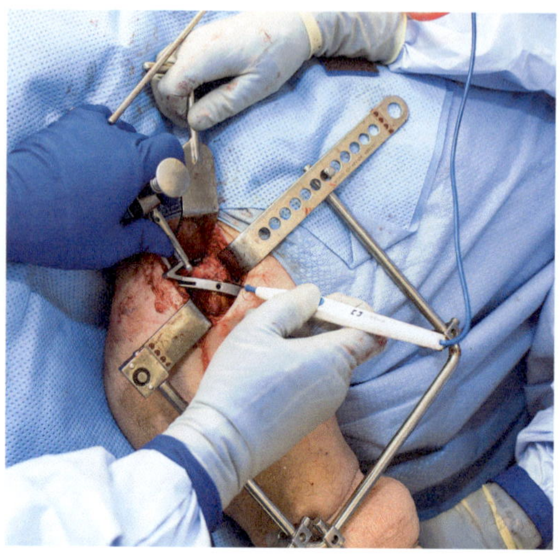

FIGURE 13.6 Maring the proximal humerus for the osteotomy

to see the humeral head by retracting the remaining rotator cuff both anterior and posterior to aid in cutting with the proper retroversion (Fig. 13.6). The osteotomy is made from lateral to medial at a 135° angle with the shaft (Fig. 13.7). The humeral head is removed and the diameter is measured. I like to do the humeral osteotomy this way instead of anterior to posterior as I do with patients with osteoarthritis and an intact rotator cuff tear as it preserves the subscapularis tendon and allows early active range of motion. Also, it is uncommon for there to be inferior humeral head osteophytes in patients with cuff arthropathy since, when present, excision of the inferior humeral head osteophytes necessitates incision of the entire subscapularis tendon to expose the osteophytes. The osteoarthritis in patients with massive rotator cuff tears is usually different than in those with an intact rotator cuff. It usually involves the superior humeral head and the superior glenoid as a result of the superior position of the humeral head. There can also be concentric glenoid wear. Loss of glenoid bone is a concern after hemiarthroplasty and if present before surgery

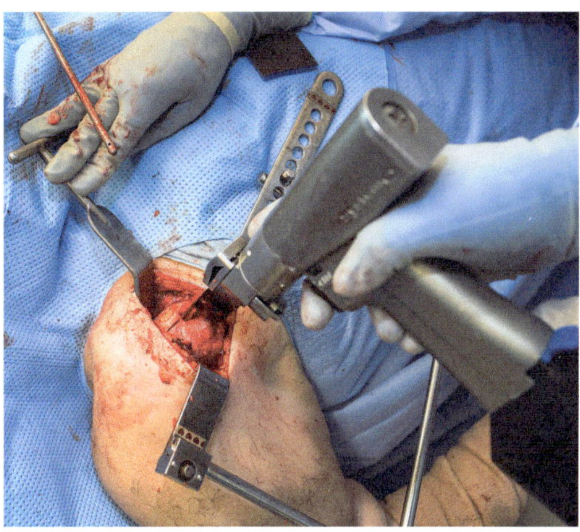

FIGURE 13.7 The shoulder is internally rotated and then and oteotomy is done from lateral to medial in 30° of retroversion

and is severe can be a contraindication to hemiarthroplasty. Progressively larger broaches are then placed down the humeral canal in line with the humeral shaft and I like to do this, on average with the arm in about 30° of external rotation relative to the table so that the broach can be inserted perpendicular to the table to match the humeral retroversion (Fig. 13.8). When the surgeon gets good fixation of the broach in the proximal humeral bone, the broaching can stop as good proximal cancellous humeral bone will provide good fixation and endoseal contact with the humerus is not necessary. The head component is matched to the diameter of the humeral head that was resected. The thickness of the humeral head prosthesis can be judged as being on average three-fourths of the radius. If the shoulder has good passive range of motion and the humeral head can be translated to the rim of the glenoid, the trial components can be removed and a prosthesis with a surface for bone ingrowth can be impacted in place. Morselized cancellous bone from the humeral head can be placed in the endoseal canal of the humerus before the prosthesis to aid in fixation. It is important that the greater tuberosity is a bit below the top of the humeral head to minimize

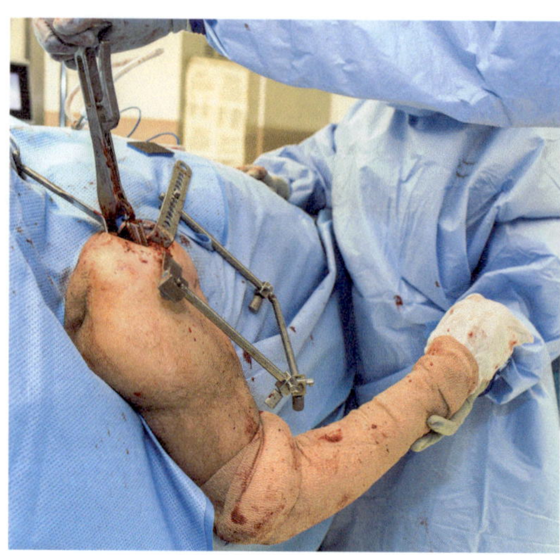

FIGURE 13.8 Inserting the humeral broach

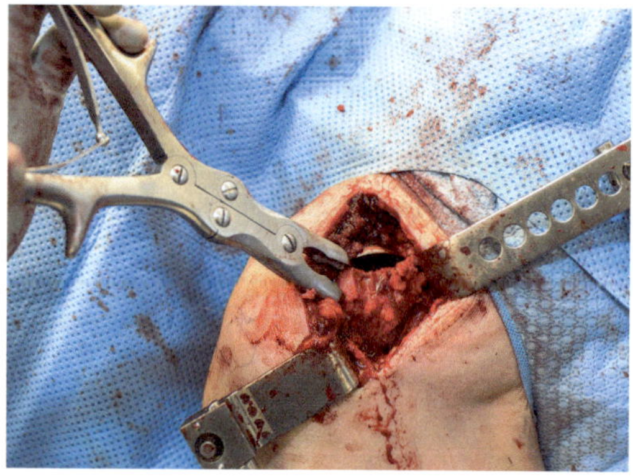

FIGURE 13.9 Tuberoplasty (debridement of about 7 mm of the height of the greater tuberosity)

impingement of the greater tuberosity on the acromion with shoulder elevation. So, a tuberoplasty is done by debriding the bone of the top of the greater tuberosity (Fig. 13.9) so that the prosthesis is about 7 mm higher than the greater tuberosity (Fig. 13.10).

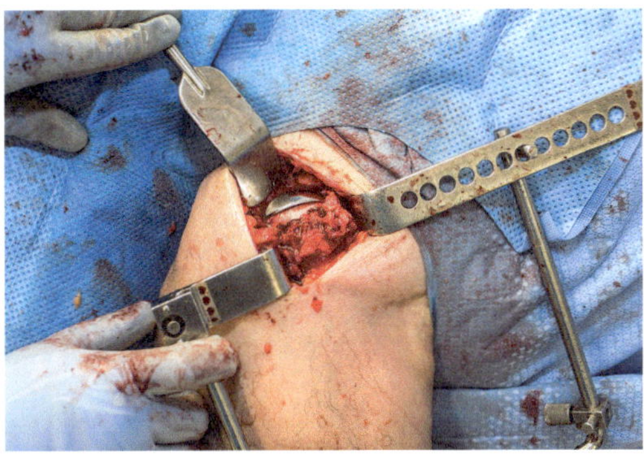

FIGURE 13.10 The prosthesis in place after the tuberoplasty

If the procedure was done through the rotator cuff tear the deltopectoral interval is closed followed by the skin. If any of the subscapularis tendon was incised to do the procedure, it is repaired to the lesser tuberosity with running/locking sutures and then the skin is closed.

Supervising the rehabilitation is important for a successful outcome. If the subscapularis tendon was not incised, a sling is used for comfort and the patient does pendulum exercises and then begins active ROM and stretching to diminish stiffness as soon as it is comfortable to do so, usually 7–10 days postoperative. Postoperative AP (i.e., Grashey) (Fig. 13.11a) and axillary lateral (Fig. 13.11b) radiographs done a week after surgery revealed good alignment of the prosthesis. If the subscapularis tendon was incised and repaired, the patient stays in the sling long enough for the early healing, 2–4 weeks depending on how good was the repair. Strengthening is begun 3 months postoperative.

Outcome

This 62-year-old gentleman recovered uneventfully. At 4 months postoperative, he had little pain and was sleeping normally. He had full range of motion with forward flexion to 150°, external rotation with the arm at the side to 40° and internal

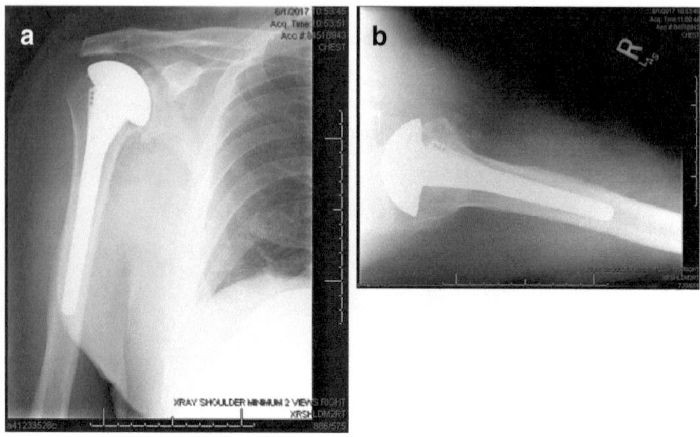

FIGURE 13.11 (**a, b**) Postoperative radiographs

rotation to L1, and strength of 4/5 to abduction and external rotation and 5/5 to internal rotation, similar to preoperative.

Literature Review

Initial treatment of cuff arthropathy is nonoperative. The usual indication for surgery is symptoms that persist over several months of nonoperative treatments. Indications for hemiarthroplasty are good shoulder function with cuff arthropathy, that is, glenohumeral joint osteoarthritis and a massive rotator cuff tear. Superior positioning of the humeral head on the glenoid is usual. A high rate of glenoid loosening after traditional total shoulder arthroplasty [1] initially led surgeons to hemiarthroplasty as surgical treatment for the patient with cuff arthropathy. For those with good shoulder function and an intact coracoacromial arch [2] who are young and/or want to maintain activity levels greater than those recommended after reverse total shoulder arthroplasty, hemiarthroplasty has high patient satisfaction. Pain is diminished by two-thirds on average [3]. Elevation to 90° or more is a prerequisite for this surgery [4] and these patients have intact teres minor and at least a portion of the subscapularis tendon that is intact. Interestingly those with less preoperative range of passive external rotation do better than those with more external rotation [5] probably because those with osteoarthritis being a large portion of their problem do better than those with symptoms being more from the rotator cuff tear. Those who have hemiarthroplasty for cuff tear arthropathy do not do as well as those with an intact rotator cuff tear [6] as weakness usually in abduction and external rotator persists and a few have worse function after hemiarthroplasty done for cuff arthropathy [7]. Specifically about 10% lose strength and some of them are unable to lift the arm overhead afterwards. Survivorship at a decade is about 80% compared to about 90% when the rotator cuff is intact [8]. Other complications include persistent pain, stiffness, aseptic loosening, infection, and deep vein thrombosis. Glenoid erosion that occurs over time is the most common complication [9] and can occur in the acromion as well but this has very rarely been a problem for the patient in my experience. A variety of soft tissues for resurfacing the glenoid have been tried but none has proved durable. Hemiarthroplasty is not difficult, complications are few, and it has proved to be durable over the several decades when done for cuff arthropathy.

Clinical Pearls/Pitfalls

- The key to the management of cuff arthropathy is patient selection. Those with good function can be treated with hemiarthroplasty as long as they are satisfied with pain relief of two-thirds on average and a small risk of losing function afterwards.
- The surgery can be done without incising the rotator cuff in the majority of patients.
- Rehabilitation can begin as soon as comfortable. It is important not to immobilize the arm for a prolonged period of time after the surgery as weakness can ensue that increases the chance of function being worse.
- It is important to counsel the patient about bone erosion and although rare there is a chance that function will be worse after hemiarthroplasty done for cuff arthropathy.

References

1. Feeley BT, Gallo RA, Craig EV. Cuff tear arthropathy: current trends in diagnosis and surgical management. J Shoulder Elb Surg. 2009;18(3):484–94. doi:10.1016/j.jse.2008.11.003. Review. PMID: 19208484

2. Field LD, Dines DM, Zabinski SJ, Warren RF. Hemiarthroplasty of the shoulder for rotator cuff arthropathy. J Shoulder Elb Surg. 1997;6(1):18–23. PMID: 9071678

3. Gartsman GM, Roddey TS, Hammerman SM. Shoulder arthroplasty with or without resurfacing of the glenoid in patients who have osteoarthritis. J Bone Joint Surg Am. 2000;82(1):26–34. PMID: 10653081

4. Goldberg SS, Bigliani LU. Hemiarthroplasty for the rotator cuff-deficient shoulder. Surgical technique. J Bone Joint Surg Am. 2009;91(Suppl 2 Pt 1):22–9. doi:10.2106/JBJS.H.01379. PMID: 19255197

5. Somerson JS, Sander P, Bohsali K, Tibbetts R, Rockwood CA Jr, Wirth MA. What factors are associated with clinically important improvement after shoulder hemiarthroplasty for cuff tear arthropathy? Clin Orthop Relat Res. 2016;474(12):2682–8. PMID: 27530396

6. Matsen FA 3rd, Russ SM, Vu PT, Hsu JE, Lucas RM, Comstock BA. What factors are predictive of patient-reported outcomes? A prospective study of 337 shoulder arthroplasties. Clin Orthop Relat Res. 2016;474(11):2496–510. PMID: 27457623

7. Williams GR Jr, Rockwood CA Jr. Hemiarthroplasty in rotator cuff-deficient shoulders. J Shoulder Elb Surg. 1996;5(5):362–7. PMID: 8933458

8. Gadea F, Alami G, Pape G, Boileau P, Favard L. Shoulder hemiarthroplasty: outcomes and long-term survival analysis according to etiology. Orthop Traumatol Surg Res. 2012;98(6):659–65. doi:10.1016/j.otsr.2012.03.020. PMID: 22944393

9. Al-Hadithy N, Domos P, Sewell MD, Naleem A, Papanna MC, Pandit R. Cementless surface replacement arthroplasty of the shoulder for osteoarthritis: results of fifty Mark III Copeland prosthesis from an independent center with four-year mean follow-up. J Shoulder Elb Surg. 2012;21(12):1776–81. doi:10.1016/j.jse.2012.01.024. PMID: 22572402

Chapter 14
Reverse Total Shoulder Arthroplasty for Cuff Arthropathy

Patrick J. McMahon

Case Presentation

The patient is a 78-year-old active male with a 5-year history of worsening right shoulder pain. There was no specific injury when the shoulder problems began. When I saw him he had persistent moderate, achy constant shoulder pain that was worse with activities and awakened him a night. About a year prior he had lost the ability to lift his arm. He was treated with physical therapy and two cortisone injections in the sub-acromial space that has each resulted in diminished pain for 3–4 weeks before the pain had recurred.

On physical examination, he stood 6 ft tall and weighed 170 pounds. He had diminished active range of motion of the right shoulder and pain with motion. Specifically the active forward flexion was to 50°, the external rotation was to 30°, and the internal rotation was to L3. There was moderate crepitus with motion. He had passive forward flexion to 120°.

P.J. McMahon, M.D.
Orthopedics and Rehabilitation,
Department of Bioengineering, University of Pittsburgh,
2100 Jane St., Pittsburgh, PA 15203-2076, USA
e-mail: mcmahonp@upmc.edu

© Springer International Publishing AG 2018
P.J. McMahon (ed.), *Rotator Cuff Injuries*,
DOI 10.1007/978-3-319-63668-9_14

The external and internal rotations were the same passively as they were actively. He had diffuse mild tenderness of the shoulder and none specifically at the acromioclavicular and sternoclavicular joints. The right shoulder strength was diminished in abduction, rated as 2/5 with pain, but was good in external rotation, 4/5, and in internal rotation, 5/5. I did not do impingement or instability testing.

The true AP (i.e., Grashey) (Fig. 14.1a) and axillary lateral (Fig. 14.1b) radiographs of the patient's right shoulder revealed that the humeral head was superior on the glenoid and was bone-on-bone against the glenoid and the acromion. As the patient had failed nonsurgical treatment, and had persistent constant pain and poor shoulder function, we discussed the risks and benefits of nonoperative and operative treatments and he chose reverse TSA.

Diagnosis/Assessment

The patient's history, physical, and imaging findings are consistent with the diagnosis of rotator cuff arthropathy with pseudoparalysis in elevation. He had sufficient strength in external and internal rotation. Initial treatment was nonoperative including rehabilitation and NSAIDs. A subacromial

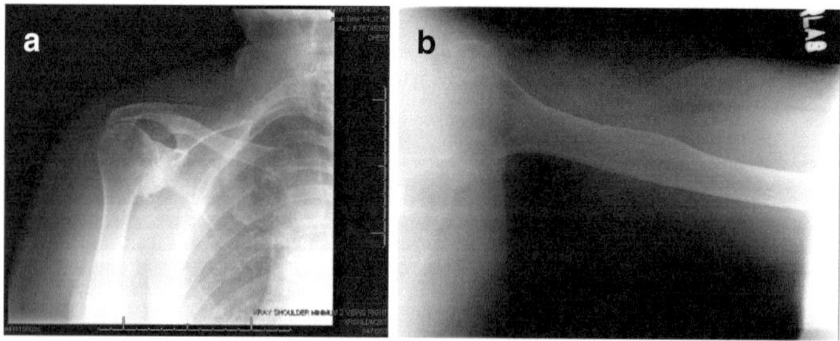

FIGURE 14.1 (**a** and **b**) The true lateral (Grashey) and axillary lateral radiographs of the patient's right shoulder revealed that the humeral head was superior on the glenoid and was bone-on-bone against the acromion and there was moderate AC joint osteoarthritis

injection of lidocaine and cortisone that resulted in immediate diminished pain and persisted for several weeks can be helpful in ruling out other causes of shoulder pain such as cervical radiculopathy and malingering. The usual indication for surgery is symptoms that persist over several months of nonoperative treatments in those with inability to lift the arm against gravity, known as pseudoparalysis in those with glenohumeral joint osteoarthritis and superior positioning of the humeral head on the glenoid. The osteoarthritis in patients with massive rotator cuff tears is usually different than those with an intact rotator cuff. The osteoarthritis usually involves the superior humeral head and the superior glenoid as a result of the superior position of the humeral head. Alternatively there can be concentric glenoid wear. Loss of glenoid bone can make positioning of the glenoid component more difficult and sometimes can make it impossible if it is severe. Inferior humeral head osteophytes, common in those with an intact rotator cuff, are uncommon in rotator cuff arthropathy. It is important to assess the acromion as it is sometimes thin, making it more prone to fracture after reverse TSA and the patient should be aware of this risk. When there is AC joint osteoarthritis as with this patient, I have been successful using the absence of tenderness at the AC joint and the absence of pain at the AC joint with cross-body motion, as is usually the case, in leaving the AC joint alone. When I started doing reverse TSA in the early 2000s I did it only in those more than 70 years of age. I now do the surgery in younger patients with good results [1, 2] but the vast majority of my patients with reverse TSA continue to be elderly.

Management

With the patient in the Fowler's position and the arm on a Mayo Stand a deltopectoral incision was made (Fig. 14.2). The deltopectoral interval was split and the clavipectoral fascia was incised lateral to the conjoined tendon. A self-retaining

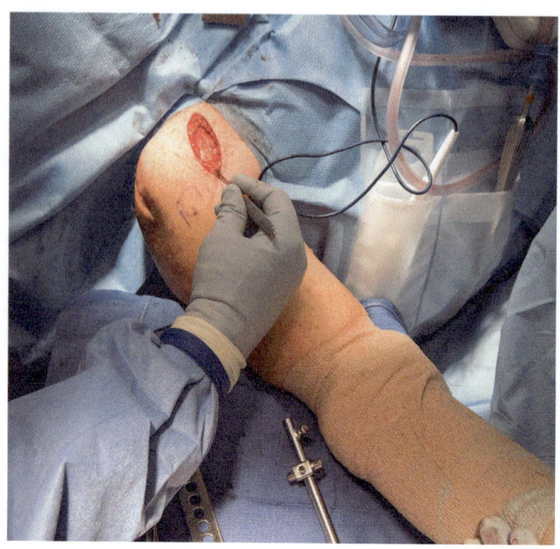

Figure 14.2 Surgical incision

retractor was placed with one side under the conjoined tendon and the other under the deltoid tendon. With the arm at the side, the shoulder was then externally rotated to expose the subscapularis tendon insertion on the lesser tuberosity. As the superior two-thirds of the subscapularis tendon was not torn it was peeled off the lesser tuberosity (Fig. 14.3). A Fukuda retractor was placed into the joint and the shoulder was extended and externally rotated to expose the humeral head. The shoulder was pushed superior to expose more of the humeral head. The long head of the biceps tendon is almost always torn and in the rare instance when it is not a tenodesis can be done just below the bicipital groove. I used an intramedullary guide and a proximal humeral cutting guide to aid in the humeral osteotomy. The intramedullary guide was placed into the lateral humeral head 9 mm posterior to the bicipital groove which is the average. It is sometimes difficult to find the junction of the lateral humeral head and the greater tuberosity when the cuff arthropathy is chronic and the proximal humerus has a "bald eagle" appearance. Then a starting point is made so that the intramedullary guide will go

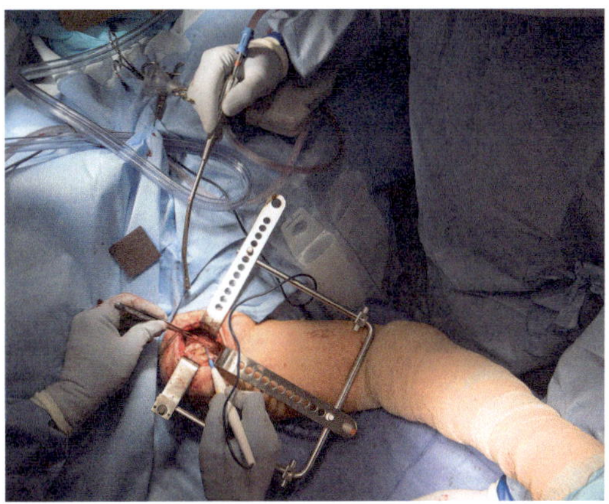

FIGURE 14.3 Exposure of the lesser tuberosity with the arm in external rotation

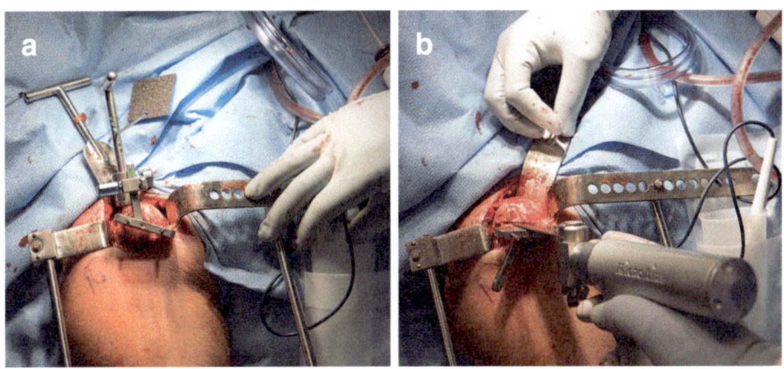

FIGURE 14.4 (**a**) Intramedullary guide for the humeral osteotomy. (**b**) Osteotomy of the humeral head

straight down the humeral shaft. I positioned the guide in about 20° of retroversion and an osteotomy was made from anterior to posterior at a 155° angle with the shaft (Fig. 14.4). The humeral head was removed and the diameter was measured. Inferior humeral head osteophytes, although unusual, were removed with a rongeur. I then directed my attention to the glenoid. With the shoulder in abduction and external rotation the humeral osteotomy was placed posterior to the glenoid so that the surface of the humeral osteotomy was 90° to the surface of the glenoid (Fig. 14.5). If it will not stay, I retract the humerus with a Sonnabend or a Fukuda retractor. As the anterior capsule was intact it was incised at its insertion onto the labrum with a scalpel. An axillary nerve tug test was done by placing a finger along the inferior margin of the subscapularis muscle about 6 cm medial to the conjoined tendon while the deltoid muscle was tugged laterally. The axillary nerve was felt to tighten. It can be exposed and tagged. The inferior capsule was incised with a Bovie. The Bovie is used so that if it is close there will be stimulation of the axillary nerve alerting me. If there is any question of axillary nerve injury the tug test is repeated. A forked retractor was placed on the anterior glenoid neck. A finger was placed inferior to the glenoid to palpate the lateral border of the scapula. Sometimes a 1/2 in. periosteal elevator is used to remove the origin of the long head of the triceps tendon from the inferior glenoid if it prevents palpation of the lateral border of the scapula. A forked retractor was also placed on the lateral border of the scapula. A starting point was made so that the glenoid component will

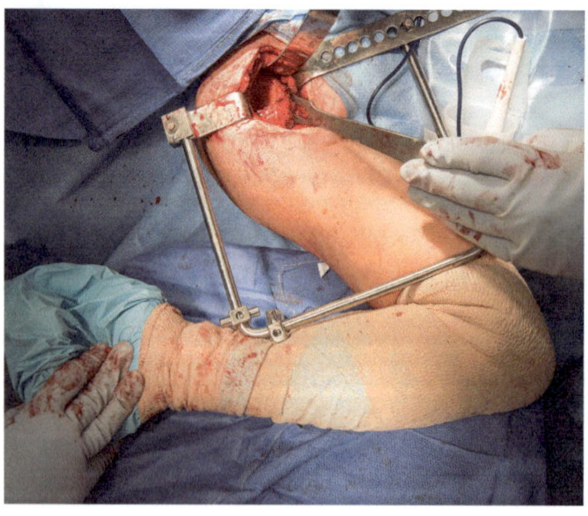

FIGURE 14.5 The humeral head osteotomy is placed behind the glenoid and the arm placed in abduction and external rotation for exposure of the glenoid

overhand the inferior glenoid by about 7 mm. This is usually a bit inferior to the center of the glenoid but varies depending on the glenoid size. The glenoid was reamed (Fig. 14.6) as was the hole for the center peg. The glenoid baseplate was impacted in place with its inferior hole aligned with the lateral border of the scapula. The inferior screw is the most important and I like it to be a locking screw at least 30–42 mm in length with good cortical fixation at its tip. I direct it posterior so that it exits the scapula at the infraspinatus fossa and not the subscapularis fossa. Anterior and posterior screws were placed. If needed, the superior screw is also a locking screw that I try to place into the base of the coaracoid so it does not exit the posterior glenoid where it may weaken the base of the scapula spine and contribute to scapula spine fracture. A trial glenosphere was placed on the glenoid baseplate. The humerus was then again dislocated in extension and external rotation. The humeral reaming guide was placed down the humeral canal in line with the humeral shaft (Fig. 14.7) and the proximal humerus was reamed. I prefer to cement the humeral prosthesis so I then placed a cement restrictor down the canal so that

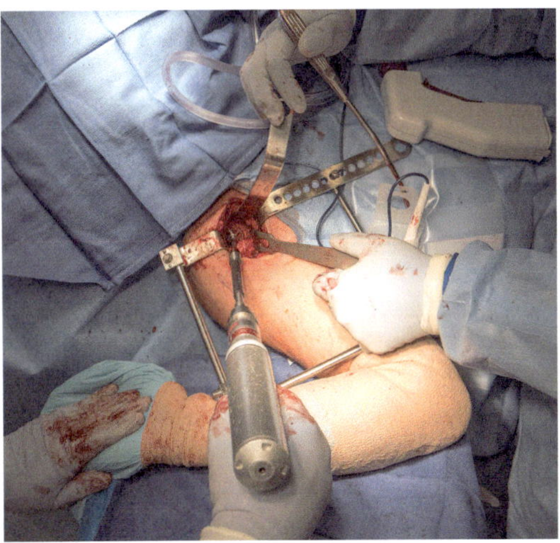

FIGURE 14.6 The glenoid is reamed for the glenoid components

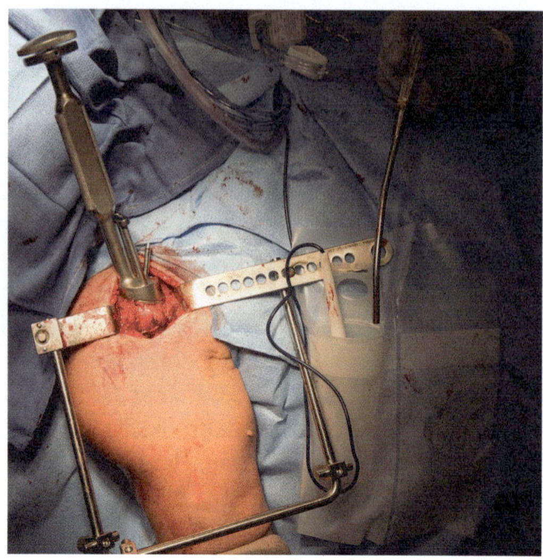

FIGURE 14.7 The humeral reaming guide is inserted in line with the humeral shaft

it was a centimeter or two below the prosthesis. For an uncemented humeral stem the surgeon can place the humeral trial so that there is good fixation in the humeral bone. I prefer to place as large a humeral cup as will fit to diminish impingement and to maximize range of motion. The prosthesis is reduced tightly so that there is only a millimeter or two of inferior shuck. As the shoulder had good passive range of motion and the arm could be placed at the side without the humeral prosthesis lifting off the trial glenosphere, the trial components were removed and the glenosphere impacted onto the glenoid baseplate so that it overhung the inferior glenoid bone by about 7 mm. A mildly lateral-based glenoid design may be more effective than prosthesis positioning in diminishing scapula notching [3]. A glenosphere with the Morse taper hole eccentric to its center can also aid in its placement. The humeral prosthesis was then cemented in place (Fig. 14.8). If the humeral component is not cemented, morselized cancellous bone from the humeral head can be placed in the canal of the humerus before the prosthesis to aid in fixation if needed. The subscapularis tendon was sewn back

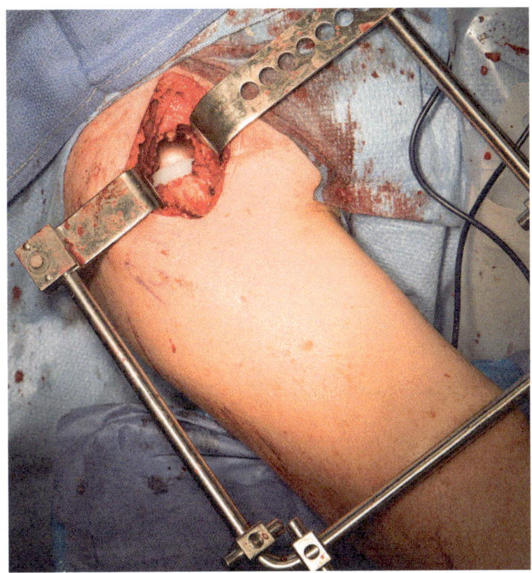

FIGURE 14.8 The completed prosthesis in place

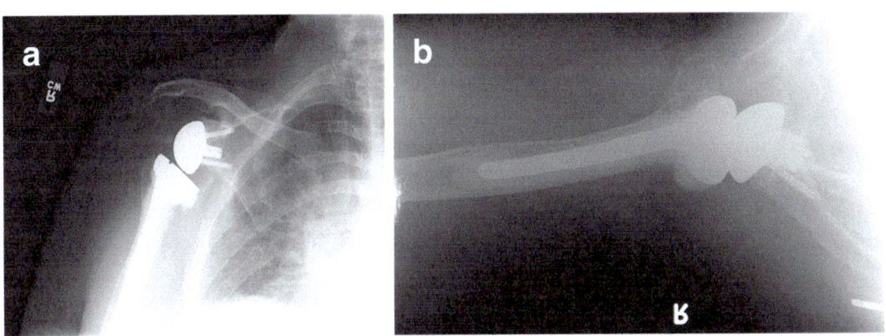

FIGURE 14.9 The true lateral (i.e., Grashey), (**a**) and axillary lateral, (**b**) radiographs after reverse TSA

to the lesser tuberosity with sutures through bone and running, locking sutures in the tendon. The deltopectoral interval was closed followed by the skin.

Supervising the rehabilitation is important for a successful outcome. A sling was used for comfort and the patient did pendulum exercises. Postoperative radiographs demonstrated the position of the reverse TSA (Fig. 14.9a, b). Four weeks postoperative the patient began active ROM. Strengthening was begun 3 months postoperative. Patient satisfaction is high with reverse TSA with about 85% pain relief and two-thirds of the normal range of motion being restored on average.

Outcome

This 78-year-old gentleman recovered uneventfully. At 3 months postoperative, he had little pain, was sleeping normally, and had forward flexion to 140°, external rotation with the arm at the side to 10°, and internal rotation to L5. He had strength of 4/5 to abduction and external rotation of 5/5 to internal rotation.

Literature Review

Reverse TSA is an effective treatment for those with rotator cuff arthropathy and pseudoparalysis. These are usually elderly patients that on average get about two-thirds to three-quarters of their usual range of motion in elevation. It is not so successful in helping with external and internal rotation with the arm at the side. Instead these motions are often limited after reverse TSA so that, as in this case they are worse than preoperative. Most patients do not have a problem sacrificing external and internal rotation with the arm at the side so that they can lift their arm overhead. In addition to preoperative weakness in elevation, some patients have weakness in external rotation of the abducted shoulder that reverse TSA does not help, so in those patients a latissimus dorsi transfer as described in Chap. 15 is helpful. Complications after reverse TSA for cuff arthropathy occur in about 10% of patients and include persistent pain, stiffness or weakness, hematoma, dislocation, acromion and scapula spine fracture [4], particulate debris, aseptic loosening, heterotopic bone [5], and infection. Some of these complications such as acromion and scapula spine fracture and recurrent dislocations are very difficult to treat and often lead to a poor outcome. Fracture and dissociation of the glenoid components, which were among my concerns when I started to do reverse TSA, have thankfully turned out to be rare.

Clinical Pearls/Pitfalls

- Patient selection is important in the management of cuff arthropathy with pseudoparalysis. Those with pain and poor function can be treated with reverse TSA with excellent percent pain relief and two-thirds restoration of motion, on average.
- Rehabilitation should be supervised to minimize subscapularis tendon rupture and allow for glenoid component fixation.
- Complications occur in about 10% of patients and it is important to inform the patient of them before surgery as some of them are very difficult to treat and lead to a poor outcome.

References

1. Otto RJ, Clark RE, Frankle MA. Reverse shoulder arthroplasty in patients younger than 55 years: 2- to 12-year follow-up. J Shoulder Elbow Surg. 2016; doi:10.1016/j.jse.2016.09.051. pii: S1058–2746(16)30492-X. [Epub ahead of print], PMID: 28034540
2. Samuelsen BT, Wagner ER, Houdek MT, Elhassan BT, Sánchez-Sotelo J, Cofield R, Sperling JW. Primary reverse shoulder arthroplasty in patients aged 65 years or younger. J Shoulder Elbow Surg. 2017;26(1):e13–7. doi:10.1016/j.jse.2016.05.026. PMID: 27522342
3. Huri G, Familiari F, Salari N, Petersen SA, Doral MN, McFarland EG. Prosthetic design of reverse shoulder arthroplasty contributes to scapular notching and instability. World J Orthop. 2016;7(11):738–45. PMID: 27900271
4. Mayne IP, Bell SN, Wright W, Coghlan JA. Acromial and scapular spine fractures after reverse total shoulder arthroplasty. Shoulder

Elbow. 2016;8(2):90–100. doi:10.1177/1758573216628783. PMID: 27583005
5. Verhofste B, Decock T, Van Tongel A, De Wilde L. Heterotopic ossification after reverse total shoulder arthroplasty. Bone Joint J. 2016;98-B(9):1215–21. doi:10.1302/0301-620X.98B9.37761. PMID: 27587523

Chapter 15
Adding a Latissimus Dorsi Tendon Transfer to Reverse Shoulder Arthroplasty

Donavan Kip Murphy, Justin Walden, and Tom R. Norris

Case Presentation

A very pleasant right-hand-dominant 84-year-old gentleman with a history of coronary artery disease presented with right-shoulder dysfunction that has significantly affected his activities of daily living. He was a retired clerical worker but remained active and prior to a fall several months ago states that he was able to use his right arm with ease and only experienced minimal aching and pain in the right shoulder. The patient couldn't remember the circumstances or details of his fall, but since that time he was unable to lift his right arm. He initially presented to his primary care physician who felt that he suffered from a shoulder strain and he subsequently was instructed to ice his shoulder and rest his arm in a sling. Following a period of rest, the patient reported continued

D.K. Murphy, M.D., M.B.A. (✉) • J. Walden, M.D.
T.R. Norris, M.D.
San Francisco Shoulder Elbow and Hand Clinic,
2351 Clay St, Suite 510, San Francisco, CA 94115, USA
e-mail: Kipmurphy@gmail.com; justinkwalden@gmail.com;
trnorris@tomnorris.com

© Springer International Publishing AG 2018
P.J. McMahon (ed.), *Rotator Cuff Injuries*,
DOI 10.1007/978-3-319-63668-9_15

pain and weakness and was referred to the senior author for evaluation and treatment.

He complained of nagging, aching, and throbbing pain that was more severe with use. He reported grinding with shoulder movement. He also complained of night pain and difficulty sleeping. This had greatly affected him as he was unable to use his arm to eat, dress himself, or comb his hair. Inability to use his arm above his waist has caused him a great deal of frustration.

When examined, he had significantly decreased range of motion accompanied with pain. There was atrophy of the supraspinatus and infraspinatus muscles. Active ranges of motion comparing of the right and left shoulder were forward elevation to 40 and 135°, abduction to 55 and 115°, and external rotation at his side to 25 and 70°, and external rotation in 90° of supported abduction to −20 and 80°, respectively (Fig. 15.1). Passive range of motion elicited crepitus. Strength testing revealed 1/5 power in abduction and external rotation at his side. Strength in internal rotation was normal as he had a negative belly-press test. With his arm in 90° of supported abduction and 90° of external rotation with the elbow flexed he could not maintain neutral with attempted

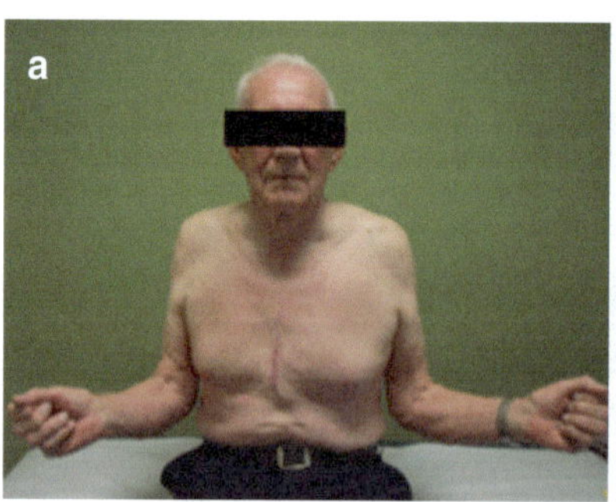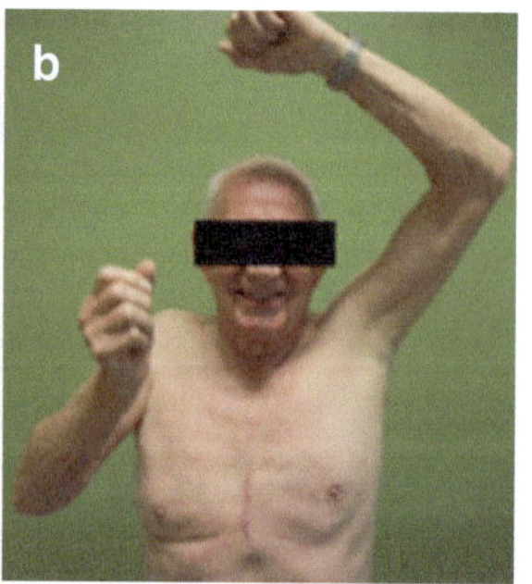

FIGURE 15.1 Preoperative clinical photos depicting limited range of motion. (**a**) External rotation at the patient's side comparing right to left was 25/75. (**b**) Abduction and forward elevation were severely limited on the patient's right. Notice the patient's right arm internally rotated as he attempts to forward elevate

external rotation and therefore he had a positive Hornblower's sign. External rotation lag of 20° was also present. Muscle contractions of his anterior, middle, and posterior deltoid were visible and he was sensate in the axillary distribution. His cervical spine, elbow, and remaining neurovascular exam was unremarkable.

Preoperative standing anterior to posterior (AP), axillary lateral, and scapular Y views showed acromioclavicular and glenohumeral subchondral sclerosis, moderate joint space narrowing, and superior migration of the humeral head with subsequent decreased acromiohumeral distance (Fig. 15.2). Magnetic resonance imaging (MRI) of his right shoulder revealed a substantial tear of the supraspinatus and infraspinatus tendons with 3.2 cm of retraction and grade 3 fatty degeneration (i.e., equal fat and muscle) of supraspinatus and infraspinatus muscles, and grade 4 fatty infiltration of teres minor (i.e., more fat than muscle) (Fig. 15.3) muscle. Having failed previous attempts at conservative management, he was ready to proceed with operative intervention.

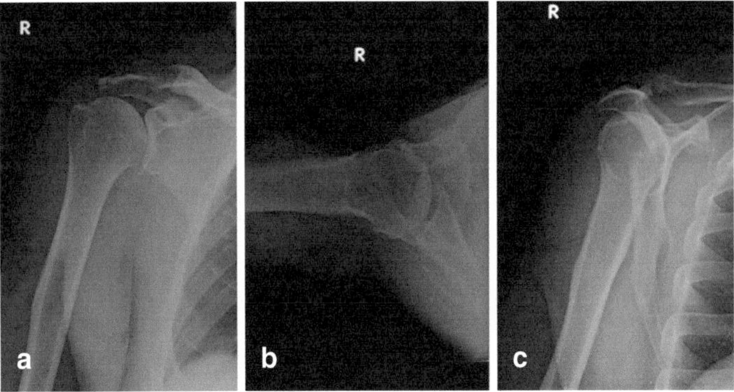

FIGURE 15.2 Preoperative standing AP, axillary lateral, and scapular Y views. AP radiograph (**a**) showing joint space narrowing, glenohumeral subchondral sclerosis, and superior migration of the humeral head with subsequent decreased acromiohumeral distance. Axillary lateral view (**b**). Scapular Y view (**c**)

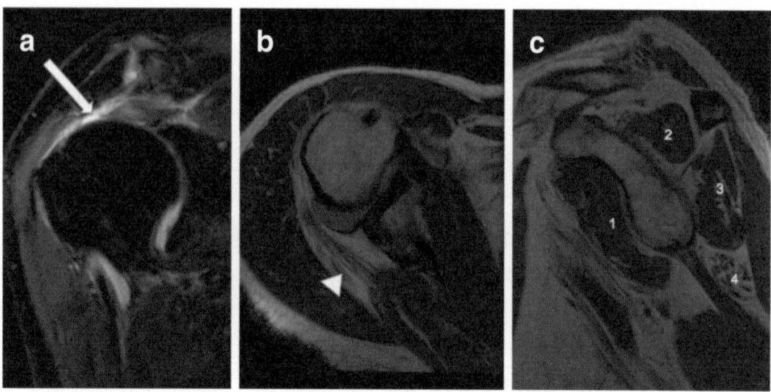

Figure 15.3 Preoperative MRI with coronal, axial, and sagittal views. Coronal view showing severe acromioclavicular and glenohumeral osteoarthritis with a substantial tear of the supraspinatus and infraspinatus tendons with retraction (*arrow*) (**a**). Axial cut demonstrating severe fatty degeneration of the infraspinatus (*arrowhead*) (**b**). Corresponding sagittal MRI showing subscapularis (**c**), (1), grade 3 fatty degeneration of the supraspinatus (2) and infraspinatus (3) muscles, and grade 4 fatty degeneration of the teres minor (4). The patient's MRI also showed severe tendinosis of the long head of the biceps tendon (not shown)

Diagnosis/Assessment

The patient's history and physical examination are consistent with rotator cuff tear arthropathy and pseudoparalysis of both forward elevation and external rotation. His external rotation weakness, lag deficit, and positive Hornblower's sign are clinical findings indicative of rotator cuff tear involving the external rotators including the teres minor muscle. The findings of grade 3 and 4 fatty infiltration of the supraspinatus, infraspinatus, and teres minor muscles on MRI are poor prognostic indicators for rotator cuff repair. RSA is indicated for this elderly man with a severe rotator cuff tear and GH joint osteoarthritis and will address the pseudoparalysis of forward elevation but will not restore active external rotation. Without active shoulder external rotators (infraspinatus and teres minor), forward elevation after RSA results in the arm internally rotating toward the trunk and activities of daily living such as combing his hair, brushing his teeth, and eating remain difficult. We give special consideration to the restoration of external rotation in this patient undergoing RSA, and we want to emphasize that to do so, it was important to look for the deficits in external rotation strength preoperatively.

Improvement in active external rotation in patients with massive rotator cuff tears was reported following LD transfers. The history of this begins with Joseph L'Episcopo who described the technique of LD and TM transfer in children with obstetrical palsy in 1934 [1]. He utilized a double-incision technique to transfer both the LD and TM tendons laterally and posteriorly on the humerus effectively changing their function from internal to external rotators. Recently, promising results were reported with LD transfers combined with RSA in patients with pseudoparalysis of both elevation and external rotation. The technique for doing so was described with a single deltopectoral incision [2].

Management

The patient was placed in the beach-chair position, and the surgical field was prepped with ChloraPrep. Following completion of draping, the free arm was placed in a McConnell arm holder to help with positioning. A deltopectoral incision was utilized, and the subdeltoid, subcoracoid, and subacromial spaces were cleared of adhesions. There was massive rotator cuff tear and retraction of supraspinatus, infraspinatus, and superior 3/4 of the teres minor tendons. The subscapularis was intact.

Working distally, the pectoralis major tendon insertion on the lateral border of the inferior bicipital groove was exposed and the upper half of the pectoralis major was released and tagged (Fig. 15.4). Following release and external rotation of the humerus, the LD and TM are visualized immediately medial to the biceps groove and tagged as a unit with non-absorbable sutures at their proximal and distal insertion

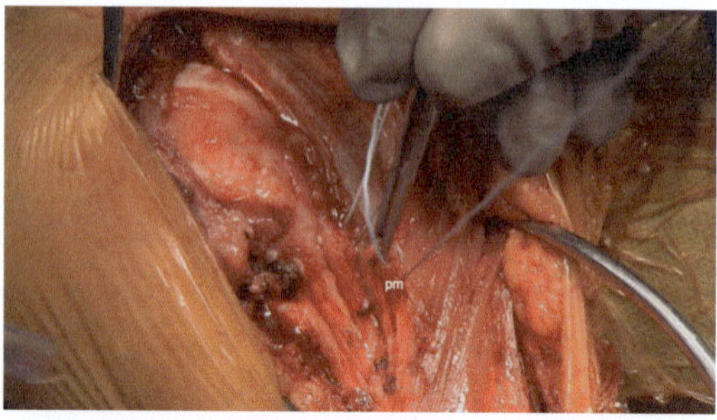

FIGURE 15.4 Intraoperative photograph after the upper one halve of the pectoralis major (*pm*) has been released. The superior and lateral corner is tagged with a permanent suture

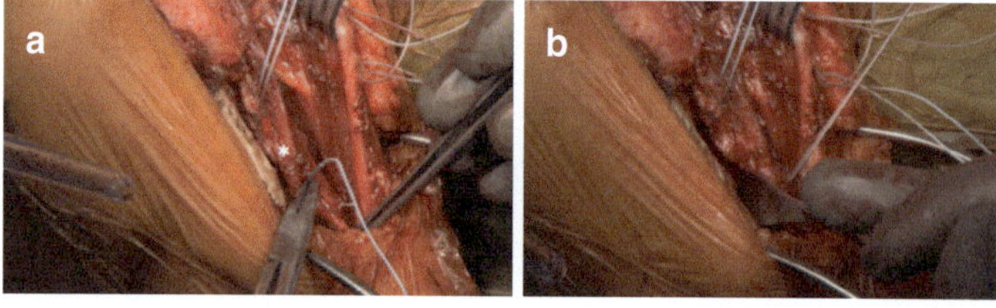

FIGURE 15.5 Intraoperative photograph of the LD and TM (*asterisk*) being tagged as a single unit (**a**). A Cobb elevator is then utilized to elevate the distal insertions of the LD and TM from the humerus (**b**)

sites (Fig 15.5a). The insertions are released. Drill holes are placed in the biceps groove at the top and bottom of the pectoralis insertion for later repair of the pectoralis and tenodesis of the long head of the biceps. An elevator is used to ensure the distal release of these tendon attachments off the humerus (Fig 15.5b). The subscapularis was then tagged in the superolateral corner and a standard subscapularis peel was performed. Currently, our preference is to now do a lesser tuberosity osteotomy when adequate bone stock is available.

Following anterior and inferior glenohumeral capsular releases, the proximal humerus was brought out easily for inspection (Fig. 15.6). A Cobb elevator was then used to dissect the triceps from the posterior humerus (Fig. 15.7). This facilitated the safe posterior passage of the tendon transfers around the humerus.

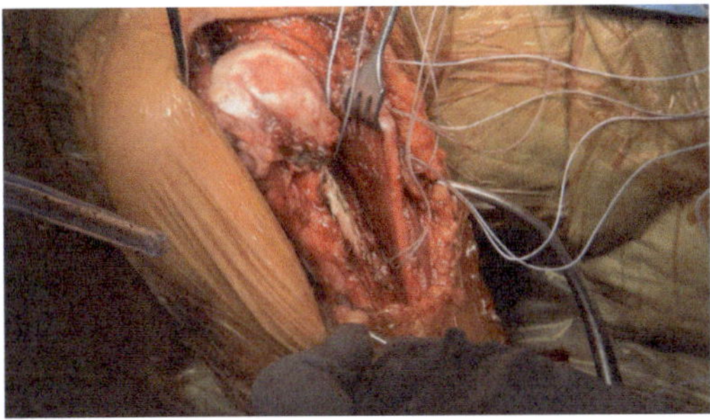

FIGURE 15.6 Intraoperative photograph of the proximal humerus brought into the field for inspection. Inspection of the humeral head surface revealed grade 3 and 4 cartilage changes

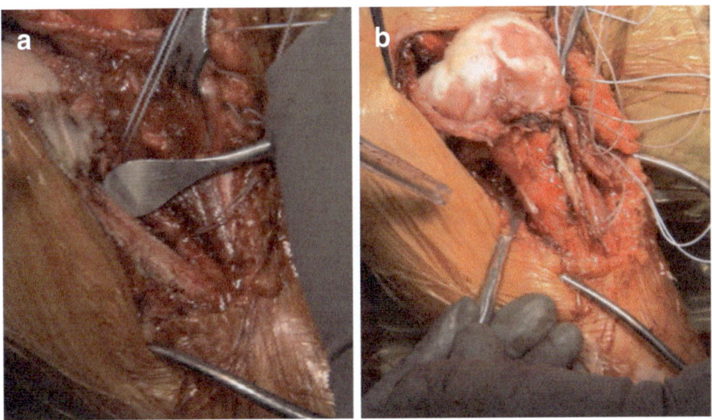

FIGURE 15.7 A Cobb is used to retract the triceps off the posterior humerus from the medial (**a**) and lateral (**b**) directions. This creates a free pathway for the tendon transfers

Then the most critical part of the procedure was to free the fibrous bands connecting the upper portions of the LD and TM from the inferior capsule and the axillary nerve. We identified the axillary nerve and marked it with a vessel loop to protect it and the fibrous bands between the LD and axillary nerve were released (Fig. 15.8). This ensured that the tendon transfer was not tethered to the axillary nerve. The radial nerve is identified on the belly of the LD but is not released as the tendon transfer moves away from the radial nerve and

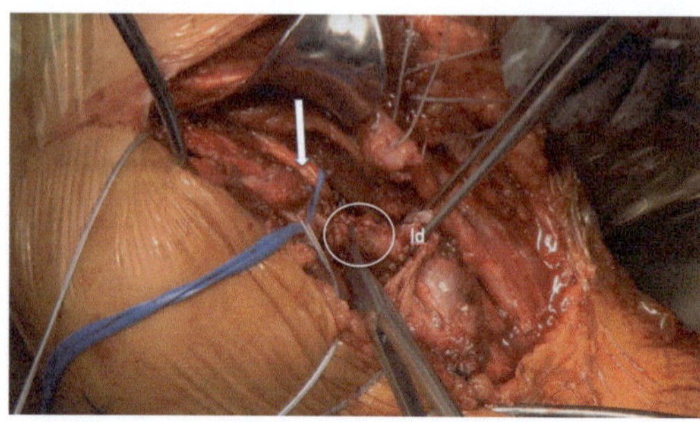

Figure 15.8 Intraoperative photograph with a vessel loop around the axillary nerve (*arrow*). Fibrous bands (*circle*) between the LD (*ld*) and axillary nerve are carefully released

will not compress it. The traction sutures were then passed posteriorly around the humerus to pull the tendons to their new insertion site at the biceps groove for later anchoring through bone tunnels along with the subscapularis.

The LD and TM tendons and muscles were then brought posteriorly around the humerus and anterior to the triceps as a supple elastic mobile unit (Fig. 15.9). Alternatively, one could bring them posterior to the triceps since the radial nerve innervates the triceps distal to the latissimus insertion on the humerus.

For the BIO-RSA (bony increased offset—reverse shoulder arthroplasty) [3], the humeral head was delivered through the incision with humeral extension and external rotation. The top of the humeral head was flattened with a saw and a hole saw was used to harvest a 29 mm diameter bone graft for later placement on the glenoid to lateralize the glenosphere and make up for any uneven glenoid wear (Fig. 15.10). Standard humeral preparation and sizing were performed and it was determined that a 90 mm long by 13 mm wide diameter conical stem gave the best press fit for the humeral stem.

The proximal humerus was then retracted posteriorly and exposure of the glenoid was obtained. Anterior and inferior glenoid capsular releases were done to mobilize the subscapularis. Inspection of the glenoid surface revealed grade 3 and 4 chondrosis. The labrum was subsequently removed and the subscapularis was elevated from the anterior scapular neck to restore excursion of the muscle. With a protective

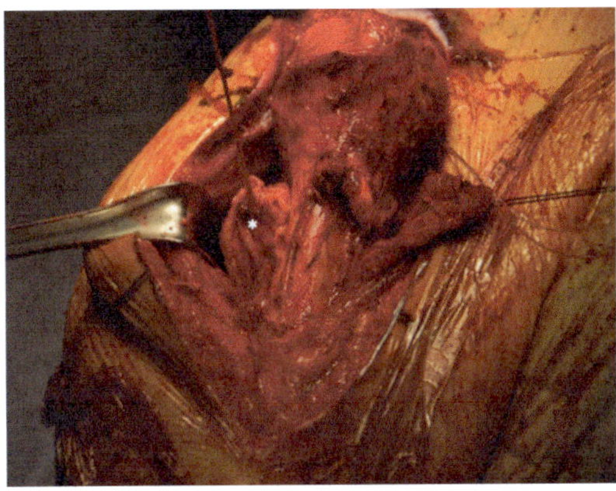

FIGURE 15.9 Intraoperative photo of the LD and TM unit (*asterisk*) being transferred posteriorly around the humerus and under the triceps as a supple elastic mobile unit

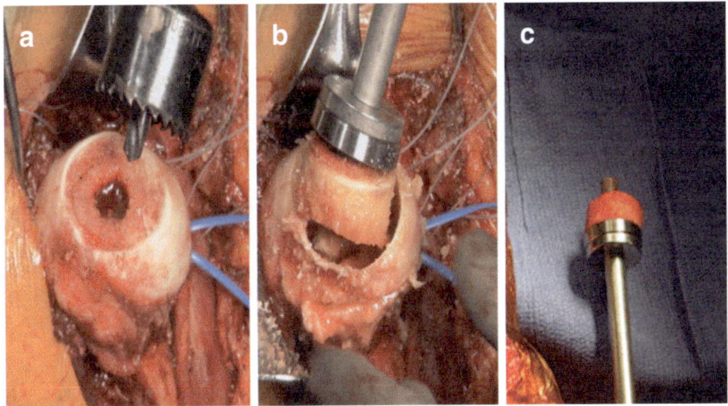

FIGURE 15.10 Intraoperative photo of the flattened humeral head (**a**). A hole saw is used to harvest a 29 mm bone graft (**b**) and prepared on the back table for later use on the glenoid (**c**)

retractor in place, the long head of the triceps was released from the inferior glenoid and the long head of the biceps was released from the superior glenoid and the intra-articular portion of the biceps was excised. The glenoid surface was measured and reamed for a 29 mm baseplate. After bone graft preparation on the back table, a 29 mm baseplate was appropriately placed over the bone graft and positioned on the prepared glenoid surface over the guide wire (Fig. 15.11). The baseplate was then fixed to the glenoid with anterior and posterior compression screws followed by superior and inferior locking screws. A 36 mm diameter glenosphere was impacted into place and securely tightened (Fig. 15.12). Alternatively, the newer threaded post baseplates with lengths up to 45 mm are available. The important principle is to make good contact with the native scapula.

Following this, the proximal humerus was again delivered through the incision with humeral extension and external

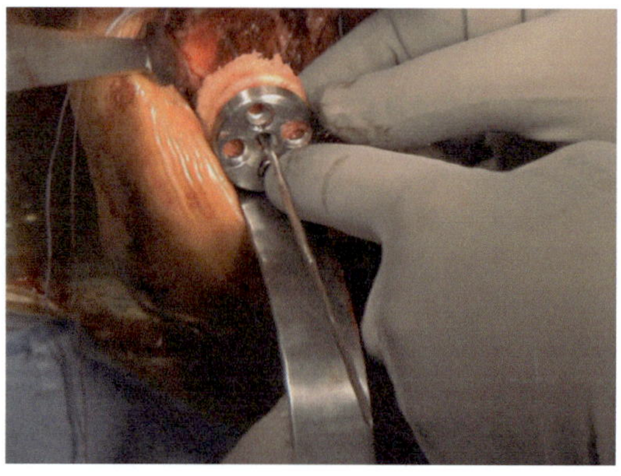

FIGURE 15.11 Intraoperative photo of baseplate and humeral autograft being placed on the glenoid

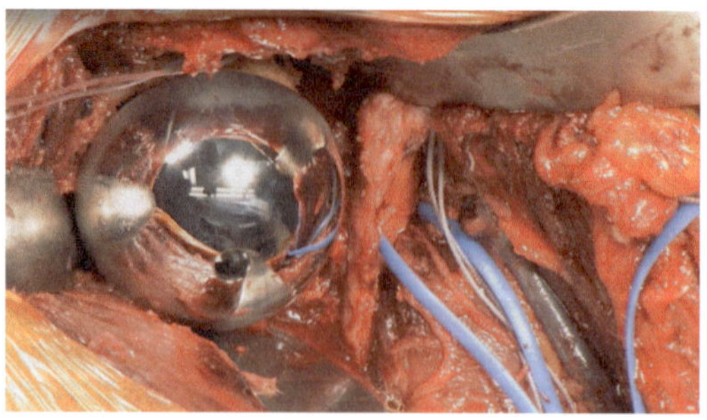

FIGURE 15.12 Intraoperative photo after the glenosphere has been placed

rotation. Drill holes were made in the humerus at the biceps groove and medial to the lesser tuberosity. Loops of sutures were passed through these holes and in the previously drilled holes at the pectoralis insertion. The humeral stem was passed down through the loops of the preplaced sutures (Fig. 15.13). This technique allows the prosthesis to serve as a suture anchor for the subscapularis, pectoralis major, LD, and TM repairs. The looped intramedullary sutures were pulled tight around the humeral prosthesis before final impaction

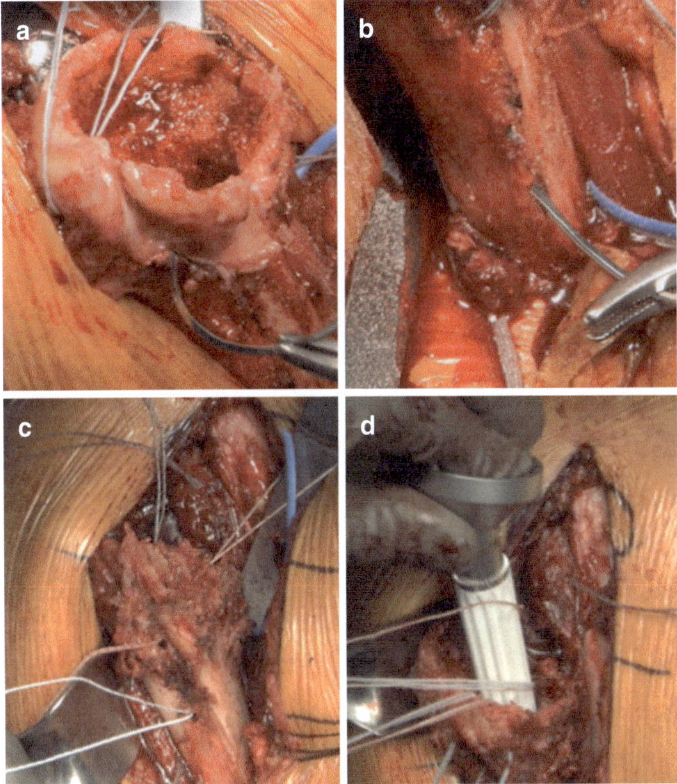

FIGURE 15.13 Intraoperative photo of looped suture passage through drill holes in the medial aspect of lesser tuberosity, lateral to bicipital groove, and at pectoralis insertion (**a–c**). Excellent fixation of the subscapularis and transferred TM and LD is obtained by passing the humeral stem through the looped sutures in the humeral canal (**d**)

into place. Following humeral stem placement, a #6 lateral spacer was impacted in the top of the humeral component and the humerus was reduced on the glenosphere. With the arm held in external rotation at the patient's side, the LD and TM are tied to the lateral portion of the biceps groove (Fig. 15.14). The repair was augmented by repair of the pectoralis major tendon to the transferred muscle unit (Fig. 15.15). Thus, this repair provided bony contact and tendon-to-tendon contact for healing. The subscapularis was then repaired to the upper portion of the lesser tuberosity with previously placed bone tunnel looped sutures (Fig. 15.15).

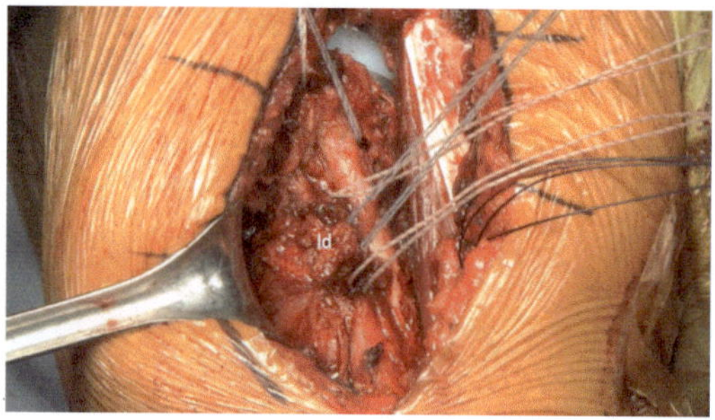

FIGURE 15.14 Intraoperative photo of the LD and TM unit (*ld*) is sutured to the humeral shaft with previously passed sutures

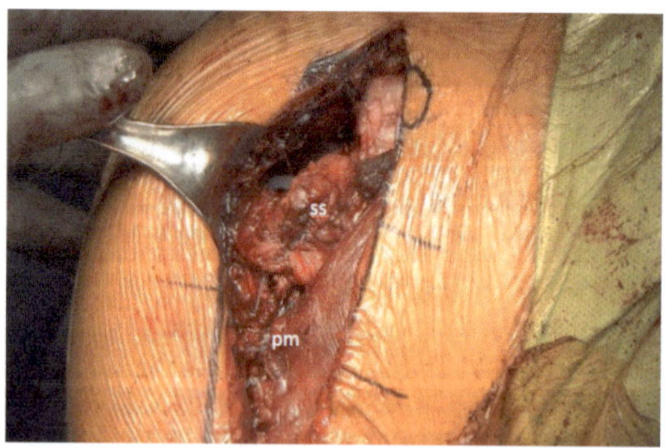

FIGURE 15.15 Intraoperative photo after the pectoralis major (*pm*) and subscapularis (*ss*) is repaired back to its insertion and to the transferred LD and TM

The wound was then closed in a layered fashion over two drains. The patient was awakened from anesthesia and transferred to the recovery room in stable condition. He was subsequently admitted to the hospital for pain control and postoperative physical therapy.

Outcome

This 84-year-old gentleman with pseudoparalysis of forward elevation and external rotation in the setting of glenohumeral osteoarthritis recovered uneventfully. Immediately in the postoperative period the patient was placed in an external rotation brace worn for 6 weeks with removal only for maintaining hygiene. Active elbow and wrist motion was allowed. After 6 weeks, he was weaned the brace and active range-of-motion exercises were initiated with a physical therapist. After 12 weeks he began active and passive internal rotation and progressive strengthening of all shoulder muscles. Physical therapy was continued for 6 months after surgery followed by his continuing a home exercise program for 1 year after the procedure. Follow-up postoperative radiographs showed excellent component alignment with incorporation of the autograft bone to the glenoid (Fig. 15.16). Motion of his right

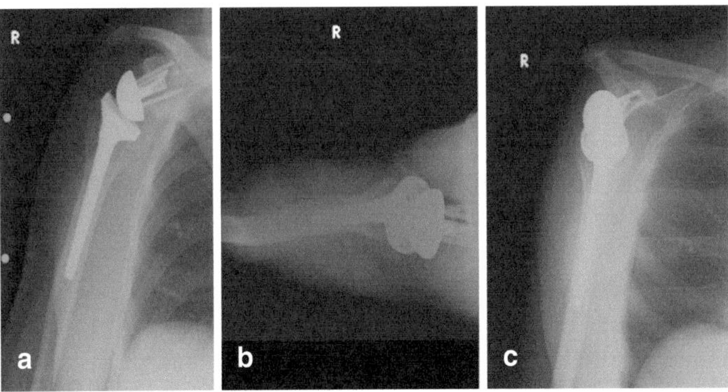

FIGURE 15.16 Postoperative radiographs show appropriate alignment of reverse total shoulder components including AP (**a**), axillary lateral (**b**) and Y scapular (**c**) views

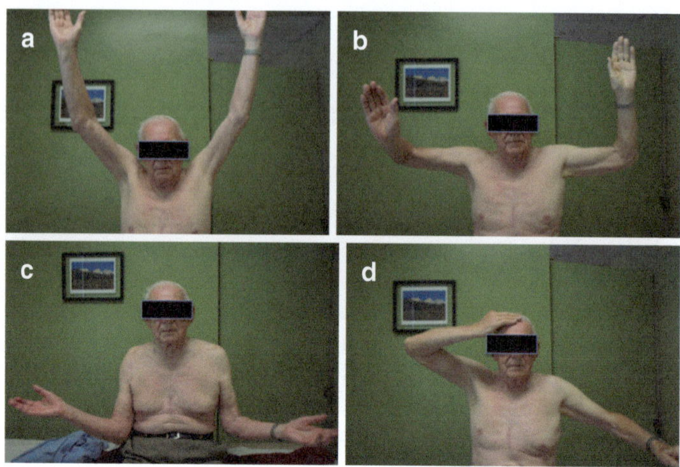

FIGURE 15.17 Clinical photographs of the patient's motion at 2 years. Comparing right to left, forward elevation was 125/140° (**a**), external rotation in 90° of abduction was 15/70° (**b**), external rotation at his side was 60/60° (**c**), and the patient could easily reach the top of his head with his elbow held to the side (**d**)

and left side at 2 years postoperatively revealed forward elevation was 125 and 140°, external rotation in 90° of abduction was 15 and 70°, and external rotation at his side was 60 and 60°, respectively, and he could easily reach the top of his head with his elbow held to the side (Fig. 15.17).

Literature Review

Reverse shoulder arthroplasty in patients with pseudoparesis is effective at restoring forward elevation and abduction while providing diminishing pain but it does not restore external rotation when both the infraspinatus and teres minor are absent or severely fatty infiltrated [4, 5]. In 2007, Gerber and colleagues reported promising preliminary results of improved forward elevation and external rotation in 12 patients with pseudoparesis when they were treated with a two-incision technique for a combined RSA and LD transfer [6]. Not only active elevation but also active external rotation were improved significantly. Gerber and colleagues later described their experience with such patients in a larger patient cohort [7] and reported significantly improved active external rotation, Constant scores and mean subjective shoulder values of the combined procedure did not deteriorate between 2 and 5 years postoperatively. We have been equally satisfied with our results of RSA and LD and TM transfer with the technique described in patients with pseudoparesis of forward elevation and external rotation. Restoring active external rotation allows the patient to control the arm in space and thereby prevent obligatory internal rotation leading to a Hornblower's sign [8]. Our patients have been able to return to activities of daily living leading to increased patient satisfaction postoperative.

While our patients have done well, long-term radiographic follow-up has caused concern as we have frequently observed lateral humeral meta-diaphyseal thinning (Fig. 15.18). Despite this observation, no negative outcome correlation has been seen clinically. It is possible that this osteolysis is related to the pressure from the tendon-muscle unit as it courses

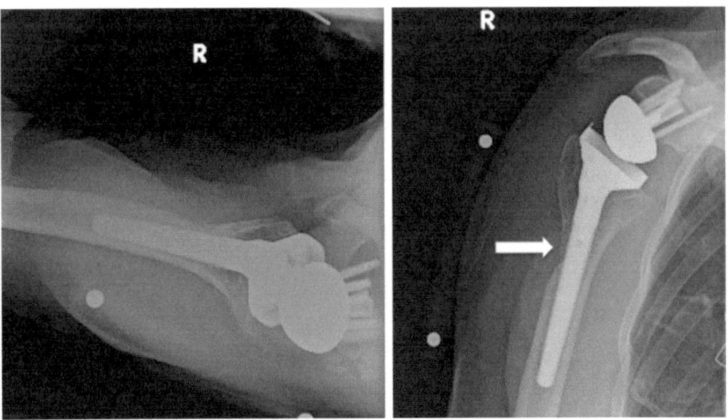

FIGURE 15.18 Five-year postoperative radiograph of a patient that had undergone RSA with LD and TM transfer. Lateral meta-diaphyseal cortical thinning is seen (*arrow*)

around the humerus or from vascular compromise with dissection. This may be avoidable by modifying our technique so that less tension is transferred by altering the insertion site. Boileau et al. have described a technique similar to ours but decreases the travel distance of the transfer with the use of transosseous sutures [9]. In their report of 17 patients with combined loss of active elevation and external rotation, mean active elevation increased from 74° preoperatively to 149° postoperatively, and external rotation increased from −21 to 13°. The authors also reported significant improvement in patient satisfaction, subjective shoulder value, Constant-Murley scores, and activities of daily living.

In summary, for the patient in this case with advanced glenohumeral osteoarthritis, and pseudoparesis of both forward elevation and external rotation, a good outcome was achieved by the addition of LD and TM tendon transfer to RSA. A video of our operative technique is available online [10].

Clinical Pearls/Pitfalls

- Preoperative clinical identification of functional loss of external rotation is critical when planning RSA.
- Keep tendons of LD and TM as a unit with interlocking sutures.
- Freeing the upper border of LD/TM from inferior capsule and axillary nerve, and reattachment of the tendon unit without superior transfer minimizes the risk of axillary nerve compression.
- Postoperative immobilization in external rotation protects the transferred tendons.

References

1. L'Episcopo JB. Tendon transplantation in obstetrical paralysis. Am J Surg. 1934;25:122–5.
2. Boileau P, Chuinard C, Roussanne Y, Neyton L, Trojani C. Modified latissimus dorsi and teres major transfer through a

single delto-pectoral approach for external rotation deficit of the shoulder: as an isolated procedure or with a reverse arthroplasty. J Shoulder Elb Surg. 2007;16:671–82.

3. Boileau P, Moineau G, Roussanne Y, Oshea K. Bony increased-offset reversed shoulder arthroplasty: minimizing scapular impingement while maximizing glenoid fixation. Clin Orthop Relat Res. 2011;469(9):2558–67.

4. Boileau P, Watkinson DJ, Hatzidakis AM, Hovorka I. The grammont reverse prosthesis: results in cuff tear arthritis fracture sequelae and revision prosthesis. J Shoulder Elb Surg. 2006;15:527–40.

5. Werner CML, Steinmann PA, Gilbart M, Gerber C. Treatment of painful pseudoparesis due to irreparable rotator cuff dysfunction with the Delta III reverse ball-and-socket total shoulder prosthesis. J Bone Joint Surg Am. 2005;87:1476–86.

6. Gerber C, Pennington SD, Lingenfelter EJ, Sukthankar A. Reverse Delta-III total shoulder replacement combined with latissimus dorsi transfer. A preliminary report. J Bone Joint Surg Am. 2007;89:940–7.

7. Gerber C, Puskas GJ, Catanzaro S. Clinical outcome of reverse total shoulder arthroplasty combined with latissimus dorsi transfer for the treatment of chronic combined pseudoparesis of elevation and external rotation of the shoulder. J Shoulder Elb Surg. 2014;23:49–57.

8. Walch G, Boulahia A, Calderone S, Robinson AHN. The 'dropping' and 'hornblower's' signs in evaluation of rotator cuff tears. J Bone Joint Surg Br. 1998;80:624–8.

9. Boileau P, Rumian AP, Zumstein MA. Reversed shoulder arthroplasty with modified L'Episcopo for combined loss of active elevation and external rotation. J Shoulder Elb Surg. 2010;19:20–30.

10. Norris TR. Latissimus dorsi/teres major transfers for external rotation in BIO-RSA. http://www.vumedi.com/node/54200. https://www.vumedi.com/video/latissiumus-dorsi-teres-major-transfers-for-external-rotation-in-bio-rsa/

Chapter 16
Adding a Bone Graft to Reverse TSA

Jesse W. Allert and Mark A. Frankle

Case Presentation

The patient is a 79-year-old active male with a 17-year history of progressive right shoulder pain. A retired police officer, the patient recalls several injuries over the course of his career, all of which were managed conservatively and none of which are acute. The patient now lives alone and finds himself unable to elevate his arm over his head. He is also unable to sleep without waking numerous times from pain in the shoulder. After failed conservative management, the patient was indicated for reverse total shoulder arthroplasty.

J.W. Allert, M.D. • M.A. Frankle, M.D. (✉)
Shoulder and Elbow Service, Florida Orthopaedic Institute,
Tampa, FL, USA
e-mail: mfrankle@floridaortho.com

© Springer International Publishing AG 2018
P.J. McMahon (ed.), *Rotator Cuff Injuries*,
DOI 10.1007/978-3-319-63668-9_16

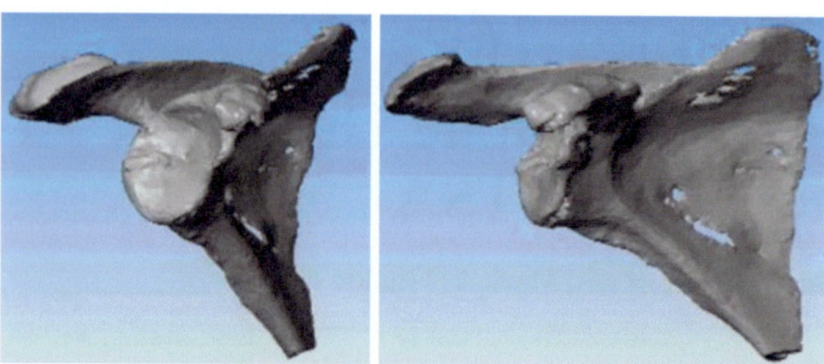

FIGURE 16.1 Three-dimensional reconstruction of routine preoperative CT imaging. With advanced imaging, the superior bone loss can be better quantified and utilized for preoperative planning

On physical examination, the patient appears younger than stated age and is right hand dominant. He has forward elevation to 60° and external rotation to neutral. He has significant crepitus and pain throughout range of motion and has noticeable weakness in flexion and external rotation.

Four radiographic views show superior migration of the humeral head in association with superior wear of the glenoid, consistent with advanced rotator cuff arthropathy. As part of routine preoperative evaluation, the patient received computed tomography with axial, coronal, and sagittal imaging. The supplemental 3D imaging can be seen in Fig. 16.1.

Diagnosis/Assessment

The patient's history, physical, and radiographic findings are consistent with the diagnosis of rotator cuff arthropathy. While there are many options for patients with a massive rotator cuff tear, this patient had notable superior migration with glenohumeral arthritis, making him an excellent candidate for reverse total shoulder arthroplasty. The uncontained defect of the superior glenoid is discussed as part of the patient's preoperative planning, and in this case it was determined that the patient may require intraoperative grafting to optimize glenoid positioning and fixation.

Management

A routine deltopectoral approach was performed. The subdeltoid, subacromial, and subcoracoid spaces were released. A subscapularis tendon peel off of the lesser tuberosity was performed and the appropriate humeral head cut was made. A standard circumferential release was completed along the rim of the glenoid, taking care to protect the axillary nerve. In this case, the glenoid revealed the expected uncontained superior defect.

Using the CT imaging and the visualized inferior glenoid as a guide, the 2.5 mm drill bit was used to drill bicortical until the tip exited the anterior scapula (Fig. 16.2). The hole was measured to assure an adequate depth of greater than 25 mm. Along the same trajectory as the drill bit, a 6.5 mm guide tap was placed (Fig. 16.3). This was used as a guide for reaming. The native inferior glenoid was reamed down to cortical bone, while the superior defect was left untouched (Fig. 16.4). The surface bone of the defect can be prepared with a motorized burr to provide a roughened surface to receive the graft.

On the back table, the humeral head was prepared and shaped to match the defect. The cartilaginous surface serves as the outer portion of the glenoid, while the remainder of the

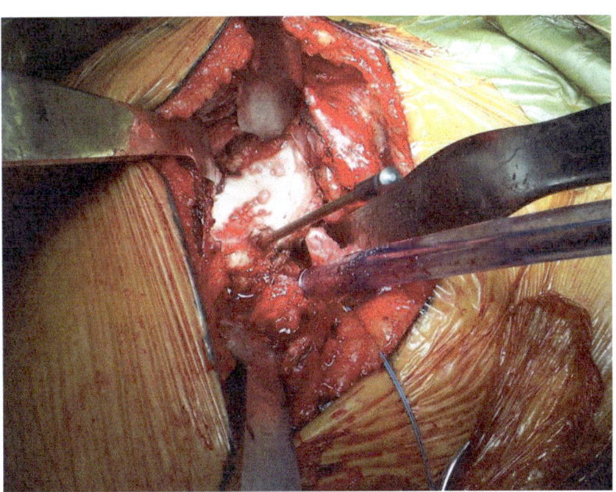

FIGURE 16.2 Right shoulder with drill bit placed in the center of the glenoid

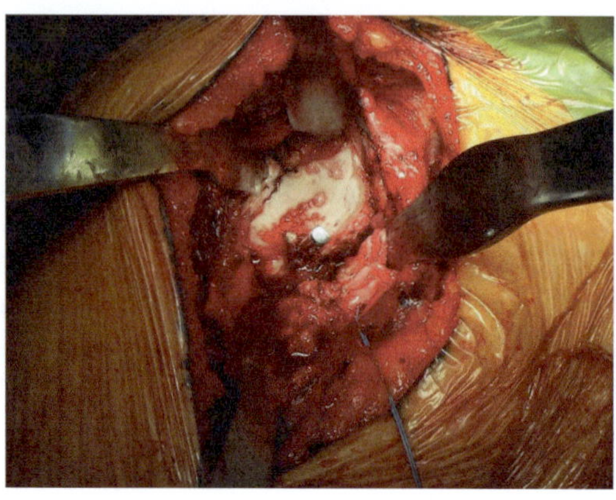

FIGURE 16.3 The tap is inserted along the same trajectory as the drill bit

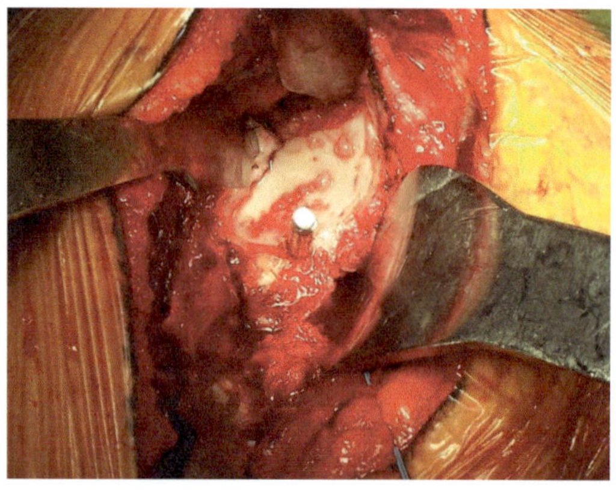

FIGURE 16.4 The inferior portion of the glenoid is reamed to bleeding bone. The superior portion with significant bone loss is noted and used as a guide to shape autograft from the humeral head cut

head is prepared to later receive the baseplate. First, the graft is fixed to the native glenoid using multiple Kirschner wires that will not obstruct placement of the reamer (Fig. 16.5). Once the autograft is securely fixed, it was reamed to the same

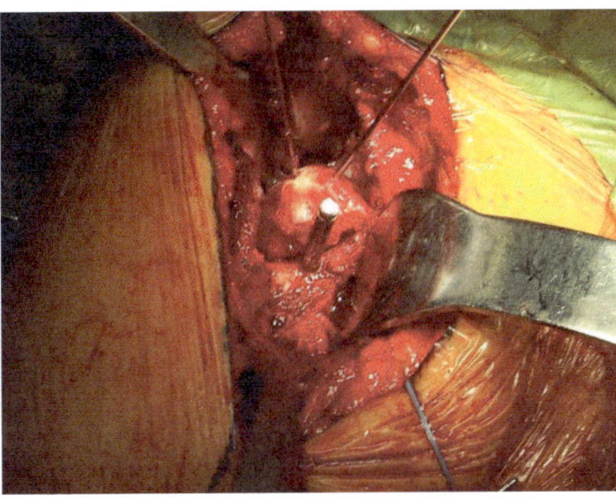

FIGURE 16.5 The humeral head autograft is inserted using multiple points of fixation

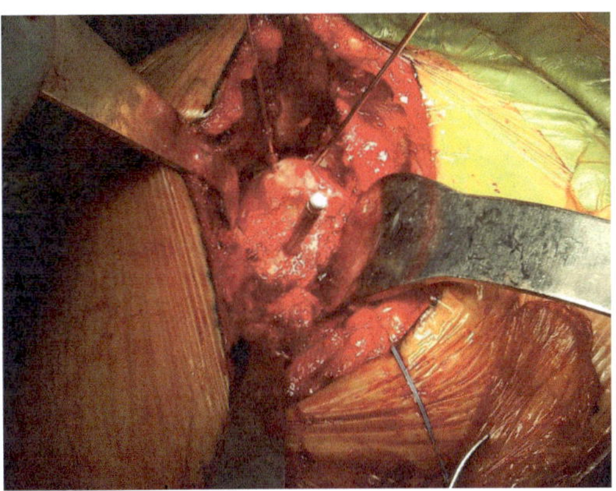

FIGURE 16.6 The graft is reamed to the depth of the previously reamed native glenoid

depth as the previously reamed native glenoid (Fig. 16.6). The baseplate was then placed, the wires removed, and peripheral screws placed (Fig. 16.7). A glenosphere that was hooded to cover more of the baseplate was impacted directly onto the graft to enhance both fixation and compression (Fig. 16.8).

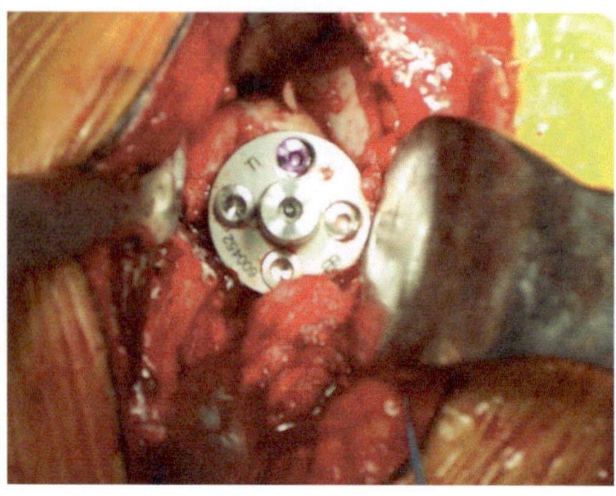

FIGURE 16.7 Baseplate is placed along with peripheral screws

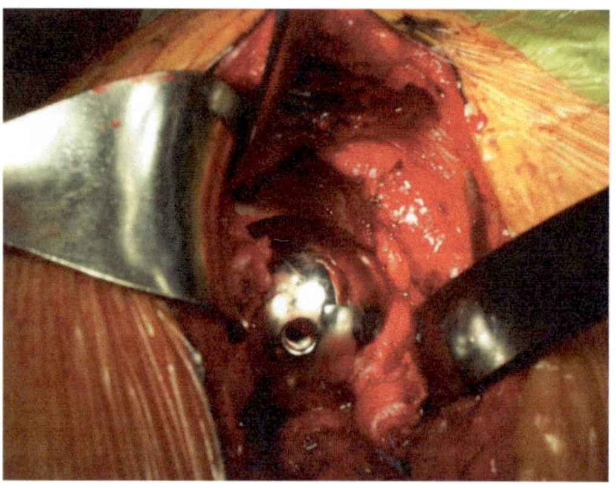

FIGURE 16.8 Glenosphere placement

Outcome

This 79-year-old male with significant limitation in preoperative range of motion went on to have forward flexion to 150°. At 5 years postoperative, his glenoid shows no radiographic evidence of glenoid component loosening (Fig. 16.9).

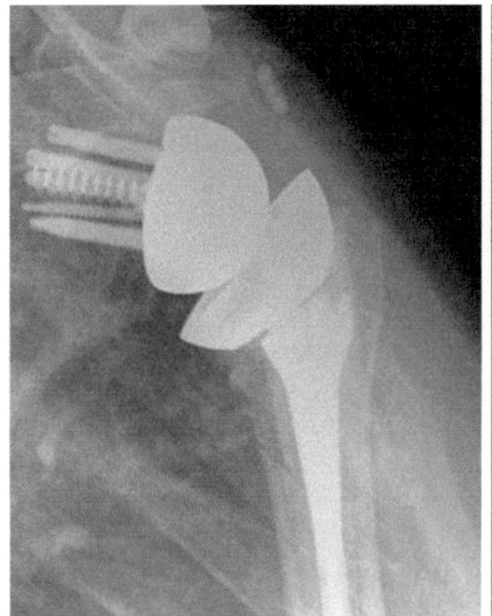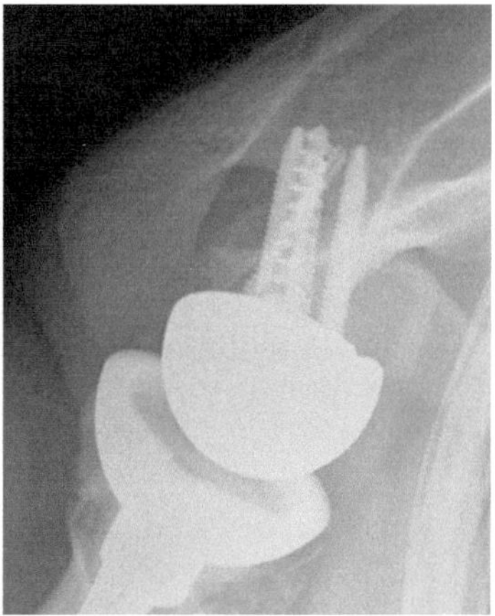

FIGURE 16.9 Postoperative x-ray imaging

Literature Review

Much has been written with regard to bone deficiency in the anatomic total shoulder arthroplasty and arthroplasty in the revision setting. There is however much less documented with regard to bone grafting in primary reverse total shoulder arthroplasty [1, 2]. Techniques include preferential reaming, bone grafting, and using custom or patient-specific instrumentation. While preferential reaming of the "high side" in this case may aid in correcting version, it would medialize the implant and remove more bone. Significant medialization can play a role in a more notable cosmetic deformity and even alter the compressive forces of the deltoid and increase dislocation rates [3–6].

In primary reverse total shoulder arthroplasty, the native humeral head can provide an excellent source of autograft without increasing morbidity. This autograft is frequently prepared as cancellous bone chips and when there is no bone loss is placed in the intramedullary canal of the humerus to enhance fixation of the humeral stem. In the setting of glenoid bone loss, a structural allograft can be created and compressed at the implant-bone interface to increase surface area and fixation. Glenoid bone stock can be maintained and the autograft can be reamed alongside the native glenoid.

Clinical Pearls/Pitfalls

- Maintain multiple points of fixation of the graft to native bone during reaming. This will keep the graft from spinning and being damaged by the reamer.
- A hooded glenosphere may be used to aid in graft compression. The hood can be oriented directly over the graft and impacted, providing additional compressive forces in addition to the baseplate.
- Err on oversizing the graft during preparation. A larger graft can always be further pared down after fixation. Undersizing the graft can decrease structural integrity and make it susceptible to inadequate fixation or breaking during preparation.
- Initially the 6.5 mm tap can be used on power to better find the trajectory of the previously placed 2.5 mm drill bit. Once the tap engages, a t-handle can be used manually to get a more tactile feel of the glenoid bone stock. As a guide that the bone is stout enough, some resistance should be detected while turning the t-handle.

References

1. Frankle MA, Teramoto A, Luo ZP, Levy JC, Pupello D. Glenoid morphology in reverse shoulder arthroplasty: classification and surgical implications. J Shoulder Elb Surg. 2009;18(6):874–85. doi:10.1016/j.jse.2009.02.013.
2. Klein SM, Dunning P, Mulieri P, Pupello D, Downes K, Frankle MA. Effects of acquired glenoid bone defects on surgical technique and clinical outcomes in reverse shoulder arthroplasty. J Bone Joint Surg Am. 2010;92(5):1144–54. doi:10.2106/JBJS.I.00778.

3. Boileau P, et al. Grammont reverse prosthesis: design, rationale, and biomechanics. J Shoulder Elbow Surg. 2005;14(1 Suppl S):147S–61S.
4. Klein S, Levy JC, Holcomb JO, Pupello D, Frankle MA. Treatment of advanced rotator cuff dysfunction with reverse shoulder arthroplasty. Minerva Ortop Traumatol. 2009;60(1):29–46.
5. Gagey O, Hue E. Mechanics of the deltoid muscle. A new approach. Clin Orthop Relat Res. 2000;375:250–7.
6. Norris T, Kelly JD, Humphrey CS. Management of glenoid bone defects in revision shoulder arthroplasty: a new application of the reverse total shoulder prosthesis. Tech Shoulder Elb Surg. 2007;8(1):37–46.

Chapter 17
Rotator Cuff Repair with Patch Tissue

Surena Namdari, Joseph Abboud, and Gerald R. Williams

Although a structurally intact repair is not a requisite for satisfactory outcomes, many studies have demonstrated the clinical benefits of achieving healing [1–5]. A rotator cuff repair may fail for many reasons but can broadly be characterized into two categories: first, an inability of the repair to withstand the mechanical loads seen by the tendon prior to healing, and second, an inability to achieve an adequate biologic healing response at the repair site. One of the strategies to improve healing rates during revision rotator cuff repairs includes the use of graft augmentation. Grafts, in

S. Namdari, M.D., M.Sc. • J. Abboud, M.D.
G.R. Williams, M.D. (✉)
Department of Shoulder and Elbow Surgery, Rothman
Institute—Thomas Jefferson University, Philadelphia, PA, USA
e-mail: grwjr@me.com

© Springer International Publishing AG 2018
P.J. McMahon (ed.), *Rotator Cuff Injuries*,
DOI 10.1007/978-3-319-63668-9_17

theory, may improve healing rates and outcomes by addressing these two modes of failure. A graft can act as a load-sharing device to diminish the stress experience by the native tissue prior to healing. Additionally, a graft can act as a scaffold to allow for cellular ingrowth, potentially leading to a more robust healing response.

Case Presentation

A 67-year-old male presented with 2 years of right-shoulder pain that had worsened after a fall 9 months ago. The patient had undergone two subacromial cortisone injections and 6 months of physical therapy without substantial relief of pain or restoration of range of motion. The patient's medical comorbidities included diabetes, hypertension, and hypercholesterolemia. The patient had previously undergone an open rotator cuff repair in 2004 on the same shoulder. He complained of difficulty sleeping and difficulty with overhead activities, particularly involving his occupation as an auto body mechanic.

On physical examination, the patient had a well-healed surgical incision without signs of erythema, induration, or drainage. His active forward elevation, active abduction, and active external rotation were 135°, 120°, and 45°, respectively. Passive forward elevation, passive external rotation, and internal rotation behind the back were 165°, 70°, and T10, respectively. With manual muscle testing, the patient had 4/5 strength with resisted flexion, abduction, and external rotation. The patient had a negative abdominal compression test and no external rotation lag sign.

Diagnosis

In addition to the clinical examination, plain radiographs and advanced imaging techniques are important for both diagnosis of rotator cuff tears and for identifying factors that may predict failure of structural healing. Initial evaluation of any patient with suspected rotator cuff pathology should include standard plain radiographs. This typically includes an AP view in the plane of the scapula (Grashey) and an axillary view at a minimum. Other views are often obtained as well, based upon the preference of the treating surgeon. The Grashey view allows for the best assessment of joint space loss as this view is taken in the plane of the joint line. Additionally, it can provide an assessment of the position of the humeral head relative to the glenoid to assess for any superior migration of the head indicative of a rotator cuff tear. Taking this radiograph in 30° of shoulder abduction can help identify subtle proximal humeral migration. The axillary view is important for determining the amount of glenoid deformity that may exist and the relative position of the humeral head in the anterior to posterior dimension. In this case, plain radiographs demonstrated a well-centered humeral head with sclerotic changes at the undersurface of the acromion and cystic changes in the greater tuberosity, consistent with prior open rotator cuff repair (Fig. 17.1).

MRI is the most common tool used to assess rotator cuff integrity. MRIs provide important insight into three critical factors that can predict failure of structural healing: (1) tear size, (2) retraction, and (3) muscle atrophy. Studies have shown that larger tears [6, 7], retracted tears [8], and tears with higher grades of muscle atrophy [6, 8] are predictors of poor tendon healing. While ultrasound and CT arthrogram studies are less commonly used, they can provide similar information. In this case, selected MRI images demonstrated full thickness tears of the supraspinatus and infraspinatus tendons with retraction to the medial humeral head (Fig. 17.2). On the T1 sagittal oblique images, there was Grade 2 atrophy of the supraspinatus, superior infraspinatus, and upper subscapularis. Additionally, there was an upper border subscapularis tear and medial subluxation of the biceps tendon.

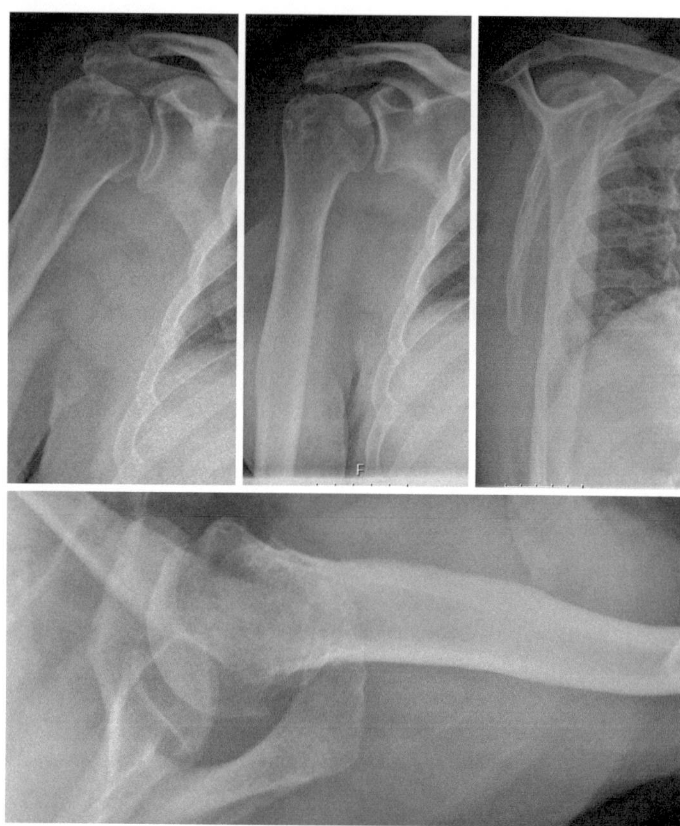

Figure 17.1 Plain radiographs demonstrating a centered glenohumeral joint, cystic changes in the greater tuberosity, and sclerosis of the undersurface of the acromion

Management

The decision to proceed with dermal augmentation of a rotator cuff tear is multifactorial. We typically consider preoperative patient-specific factors and both radiographic and intraoperative tear-specific factors when considering dermal augmentation. With regard to patient-specific factors, we consider patients older than 65 years of age, those undergoing revision repairs, smokers, and those with degenerative tears

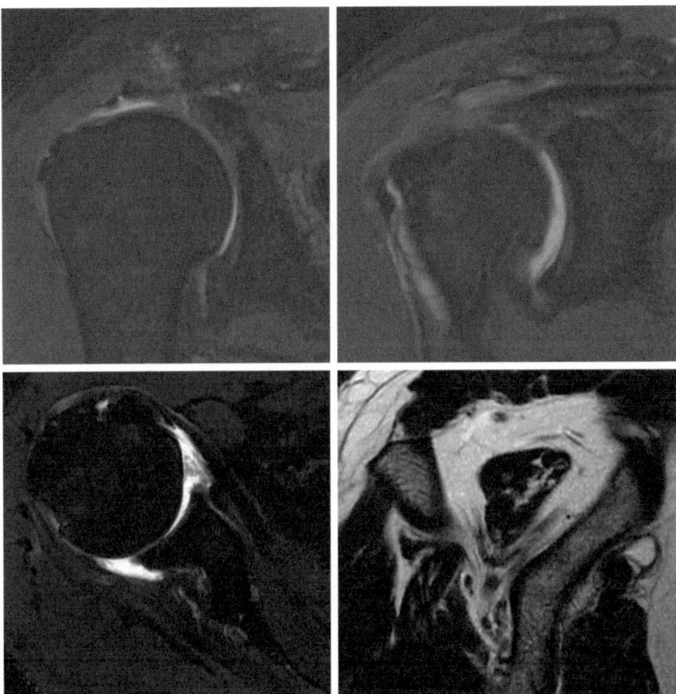

FIGURE 17.2 MRI views demonstrating a rotator cuff tear involving the supraspinatus, infraspinatus, and upper border of the subscapularis. There is also medial subluxation of the biceps tendon and evidence supraspinatus muscle atrophy

to be at greatest risk for repair failure. In terms of tear-specific factors, we consider massive tears, retracted tears, those with fatty atrophy, and tears with poor intraoperative tendon quality to be appropriate for dermal augmentation. In our practice, the intraoperative assessment of the tendon quality and its perceived ability to hold suture without "pull-through" is the most substantial factor when deciding to augment a repair with a dermal allograft patch.

There is biomechanical data to suggest that dermal or fascial grafts reduce the cyclic gapping and increase the ultimate load to failure at the repair site [9–13]. Both biologic and synthetic grafts are commercially available (Table 17.1).

TABLE 17.1 The most popular commercially available scaffolds

Product	Company	Source	Cross-linking
Artelon and sportmesh	Artimplant AB, Sweden and Biomet Sports	Polyurethane urea polymer	Not applicable
Bio-blanket	Medicine (IN, USA) Kensey Nash	Bovine dermis	Yes
Cuff Patch	Corporation (PA, USA) Arthrotek (IN, USA)	Porcine SIS	Yes
Gore-Tex patch WL	Gore and associates,	Polytetrafluoroethylene (ePTFE)	Not applicable
GraftJacket	Flagstaff (AZ, USA) Wright Medical (TN, USA)	Human cadaver dermis	No
	Dijon (France)	Terephthalic polyethylene, polyester	Not applicable
Permacol	Zimmer (IN, USA)	Porcine dermis	Yes
Restore	DePuy Orthopedics (IN, USA)	Porcine SIS	No
Arthroflex	LifeNet Health, Virginia Beach, VA	Acellular human dermal extracellular matrix	Yes
TissueMend	Stryker Orthopedics (NJ, USA)	Fetal bovine dermis	Yes

SIS small intestine submucosa

Biologic grafts can vary in their tissue of origin (human, bovine, porcine, or equine dermis) as well as their postharvest processing techniques. Postharvest processing can influence the sterility and mechanical properties of the graft. Grafts can undergo acellularization (removal of cellular and genetic material from the graft), lyophilization (drying process used to improve product shelf life), lamination (layering of multiple sheets of tissue to improve material properties), and/or cross-linking (improves stiffness and material properties of the graft). A comprehensive review of all available graft options is beyond the scope of this chapter which will focus on human dermal graft augmentation. (Can you write a sentence why you prefer the dermal graft?)

We prefer to perform arthroscopic rotator cuff repair in the beach-chair position. After diagnostic arthroscopy and treatment of any concomitant shoulder pathology, the rotator cuff tendon is debrided and mobilized. In our practice, tears must be reducible to at least the medial aspect of the rotator cuff footprint, with minimal tension, in order to consider a repair and dermal augmentation as there must be improvement of the normal muscle tension that has diminished with the tear, for the muscle to function after repair.

In this case, a debridement of degenerative labrum fraying, a biceps tenodesis, and an upper border subscapularis repair were performed prior to proceeding with the posterior-superior rotator cuff repair (Fig. 17.3). Two double-suture-loaded anchors were placed arthroscopically at the medial aspect of the greater tuberosity, and sutures were passed through the native tendon in a horizontal mattress configuration (Fig. 17.4). We performed acellular dermal extracellular matrix graft augmentation by the double row technique previously described by Chalmers et al. [14]. We used a posterolateral viewing portal, an 8.25 mm cannula in the anterolateral portal, and a 5.5 mm cannula anteriorly. The anterior-to-posterior and medial-to-lateral dimensions of the residual cuff and footprint were measured with a graduated

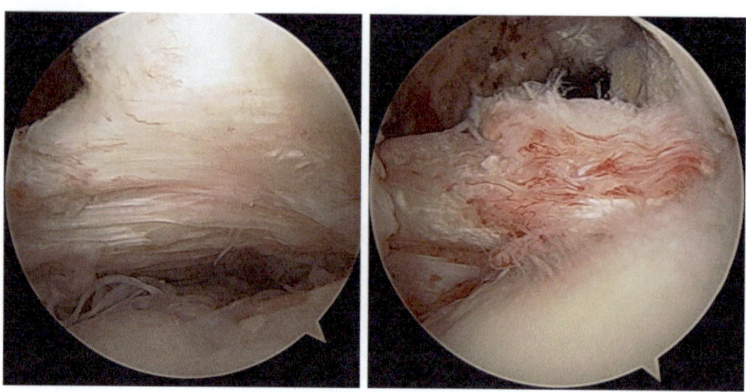

FIGURE 17.3 Arthroscopic views from a posterior-viewing portal demonstrating an upper border subscapularis tear and its subsequent repair

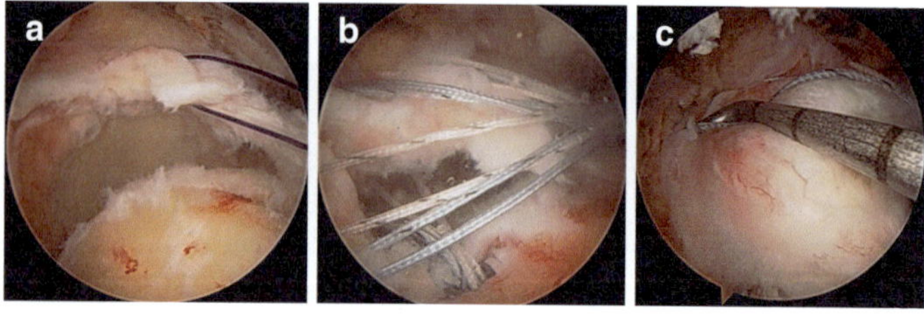

FIGURE 17.4 (**a**) Posterior superior rotator cuff tear as viewed from the posterolateral portal. (**b**) Passage of all sutures from two anchors through the rotator cuff in a horizontal mattress configuration. (**c**) Graduated probe utilized to size the graft

probe or arthroscopic measuring device (Fig. 17.4). The human dermal patch (Arthroflex, Arthrex, Naples Fl) was cut to fit the dimensions of the rotator cuff medially and the footprint laterally. The anterior limb of the anterior mattress suture was brought through the anterior cannula, and the posterior limb of the posterior mattress suture was brought through the posterior portal. The remaining sutures were

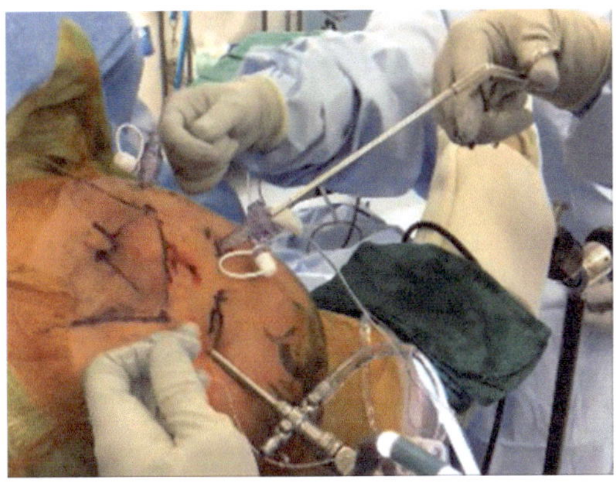

FIGURE 17.5 The graft is rolled and fed into the lateral cannula by gentle tension on the free limbs of suture through the anterior and posterior portals

then brought through the lateral cannula, from anterior to posterior sequentially, and passed through the medial border of the patch in the same order as they were passed through the rotator cuff. A mulberry knot was tied behind the patch for the anterior and posterior corners. These knots allowed the corner sutures to drag the patch into the subacromial space. The patch was then rolled and fed into the lateral cannula by gentle tension on the free limbs of suture through the anterior and posterior portals (Fig. 17.5). Once the patch was unraveled, and the mulberry knots were secured, the medial-row sutures were retrieved sequentially out of the lateral portal and tied. The lateral humeral cortex was then cleared of soft tissue, the patch was temporarily held in the proper orientation with spinal needles to prevent bunching, and one suture limb from each knot of the medial row was placed into independent knotless lateral-row anchors (Fig. 17.6).

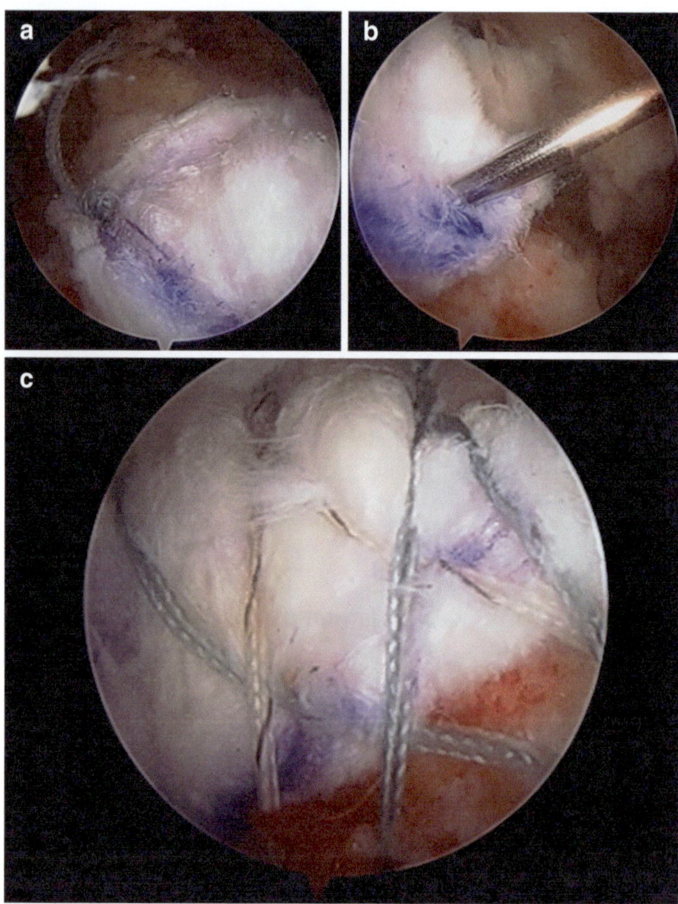

FIGURE 17.6 (**a**) View of a mulberry knot placed at the posteromedial aspect of the graft and used to drag the patch into the subacromial space in the proper orientation. (**b**) Spinal needle used to
provisionally secure the lateral portion of the graft to the greater
tuberosity in preparation for lateral anchor placement, (**c**) final
repair construct with dermal augmentation of the rotator cuff repair

Outcome

The patient was immobilized in a sling for the first 6 weeks after surgery. After 6 weeks, he began a formal therapy program, focusing initially on passive range of motion followed by progressive active-assisted and active motion from 6 to 12 weeks after surgery. At 12 weeks after surgery, strengthening was progressively added to the therapy program. At 3 months after surgery, the patient had active forward elevation of 165°, active abduction of 160°, active external rotation of 60°, and internal rotation to the T12 vertebral level (Fig. 17.7). At 6

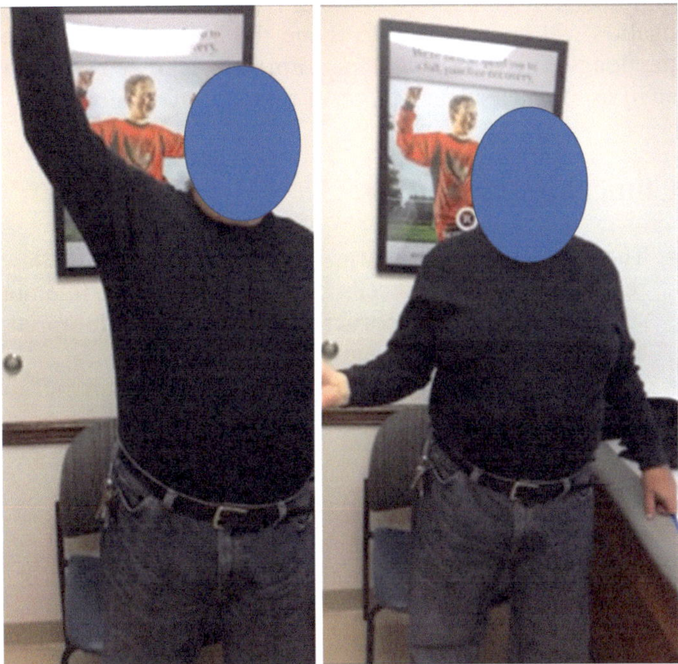

FIGURE 17.7 Postoperative active forward elevation and active external rotation at 3 months after surgery

months after surgery, the patient underwent MRI evaluation and ultrasound evaluation of the shoulder as part of a research protocol. Both studies demonstrated rotator cuff healing. At the 6-month time point, the patient had returned to his job as a mechanic without restrictions.

While some case series have demonstrated successful outcomes with dermal augmentation of revision rotator cuff repair [15] others have not demonstrated a substantial benefit to augmentation [16]. There exists in our opinion only one higher quality study on the use of grafts in rotator cuff repairs, which demonstrated a modest improvement in clinical outcomes and a 45% improvement in healing rates in the setting of primary, two-tendon rotator cuff repair [17]. Further investigation will be necessary to refine the indications, describe the long-term results, and perform a comprehensive cost analysis of patch augmentation of rotator cuff repairs.

Clinical Pearls/Pitfalls

- The graft selected for dermal augmentation should allow repopulation with host cells, be durable enough to tolerate suture fixation and forces across the rotator cuff footprint, and present no host inflammatory response.
- If it is not possible to obtain a repair of the rotator cuff to at least the medial aspect of the greater tuberosity footprint with minimal tension, dermal augmentation is not recommended.
- When retrieving sutures through the lateral portal and passing them through the dermal graft, it is critical to ensure that sutures do not cross one another within the cannula.
- Mulberry knots on the posteromedial and anteromedial aspects of the graft can ensure proper orientation and stability of the graft once it is introduced into the subacromial space.
- Spinal needles placed at the posterolateral and anterolateral portions of the graft can provide provisional fixation of the lateral aspect of the graft to the tuberosity while

sutures are passed through and tensioned within lateral-row anchors.

- A delayed rehabilitation program of 6 weeks of sling immobilization prior to initiating physical therapy is preferred in order to optimize chances of healing.

References

1. Boileau P, Brassart N, Watkinson DJ, Carles M, Hatzidakis AM, Krishnan SG. Arthroscopic repair of full-thickness tears of the supraspinatus: does the tendon really heal? J Bone Joint Surg Am. 2005;87:1229–40. doi:10.2106/JBJS.D.02035.
2. Gazielly DF, Gleyze P, Montagnon C. Functional and anatomical results after rotator cuff repair. Clin Orthop Relat Res. 1994;304:43–53.
3. Harryman DT 2nd, Mack LA, Wang KY, Jackins SE, Richardson ML, Matsen FA 3rd. Repairs of the rotator cuff. Correlation of functional results with integrity of the cuff. J Bone Joint Surg Am. 1991;73:982–9.
4. Kim KC, Shin HD, Lee WY. Repair integrity and functional outcomes after arthroscopic suture-bridge rotator cuff repair. J Bone Joint Surg Am. 2012;94:e48. doi:10.2106/JBJS.K.00158.
5. Namdari S, Donegan RP, Chamberlain AM, Galatz LM, Yamaguchi K, Keener JD. Factors affecting outcome after structural failure of repaired rotator cuff tears. J Bone Joint Surg Am. 2014;96:99–105. doi:10.2106/JBJS.M.00551.
6. Choi S, Kim MK, Kim GM, Roh YH, Hwang IK, Kang H. Factors associated with clinical and structural outcomes after arthroscopic rotator cuff repair with a suture bridge technique in medium, large, and massive tears. J Shoulder Elb Surg. 2014;23:1675–81. doi:10.1016/j.jse.2014.02.021.
7. Lapner PL, Sabri E, Rakhra K, McRae S, Leiter J, Bell K, et al. A multicenter randomized controlled trial comparing single-row with double-row fixation in arthroscopic rotator cuff repair. J Bone Joint Surg Am. 2012;94:1249–57. doi:10.2106/JBJS.K.00999.
8. Tashjian RZ, Hung M, Burks RT, Greis PE. Influence of preoperative musculotendinous junction position on rotator cuff healing using single-row technique. Arthroscopy. 2013;29:1748–54. doi:10.1016/j.arthro.2013.08.014.

9. Adams JE, Zobitz ME, Reach JS Jr, An KN, Steinmann SP. Rotator cuff repair using an acellular dermal matrix graft: an in vivo study in a canine model. Arthroscopy. 2006;22:700–9. doi:10.1016/j.arthro.2006.03.016.

10. Baker AR, McCarron JA, Tan CD, Iannotti JP, Derwin KA. Does augmentation with a reinforced fascia patch improve rotator cuff repair outcomes? Clin Orthop Relat Res. 2012;470:2513–21. doi:10.1007/s11999-012-2348-x.

11. Ely EE, Figueroa NM, Gilot GJ. Biomechanical analysis of rotator cuff repairs with extracellular matrix graft augmentation. Orthopedics. 2014;37:608–14. doi:10.3928/01477447-20140825-05.

12. McCarron JA, Milks RA, Mesiha M, Aurora A, Walker E, Iannotti JP, et al. Reinforced fascia patch limits cyclic gapping of rotator cuff repairs in a human cadaveric model. J Shoulder Elb Surg. 2012;21:1680–6. doi:10.1016/j.jse.2011.11.039.

13. Omae H, Steinmann SP, Zhao C, Zobitz ME, Wongtriratanachai P, Sperling JW, et al. Biomechanical effect of rotator cuff augmentation with an acellular dermal matrix graft: a cadaver study. Clin Biomech (Bristol, Avon). 2012;27:789–92. doi:10.1016/j.clinbiomech.2012.05.001.

14. Chalmers PN, Frank RM, Gupta AK, Yanke AB, Trenhaile SW, Romeo AA, et al. All-arthroscopic patch augmentation of a massive rotator cuff tear: surgical technique. Arthrosc Tech. 2013;2:e447–51. doi:10.1016/j.eats.2013.07.003.

15. Kokkalis ZT, Mavrogenis AF, Scarlat M, Christodoulou M, Vottis C, Papagelopoulos PJ, et al. Human dermal allograft for massive rotator cuff tears. Orthopedics. 2014;37:e1108–16. doi:10.3928/01477447-20141124-59.

16. Sears BW, Choo A, Yu A, Greis A, Lazarus M. Clinical outcomes in patients undergoing revision rotator cuff repair with extracellular matrix augmentation. Orthopedics. 2015;38:e292–6. doi:10.3928/01477447-20150402-57.

17. Barber FA, Burns JP, Deutsch A, Labbe MR, Litchfield RB. A prospective, randomized evaluation of acellular human dermal matrix augmentation for arthroscopic rotator cuff repair. Arthroscopy. 2012;28:8–15. doi:10.1016/j.arthro.2011.06.038.

Chapter 18
Use of PRP in Rotator Cuff Repair

Thierry Pauyo and James P. Bradley

Case Presentation

A 64-year-old, right-hand-dominant male golfer presented to us for evaluation of his left shoulder. He reported ongoing pain on the anterolateral aspect of his shoulder for the last 6 months. It was insidious in onset, worse at night, and with overhead activities. It was associated with stiffness and his golf swing was significantly affected. He denied any trauma and said that the shoulder problems were from overuse. He had a subacromial steroid injection 3 months ago by his primary care physician and had two courses of physical therapy, with very little improvement.

T. Pauyo, M.D., F.R.C.S.C.
University of Pittsburgh Medical Center,
3200 South Water St., Pittsburgh, PA 15203, USA

J.P. Bradley, M.D. (✉)
Burke and Bradley Orthopaedics, University of Pittsburgh
Medical Center, Suite 4010, 200 Delafield Road,
Suite 200, Pittsburgh, PA 15215, USA
e-mail: bradleyjp@upmc.edu

© Springer International Publishing AG 2018
P.J. McMahon (ed.), *Rotator Cuff Injuries*,
DOI 10.1007/978-3-319-63668-9_18

A thorough history and clinical examination are paramount in making a diagnosis of rotator cuff pathology. Cervical spine pathology can mimic rotator cuff pathology; hence, a neck examination should never be overlooked. Clinical examination showed an individual with average built and normal neck movements and negative Spurling's sign. No periscapular muscle atrophy was noted. His active and passive range of motion was normal and similar to the right shoulder. His forward flexion strength was 4/5 and external rotation was 5/5. Belly press, bear hug, and liftoff tests were negative. O'Brien's test was equivocal and no bicipital groove or acromioclavicular tenderness was noted. He had normal neurological examination of the left upper extremity.

We performed a series of shoulder radiographs including anterior-posterior (AP), scapular Y view and axillary view in this patient. With the AP radiograph, we specifically assess for any superior migration of humeral head or osseous changes at the greater tuberosity or humeral head, which can be indicative of chronic cuff pathology and the acromial shape is assessed with the scapular Y view. In this case, radiographs did not reveal any glenohumeral arthrosis or proximal migration of humeral head. Moderate acromioclavicular joint arthrosis was noted but clinically he had no tenderness to palpation.

The patient also had a magnetic resonance imaging (MRI) that revealed a full-thickness U-shaped, supraspinatus tendon tear with retraction to the glenoid and no fatty atrophy or infiltration of the rotator cuff muscles. Of note, we do not find MR arthrogram useful for routine rotator cuff assessment. Standard MRI allows detailed evaluation of rotator cuff tear pattern, tendon retraction, and amount of fatty atrophy or infiltration of the muscles. It also provides excellent assessment of the labrum, long head of bicep tendon, glenohumeral ligaments, and cysts around the joint.

Diagnosis/Assessment

This is a 64-year-old right-hand-dominant male with a history of clinical examination and diagnostic imaging consistent with a symptomatic full-thickness supraspinatus tear with retraction to level of the glenoid and normal rotator cuff muscles. The patient had already failed nonoperative treatments including 6 weeks of physical therapy and steroid injection. We discussed further treatment options. We refrained from additional subacromial injection of steroid as we think it may diminish the beneficial effects of PRP. To care for his present symptoms and diminish the risk of the future tear worsening and likely irreversible muscle changes we decided that surgery was the best next treatment. We offered him arthroscopic double-row rotator cuff repair, subacromial decompression, and PRP injection into the bone-tendon interface.

Management

During surgery, a blood sample was collected with a venipuncture and the PRP was prepared with a centrifugation process (Figs. 18.1, 18.2, 18.3, 18.4, and 18.5). After double-row rotator

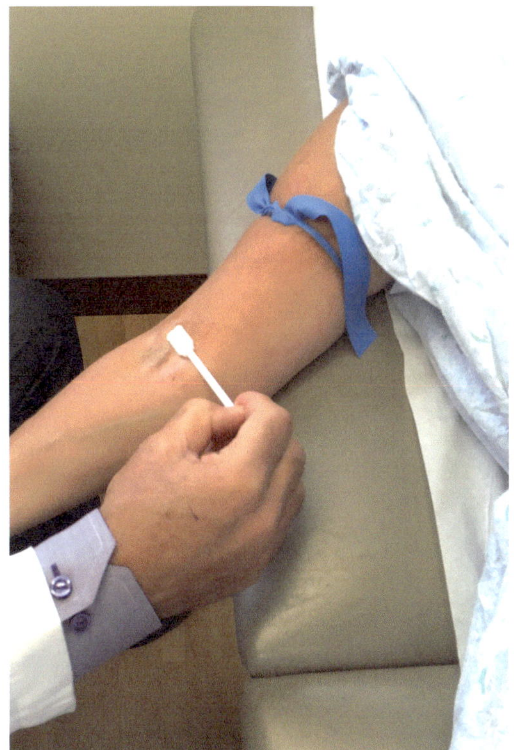

FIGURE 18.1 The arm is sterilely prepped for the venipuncture

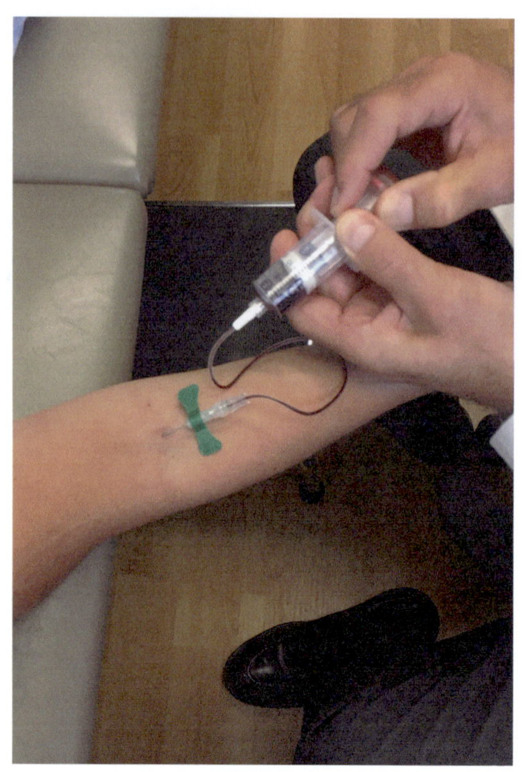

FIGURE 18.2
The blood
sample is
obtained

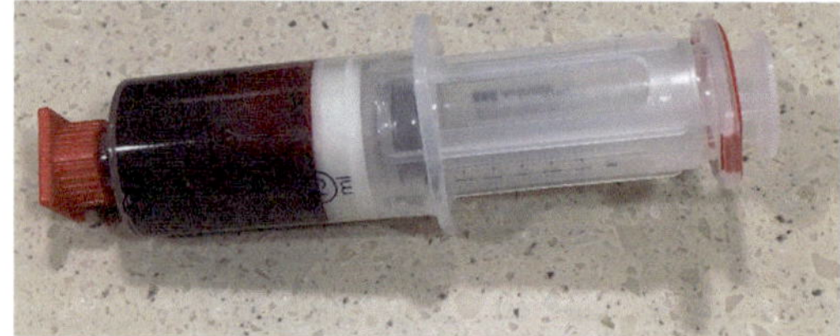

FIGURE 18.3
15 cc of blood
is collected

FIGURE 18.4 Sample
centrifuged for
5 min at 1500 rpm

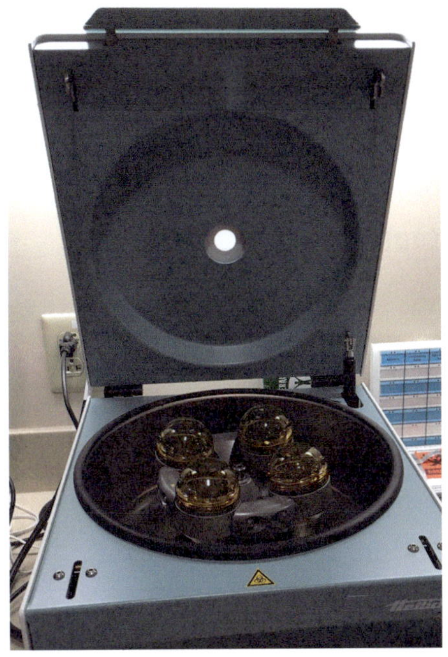

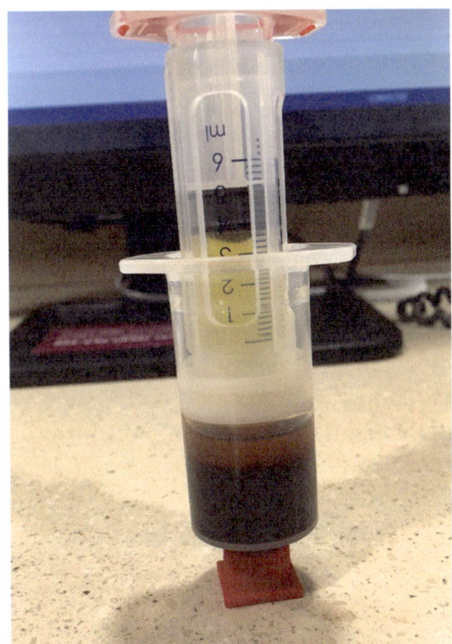

FIGURE 18.5 Platelet-
containing plasma
(*yellow* fluid)
extracted from centri-
fuged blood sample

cuff repair, that is described elsewhere in this book, a needle was placed at the bone-tendon interface. The subacromial space was evacuated of fluid and arthroscopic portals were sutured close. The PRP was then injected through the needle as the last step of the procedure.

Outcome

The patient participated in our postoperative protocol, which consists of a sling and pendulum exercises for the first 6 weeks postoperatively followed by active range of motion, and then strengthening which begins 3 months postoperatively. Six months after surgery the patient reported no pain, had normal range of motion and strength, and had returned to his usual activities including golf.

Literature Review

The healing process following rotator cuff repair is governed by a complex amalgam of biomechanical factors that has been widely studied. The rotator cuff enthesis consists of tendons, fibrocartilage, mineralized fibrocartilage (Sharpey's fibers), and lamellar bone [1]. The repair provides mechanical stability to protect and promote healing at the tendon-bone interface. The principles for healing of rotator cuff repair are twofold: (1) obtaining structural stability by achieving strong fixation while restoring the anatomic surface of the rotator cuff tendon footprint and (2) minimizing gap formation and failure of the construct by promoting and maintaining mechanical stability while the healing occurs [2]. While the outcomes after rotator cuff repair are typically good, with more than 80% regaining (normal or full) function, re-rupture rates are about 25% and can be as high as 42% [3]. Therefore, we believe that everything that can be done to promote healing should be done.

There are many factors that affect healing after rotator cuff repair ranging from patient factors, tear characteristics, soft-tissue structural problems, and repair technique and implants. Recently there has also been interest in the biology of the healing response. The biologic approach aims to optimize soft-tissue healing to improve clinical outcomes [4]. One method utilizes PRP to curb the inflammation response and supplement tendon-bone healing with growth factors.

Over the past few years, the advances in the biomechanical repair constructs of rotator cuff tear may have peaked, stimulating a growing interest in biological aids to rotator cuff healing. The biologic factors recently studied to enhance soft-tissue healing and regeneration have mainly focused on growth factors, stem cells, and PRP.

Growth factors are molecules involved in the modulation of cell growth during the signal cascade of inflammation. Their influence is paramount in the inflammatory phase of tendon healing [5]. The molecules involved include fibroblast growth factor (FGF), vascular endothelial growth factor (VEGF), platelet-derived growth factor (PDGF-β), transforming growth factor-beta (TGF-β), and insulin-like growth factor-1 (IGF-1) [6]. These growth factors are produced in great majority by fibroblast and inflammatory cells such as leukocytes and platelets [7]. During the inflammatory and repair phase of tendon healing, platelets aggregate at the site of soft-tissue injury and release an extensive amount of growth factors prompting cell migration and differentiation at the site of injury [8]. Platelets provide a colossal amount of autogenous growth factors. PRP is easy to harvest from blood and is therefore one of the most commonly used biological aids in rotator cuff repair.

PRP has been shown to decrease inflammation through inhibition of molecules such as interleukin 1B and to promote healing through modulation of TGF-B production [5, 9]. PRP is a fraction of whole blood containing very high platelet concentrations (150,000–350,000), which on activation release various growth factors. The preparation consists of obtaining whole blood from the patient with a venipuncture followed by centrifugation to concentrate the platelets. The centrifugation also concentrates growth factors above physiologic level that can then be sterilely injected at the site of the tendon-bone repair. The growth factors present in the concentrate may stimulate cell proliferation and provide a temporary matrix that fills defects in the repair and serve as a matrix for cell migration and tissue remodeling [10].

There are different classification systems to describe the final PRP concentrate. The scientific community has not adopted a universal classification system, which has led to heterogeneity in the way PRP has been described. One of the classifications contains four categories: (1) pure PRP (P-PRP) with a low content of leukocytes, (2) leukocyte-rich PRP (L-PRP) with a high content of leukocytes, (3) pure platelet-rich fibrin (P-PRF), and (4) leukocyte-rich platelet-rich fibrin (L-PRF), with a high content of leukocytes and a high-density fibrin network [11]. The role of leukocytes in the PRP is still the subject of debate as some studies have found it to have a role in the anabolic process of collagen synthesis while other studies have found it to be catabolic [10, 12, 13]. A second classification system has been described with two categories, (1) presence or (2) absence of leukocytes, and further sub-classified with (a) PRP-activated, ex vivo activation with thrombin and calcium, or (b) PRP-inactivated, in vivo activation by endogenous collagen [11, 14]. Lastly, our preference is the PAW classification that is based on three factors: [1] the absolute number of *p*latelets, [2] the type of platelet *a*ctivation, and [3] the presence or absence of *w*hite cells [15].

There are different methods of PRP delivery. Currently PRP can be administered as a liquid, in a gel or in a matrix scaffold. The liquid form of PRP can be activated by endogenous methods such as by simple agitation of platelets during centrifugation or by compression of platelets during needle delivery. Endogenous activation also has a potential for slower aggregation of platelets and release of growth factors by allowing contact with type 1 collagen in the rotator cuff tendon to operate as the activator, thereby providing a natural release pattern [16]. The liquid form can be directly administered to the tendon-bone interface of the rotator cuff repair during arthroscopic surgery or simply injected through the arthroscopic portal after evacuation of the intra-articular and subacromial fluid.

The PRP gel and matrix scaffold entail exogenous activation of platelets with the use of calcium chloride and thrombin. The scaffold may better keep the PRP in place at the repair site and possibly to create a more sustained release over the span of several days [15].

Several prospective comparative studies have examined the clinical and structural outcomes with PRP in rotator cuff repair; however the results have been conflicting. Warth et al. performed a systematic review of all level I and II studies comparing clinical and structural outcomes after rotator cuff repair with or without PRP [17]. There was no statistical differences in overall gain in outcome scores or re-tear found, but they noticed a significant gain in shoulder Constant score when PRP was applied at the tendon-bone interface compared to application on top of the repaired tendon. Most of the included studies were powered to detect large differences in outcome scores only. Other studies have indicated that there may be a decrease in re-tear rate with PRP; however, they were unable to show differences in clinical outcomes [18–20]. In a meta-analysis of 13 studies which also included a cost-effectiveness analysis, Vavken et al. found a significant reduction in re-tear rates with PRP; however, this benefit was not cost effective [21]. Another meta-analysis of eight randomized controlled studies comparing rotator cuff repair with and without PRP found no statistical difference in re-tear rates and clinical outcomes [22]. Other systematic reviews have had similar results [23–25]. Furthermore, a Cochrane review by Moraes et al. pooled 19 studies with 1088 participants on the use of PRP in not only rotator cuff but also 5 other tendon pathologies. They found no significant improvement in functional outcomes and insufficient evidence to support the use of PRP in clinical practice [26].

Hsu et al. reported that successful use of PRP varies depending on the preparation method, composition, medical condition of patient, anatomical location, and tissue type [27]. But heterogeneity of the different studies hampers comparison. There are differences in the number of doses administered and the PRP preparation including different volumes of autologous blood collected, speed and time of centrifugation, activating agent and leukocyte concentrations, final volume of PRP, and final concentration of platelets and growth factors. There are also differences in the time between PRP preparation and administration including preoperative, intraoperative, and postoperative administration. The method of administration whether image guided, arthroscopic guided, direct vision, or no guidance varies. Lastly the surgical techniques have varied between single- and double-row repairs and the postoperative rehabilitation protocols are not the same [26, 28].

Overall, studies do not support the clinical use of PRP in rotator cuff repair [29–31] but some data supports its use in a subset of patients. There may be a decrease in re-tear rates among patients treated for small- and medium-size rotator cuff [32, 33]. In a meta-analysis of five studies with 303 patients, Cai et al. found a significant difference in failure of small- to moderate-size rotator cuff repairs when PRP was not used [34]. Chahal et al., in a meta-analysis of five studies including two randomized and three nonrandomized clinical trials of 261 patients, found no difference in rotator cuff re-tear rate and functional outcomes [35]. However, in a stratified sub-analysis, they found a significant reduction in re-tears in those with PRP. In those with massive rotator cuff tears, Antuna et al. found that 28 patients had no significant difference in repairs regardless if they received PRP or not [36]. Bergeson et al. found that outcomes of patients with a combination of advance age, severe tear size, and fatty infiltration were not influenced by an inclusion of PRP scaffold with rotator cuff repair [30].

The use of PRP in rotator cuff tendinopathy has also been studied. Carr et al. studied PRP in patients undergoing arthroscopic acromioplasty for chronic rotator cuff tendinopathy in 60 patients [37]. They found no effect of PRP on clinic outcomes in this patient population. These findings are supported by another randomized controlled trial evaluating chronic rotator cuff tendinopathy, which found a limited role for PRP administration in the short term [38].

PRP can be administered preoperatively, intraoperatively, or postoperatively. It is still unclear which method yields the best effect on soft-tissue healing at the tendon-bone interface. In a review of seven meta-analyses, Saltzman et al. found that PRP injection at the time of arthroscopic intervention does not affect re-tear rate or affect functional outcome. However, there was a trend in reducing re-tear rates in a PRP scaffold construct when it was applied at tendon-bone interface, in a double-row repair, and with small- and medium-sized rotator cuff tears [39]. Furthermore, in 53 patients, Randelli et al. found a significant improvement in early functional outcomes in the intraoperative PRP-treated rotator cuff repair as compared to the control group [40].

The effect of the PRP in the postoperative phase has also been studied. Wang et al. studied 60 arthroscopic supraspinatus tendon repairs with administration of PRP at postoperative days 7 and 12 [41] and found that two distinct image-guided PRP administrations in the postoperative period did not improve early tendon-bone healing or functional recovery. As the biological effects of the growth factors in PRP on reducing inflammatory markers have been well documented [5, 9], a decrease in inflammation following the surgical procedure could potentially decrease the patient's postoperative pain. Hak et al. conducted a double-blinded placebo study that demonstrated no conclusive effect of PRP in decreasing postoperative pain after arthroscopic rotator cuff repair in a 6-week postoperative period [42]. However, Randelli et al. studied 53 patients and found improvement in pain scores at 3, 7 14, and 30 postoperative days [40].

Lastly PRP has been studied in the rehabilitation phase of tendon healing. In a randomized controlled trial, Ilhanli et al. compared the effectiveness of PRP injection versus physical therapy (PT) in the treatment of chronic partial-thickness supraspinatus tendon tears [43]. Both groups had significantly reduced pain and improved range of motion. While increases in ROM degrees were significantly higher in the PT group than the PRP group and pain with activity and at rest was also higher in the PT group than the PRP group, improvement of the DASH score was significantly better in the PRP group than the PT group.

In summary, clinical use of platelet-rich plasma remains controversial. Studies are hampered by heterogeneity in preparation protocols, timing of delivery, method and number of administration, surgical procedures, and postoperative intervention and rehabilitation protocols. There is no evidence to support the common use of PRP in rotator cuff repair. However, there may be positive effect on structural healing at the tendon-bone interface in small- to medium-size rotator cuff tear with intraoperative administration of PRP. We think it is too early to decide if PRP is helpful in rotator cuff repair. We urge clinicians to continue to assess the new studies regarding the use of PRP as an aid in rotator cuff repair.

Clinical Pearls

- PRP has been shown to decrease inflammation through inhibition of molecules such as interleukin 1B and to promote healing through modulation of TGF-B production which is proposed to affect rotator cuff healing.
- PRP can be administered intraoperatively as it may reduce re-tear rates when it is applied at the tendon-bone interface.
- While there is not a consensus that PRP is helpful in all rotator cuff repairs, it may be helpful in patients with small- and medium-size rotator cuff tears.
- PRP should not be used in unhealthy, older patients with large and massive tears and advanced fatty infiltration of the muscles.

References

1. Thangarajah T, Pendegrass CJ, Shahbazi S, Lambert S, Alexander S, Blunn GW. Augmentation of rotator cuff repair with soft tissue scaffolds. Orthop J Sports Med. 2015;3(6):2325967115587495.
2. McCormack RA, Shreve M, Strauss EJ. Biologic augmentation in rotator cuff repair--should we do it, who should get it, and has it worked? Bull Hosp Jt Dis (2013). 2014;72(1):89–96.
3. Charousset C, Bellaiche L, Kalra K, Petrover D. Arthroscopic repair of full-thickness rotator cuff tears: is there tendon healing in patients aged 65 years or older? Arthroscopy. 2010;26(3):302–9.
4. LaPrade RF, Dragoo JL, Koh JL, Murray IR, Geeslin AG, Chu CR. AAOS research symposium updates and consensus: biologic treatment of orthopaedic injuries. J Am Acad Orthop Surg. 2016;24(7):e62–78.
5. Randelli P, Randelli F, Ragone V, et al. Regenerative medicine in rotator cuff injuries. Biomed Res Int. 2014;2014:129515.
6. Wurgler-Hauri CC, Dourte LM, Baradet TC, Williams GR, Soslowsky LJ. Temporal expression of 8 growth factors in tendon-to-bone healing in a rat supraspinatus model. J Shoulder Elbow Surg. 2007;16(5 Suppl):S198–203.
7. Wahl SM, Wong H, McCartney-Francis N. Role of growth factors in inflammation and repair. J Cell Biochem. 1989;40(2):193–9.
8. Gamradt SC, et al. Platelet rich plasma in rotator cuff repair. Tech Orthop. 2007;22(1):26–33. Lippincott Williams & Wilkins
9. Namazi H. Rotator cuff repair healing influenced by platelet-rich plasma construct augmentation: a novel molecular mechanism. Arthroscopy. 2011;27(11):1456. author reply-7
10. Alsousou J, Thompson M, Hulley P, Noble A, Willett K. The biology of platelet-rich plasma and its application in trauma and orthopaedic surgery: a review of the literature. J Bone Joint Surg. 2009;91(8):987–96.
11. Dohan Ehrenfest DM, Rasmusson L, Albrektsson T. Classification of platelet concentrates: from pure platelet-rich plasma (P-PRP) to leucocyte- and platelet-rich fibrin (L-PRF). Trends Biotechnol. 2009;27(3):158–67.
12. Cross JA, Cole BJ, Spatny KP, et al. Leukocyte-reduced platelet-rich plasma normalizes matrix metabolism in torn human rotator cuff tendons. Am J Sports Med. 2015;43(12):2898–906.

290   T. Pauyo and J.P. Bradley

13. Martin P, Leibovich SJ. Inflammatory cells during wound repair: the good, the bad and the ugly. Trends Cell Biol. 2005;15(11):599–607.
14. Mishra A, Harmon K, Woodall J, Vieira A. Sports medicine applications of platelet rich plasma. Curr Pharm Biotechnol. 2012;13(7):1185–95.
15. DeLong JM, Russell RP, Mazzocca AD. Platelet-rich plasma: the PAW classification system. Arthroscopy. 2012;28(7):998–1009.
16. Harrison S, Vavken P, Kevy S, Jacobson M, Zurakowski D, Murray MM. Platelet activation by collagen provides sustained release of anabolic cytokines. Am J Sports Med. 2011;39(4):729–34.
17. Warth RJ, Dornan GJ, James EW, Horan MP, Millett PJ. Clinical and structural outcomes after arthroscopic repair of full-thickness rotator cuff tears with and without platelet-rich product supplementation: a meta-analysis and meta-regression. Arthroscopy. 2015;31(2):306–20.
18. Jo CH, Shin JS, Lee YG, et al. Platelet-rich plasma for arthroscopic repair of large to massive rotator cuff tears: a randomized, single-blind, parallel-group trial. Am J Sports Med. 2013;41(10):2240–8.
19. Jo CH, Shin JS, Shin WH, Lee SY, Yoon KS, Shin S. Platelet-rich plasma for arthroscopic repair of medium to large rotator cuff tears: a randomized controlled trial. Am J Sports Med. 2015;43(9):2102–10.
20. Jo CH, Kim JE, Yoon KS, et al. Does platelet-rich plasma accelerate recovery after rotator cuff repair? A prospective cohort study. Am J Sports Med. 2011;39(10):2082–90.
21. Vavken P, Sadoghi P, Palmer M, et al. Platelet-rich plasma reduces Retear rates after arthroscopic repair of small- and medium-sized rotator cuff tears but is not cost-effective. Am J Sports Med. 2015;43(12):3071–6.
22. Zhao JG, Zhao L, Jiang YX, Wang ZL, Wang J, Zhang P. Platelet-rich plasma in arthroscopic rotator cuff repair: a meta-analysis of randomized controlled trials. Arthroscopy. 2015;31(1):125–35.
23. Werthel JD, Pelissier A, Massin P, Boyer P, Valenti P. Arthroscopic double row cuff repair with suture-bridging and autologous conditioned plasma injection: functional and structural results. Int J Shoulder Surg. 2014;8(4):101–6.
24. Ruiz-Moneo P, Molano-Munoz J, Prieto E, Algorta J. Plasma rich in growth factors in arthroscopic rotator cuff repair: a randomized, double-blind, controlled clinical trial. Arthroscopy. 2013;29(1):2–9.
25. Maffulli N, Longo UG, Loppini M, Berton A, Spiezia F, Denaro V. Tissue engineering for rotator cuff repair: an evidence-based systematic review. Stem Cells Int. 2012;2012:418086.

26. Moraes VY, Lenza M, Tamaoki MJ, Faloppa F, Belloti JC. Platelet-rich therapies for musculoskeletal soft tissue injuries. Cochrane Database Syst Rev. 2014;4:CD010071.

27. Hsu WK, Mishra A, Rodeo SR, et al. Platelet-rich plasma in orthopaedic applications: evidence-based recommendations for treatment. J Am Acad Orthop Surg. 2013;21(12):739–48.

28. Randelli P, Cucchi D, Ragone V, de Girolamo L, Cabitza P, Randelli M. History of rotator cuff surgery. Knee Surg Sports Traumatol Arthrosc. 2015;23(2):344–62.

29. Rodeo SA, Delos D, Williams RJ, Adler RS, Pearle A, Warren RF. The effect of platelet-rich fibrin matrix on rotator cuff tendon healing: a prospective, randomized clinical study. Am J Sports Med. 2012;40(6):1234–41.

30. Bergeson AG, Tashjian RZ, Greis PE, Crim J, Stoddard GJ, Burks RT. Effects of platelet-rich fibrin matrix on repair integrity of at-risk rotator cuff tears. Am J Sports Med. 2012;40(2):286–93.

31. Castricini R, Longo UG, De Benedetto M, et al. Platelet-rich plasma augmentation for arthroscopic rotator cuff repair: a randomized controlled trial. Am J Sports Med. 2011;39(2):258–65.

32. Zhang Q, Ge H, Zhou J, Cheng B. Are platelet-rich products necessary during the arthroscopic repair of full-thickness rotator cuff tears: a meta-analysis. PLoS One. 2013;8(7):e69731.

33. Charousset C, Zaoui A, Bellaiche L, Piterman M. Does autologous leukocyte-platelet-rich plasma improve tendon healing in arthroscopic repair of large or massive rotator cuff tears? Arthroscopy. 2014;30(4):428–35.

34. Cai YZ, Zhang C, Lin XJ. Efficacy of platelet-rich plasma in arthroscopic repair of full-thickness rotator cuff tears: a meta-analysis. J Shoulder Elbow Surg. 2015;24(12):1852–9.

35. Chahal J, Van Thiel GS, Mall N, et al. The role of platelet-rich plasma in arthroscopic rotator cuff repair: a systematic review with quantitative synthesis. Arthroscopy. 2012;28(11):1718–27.

36. Antuna S, Barco R, Martinez Diez JM, Sanchez Marquez JM. Platelet-rich fibrin in arthroscopic repair of massive rotator cuff tears: a prospective randomized pilot clinical trial. Acta Orthop Belg. 2013;79(1):25–30.

37. Carr AJ, Murphy R, Dakin SG, et al. Platelet-rich plasma injection with arthroscopic acromioplasty for chronic rotator cuff tendinopathy: a randomized controlled trial. Am J Sports Med. 2015;43(12):2891–7.

38. Kesikburun S, Tan AK, Yilmaz B, Yasar E, Yazicioglu K. Platelet-rich plasma injections in the treatment of chronic rotator cuff

tendinopathy: a randomized controlled trial with 1-year follow-up. Am J Sports Med. 2013;41(11):2609–16.

39. Saltzman BM, Jain A, Campbell KA, et al. Does the use of platelet-rich plasma at the time of surgery improve clinical outcomes in arthroscopic rotator cuff repair when compared with control cohorts? A systematic review of meta-analyses. Arthroscopy. 2016;32(5):906–18.

40. Randelli P, Arrigoni P, Ragone V, Aliprandi A, Cabitza P. Platelet rich plasma in arthroscopic rotator cuff repair: a prospective RCT study, 2-year follow-up. J Shoulder Elbow Surg. 2011;20(4):518–28.

41. Wang A, McCann P, Colliver J, et al. Do postoperative platelet-rich plasma injections accelerate early tendon healing and functional recovery after arthroscopic supraspinatus repair? A randomized controlled trial. Am J Sports Med. 2015;43(6):1430–7.

42. Hak A, Rajaratnam K, Ayeni OR, et al. A double-blinded placebo randomized controlled trial evaluating short-term efficacy of platelet-rich plasma in reducing postoperative pain after arthroscopic rotator cuff repair: a pilot study. Sports Health. 2015;7(1):58–66.

43. Ilhanli I, Guder N, Gul M. Platelet-rich plasma treatment with physical therapy in chronic partial supraspinatus tears. Iran Red Crescent Med J. 2015;17(9):e23732.

Chapter 19
Partial Rotator Cuff Repair for Massive Rotator Cuff Repair

Edward A. Lin, Loukia K. Papatheodorou, and Dean G. Sotereanos

Case Presentation

A 52-year-old male reports right-shoulder pain, after an injury 6 weeks ago where he tripped and fell while playing basketball. Since then he has had posterolateral right-shoulder pain that radiates into the arm and wakes him at night. He is having difficulty lifting his arm overhead. The patient is a laborer and has been unable to work due to his injury. He has undergone a course of physical therapy for range of motion and strengthening, but he continues to have difficulty. On physical exam, there is no muscle atrophy. The patient has full passive range-of-motion right shoulder, but active forward elevation is limited to 90°. There is a positive

E.A. Lin, M.D.
Kayal Orthopaedic Center,
266 Haristown Road, Suite 107, Glen Rock, NJ, USA

L.K. Papatheodorou, M.D., Ph.D. • D.G. Sotereanos, M.D. ($\boxtimes$)
Department of Orthopaedic Surgery, University of Pittsburgh School of Medicine, Orthopaedic Specialists - UPMC 9104 Babcock Blvd, 5th floor, Pittsburgh, PA 15237, USA
e-mail: dsoterea@hotmail.com

© Springer International Publishing AG 2018
P.J. McMahon (ed.), *Rotator Cuff Injuries*,
DOI 10.1007/978-3-319-63668-9_19

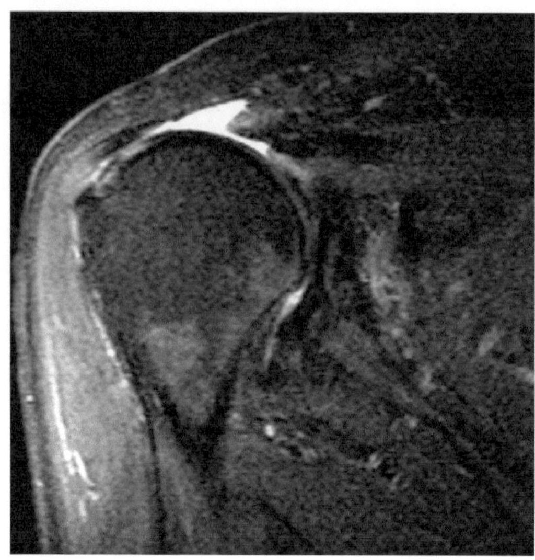

FIGURE 19.1 View of the right shoulder on MRI scan indicating a massive rotator cuff tear

drop-arm sign and a positive external rotation lag. An MRI of right shoulder demonstrates a massive retracted rotator cuff tear, involving the supraspinatus and infraspinatus tendons (Fig. 19.1). The ruptured tendon is retracted to the level of the glenoid. The tear is approximately 6 cm in length. There is no atrophy or fatty changes of the supraspinatus or infraspinatus muscle bellies. The subscapularis appears to be intact. The patient presents with profound weakness and pain and desires treatment.

Diagnosis/Assessment

The patient's history, physical, and imaging findings are consistent with the diagnosis of symptomatic massive rotator cuff tear. In elderly patients with massive rotator tears of insidious onset and abnormal MRI findings of the rotator cuff muscles, initial treatment is nonoperative including rehabilitation, NSAIDs, and avoidance of overhead activities. Because our patient is young and active and had sudden onset of symptoms after a fall and the MRI revealed normal rotator cuff muscles without atrophy or fatty infiltration, we concluded that this was an acute tear with surgery being the best chance for success.

A number of operative treatment options exist for the management of a massive rotator cuff tears. Repair can be done with either an arthroscopic or an open technique. Low- to medium-demand elderly patients with irreparable rotator cuff tears who have a significant amount of glenohumeral arthritis are usually best served by a reverse total shoulder or hemiarthroplasty prosthesis. However, in higher demand patients without joint degeneration, the solution is not quite as certain. Options include bursectomy and subacromial decompression, biceps tenotomy/tenodesis, debridement, tuberoplasty, latissimus dorsi or pectoralis transfer, and superior capsular reconstruction. All of these options are imperfect, and there is no consensus as to the superiority of one technique over another [1–4].

Management

Our patient was scheduled for urgent surgical repair of the rotator cuff of the right shoulder. Arthroscopy of the right shoulder revealed a massive rotator cuff retracted U-shaped tear. A longitudinal incision, approximately 4 cm, was made over the anterolateral acromion, beginning at acromioclavicular joint and extending laterally over the anterior acromion (Fig. 19.2). After exposure of the acromioclavicular joint, a distal clavicle excision of approximately 1 cm was performed. Then, the anterior acromion was exposed and an acromioplasty with resection of the anterior-inferior acromion to the level of the center of the clavicle was performed. After bursectomy and release of adhesions, the ruptured edge of the retracted supraspinatus and infraspinatus tendons was identified and mobilized (Figs. 19.3 and 19.4).

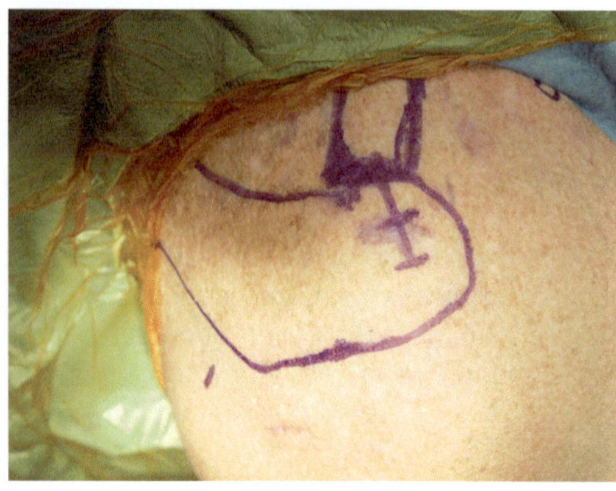

FIGURE 19.2 Longitudinal skin incision 4 cm in length begins at acromioclavicular joint and extends laterally over the anterior acromion

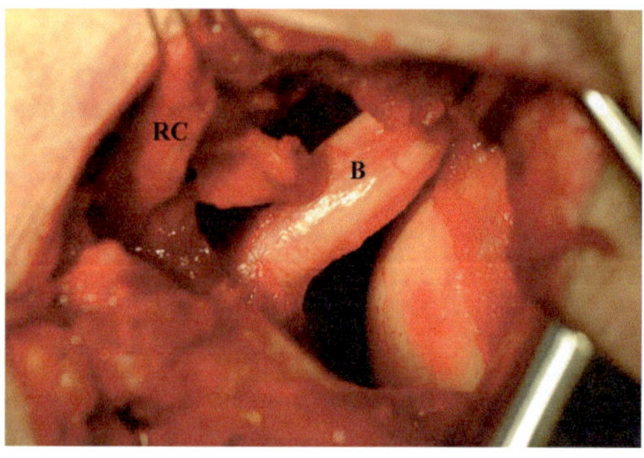

FIGURE 19.3 Intraoperative photo: Retracted massive rotator cuff tear is identified (RC: Rotator cuff, B: proximal tendon of biceps)

The tendons could not be repaired to the anatomic footprint without excessive tension. Therefore, a side-to-side margin convergence was performed. The remaining rotator cuff tissue was then partially repaired to the articular margin of the greater tuberosity without full coverage of the anatomic footprint (Fig. 19.5). The deltoid was repaired to the acromion with three transosseous sutures. Postoperatively, the patient was placed in a sling and instructed to perform pendulum exercises.

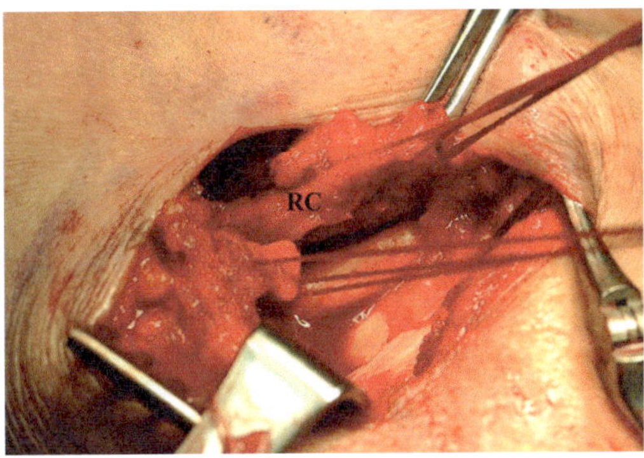

FIGURE 19.4 Intraoperative photo: After release of adhesions the retracted rotator cuff tendons are mobilized (RC: Rotator cuff)

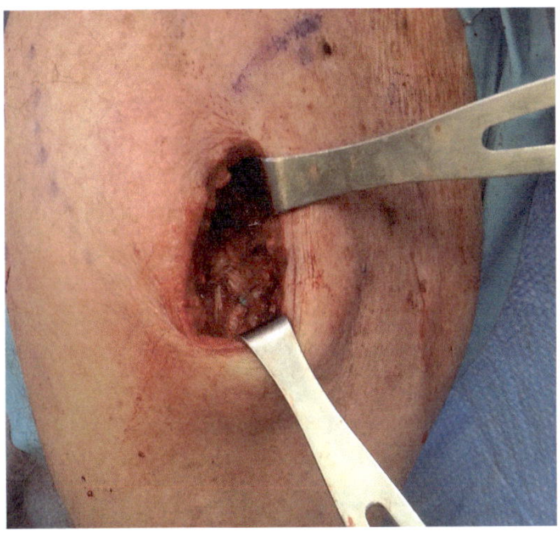

FIGURE 19.5 Intraoperative photo: Partial repair of the massive rotator cuff tear

Outcome

Physical therapy was started at 4 weeks, with a focus on reestablishing range of motion. Strengthening was initiated at 3 months. The patient was eventually able to return to full duty as a laborer, but reassigned to avoid heavy overhead activities.

Literature Review

Massive rotator cuff tears continue to be a challenging problem for the orthopedic surgeon and can result in significant pain and disability for the patient. The demands of an active, aging population require better strategies for managing larger and more disabling rotator cuff pathology. Cuff tears have been found to have a similarly negative impact on quality of life as diabetes, heart failure, hypertension, myocardial infarction, and depression [5–7]. The natural history of a cuff tear is progression of the tear, fatty degeneration, and retraction of the tendon [8–10].

Massive tears, which can be defined as a full-thickness tear greater than 5 cm in length or with involvement of two tendons, represent 10–40% of all tears and up to 80% of recurrent tears [11–13]. They are often characterized by a number of factors that make a complete primary repair difficult or impossible [14–16]. In addition to the severe tear, there is often poor tendon quality, retraction of the tendon, and extensive scarring of the torn tendon. Although it might be possible in some patients to repair a massively retracted, scarred tendon by release and mobilization of the tissues, the results are often subpar and failure rates are high, as demonstrated by MRI and ultrasonography [17]. Longstanding symptoms, an acromiohumeral interval less than 5 mm, and advanced levels of fatty infiltration of the cuff muscles may suggest a lesion that should not be fully repaired. Moreover, attempting to bring the central portion of a massive U-shaped tear back to its anatomic footprint often creates an unacceptable level of tension, so as to make the repair impossible. However, the edges of the tear near the anterior and posterior margins are often amenable for repair [18].

Partial Rotator Cuff Repair

Burkhart first introduced the concept of a partial rotator cuff repair, in which the torn rotator cuff is partially repaired, without complete coverage of the native footprint [19]. In this technique, the anterior and posterior margins of the tear are repaired, leaving the retracted central portion of the tear in place. Burkhart named this a "force couple repair," as it allows adequate balancing of the anterior and posterior forces acting on the proximal humerus [20]. Burkhart first noticed that some patients, despite having a massive rotator cuff tear, were able to maintain normal or near-normal shoulder strength and range of motion. He proposed that this was possible because the coronal and axial forces acting on the glenohumeral joint were still balanced, despite the defect within the rotator cuff. The balancing forces in the frontal plane are provided by the deltoid and subscapularis. In the axial plane, the balancing forces are from the subscapularis and infraspinatus/teres minor [21]. Therefore, complete repair of the supraspinatus might not be required for sufficient balancing of the forces. In fact, even with complete supraspinatus paralysis, 75% of abduction strength and 85–90% of external rotation strength are preserved [22]. Thus, a large defect might weaken the anterior and posterior translational forces in equal amounts, such that the resulting forces continue to maintain the humeral head in an anatomic location on glenoid surface throughout a functional range of motion [19].

Burkhart proposed that in patients with massive rotator cuff tears, achieving a partial repair could restore function by rebalancing the anterior and posterior moments acting on the glenohumeral joint [23]. Thus, this type of repair is often called a "functional repair." This also reduces the strain at the margins of the tear so that fixation will be adequate, despite being weaker than that of a complete repair. It protects the tendon-bone repair interface during healing, and allows a functional recovery despite a less-than-complete repair. Burkhart found an increase in active elevation of 90–150°

and mean 2.3 grade improvement of elevation strength in 14 patients using an open approach to achieve a partial repair [19]. He found that once the margin of the tear is fixed, it is no longer impinged under the acromion or between the rotator cable and the humeral head. Thus, shoulder motion can be achieved without pain.

Margin Convergence

Burkhart also introduced the concept of "margin convergence," also known as a "side-to-side" repair. Unlike a partial repair, in which cuff tissue is brought to bone, margin convergence involves fixation of cuff tissue to cuff tissue. It is usually performed by bringing together the retracted margins at the apex of a retracted U-shaped tear, thereby converting a massive U-shaped tear into a smaller tear. Following a margin convergence procedure, the remaining cuff tissue may or may not be fixed to bone, depending on the tension created by the repair.

Margin convergence or side-to-side repair is labeled a nonanatomic repair, since rotator cuff tissue is being fixed to other cuff tissue, rather than being brought to its anatomic location at the bony footprint on the proximal humerus. Several studies have found good clinical results and high patient satisfaction, with recurrence rates from 19 to 48% [24–26]. Bukhart et al. found excellent clinical results with massive tears and 3.5-year follow-up. In his series, he used an arthroscopic approach, and found that margin convergence of large U-shaped tears was similar to complete (tendon to bone) repair of medium-sized crescent-shaped tears [12]. In massive cuff tears, Burkhart was able to achieve an increase in forward flexion by 42–132 degrees and improvements in strength and functional scores as well.

Results of Partial Repair

There is evidence of improved clinical outcomes with partial rotator cuff repair at 3–5-year follow-up [1, 21, 27, 28]. In these studies, the partial rotator cuff repair was performed with the addition of margin convergence. Jones and Savoie found good-to-excellent results in 88% of patients. Fixation of cuff tissue onto the bony footprint did not improve long-term clinical results [29]. Van der Zwaal et al. reported good clinical results with a 19% re-tear rate at 26.5-month follow-up [24]. They used a running suture technique for their side-to-side repair [30]. Rousseau et al. found good clinical results with a 44% re-tear rate at 38-month follow-up in an elderly population (mean age 66) [25]. Nove-Josserand found an 85% satisfaction rate at 5-year follow-up with this technique [31]. They included only patients with subacromial space >7 mm and Goutallier stage 1 or 2 fatty infiltration. The recurrence rate was 17%. Duralde and Bair reported 67% of patients with good-to-excellent ASES scores with 92% satisfied with the results of partial repair [32].

Partial vs. Complete Repair vs. Debridement

Quite a few studies have suggested that a partial repair of massive rotator cuff tear results in equivalent outcomes to a complete repair. Godneneche et al. found that both partial and complete repairs gained equivalent improvements in Constant scores. However, rotator cuff strength was found to be significantly lower in the partial repairs. In addition, the re-tear rate was significantly higher in partial repairs (48.8% versus 20%). Heuberer et al. confirmed this (53% versus 29%).

A partial rotator cuff repair may result in greater functional loads on the remaining rotator cuff, thus resulting in muscular fatigue of the intact tendons [33]. Heuberer et al. prospectively analyzed 68 patients with massive rotator cuff tears and found that complete repair, partial repair, and debridement alone without repair all led to significant improvements in clinical and subjective outcomes. However with respect to strength and functional scores, complete repairs were significantly superior to both partial repairs and debridement alone. The re-tear rate for partial repairs was 29% versus 53% for complete repairs, as evaluated by

MRI. Interestingly, there was no difference between debridement and partial repairs with regard to functional and pain scores. Thus, the authors questioned whether partial repair or debridement is the preferred arthroscopic procedure in the case where a complete repair cannot be achieved. However, there is data that shoulder function deteriorates over time following a debridement [34]. Thus in the long term, partial repair may still be the preferred option, although there is limited data to support this conclusion.

Moser et al. [35] retrospectively evaluated 38 patients who underwent either complete repair, partial repair, or debridement. They found a trend towards improved motion and strength in complete and partial repairs, when compared with debridement alone. When comparing complete to partial repairs, there was a significant difference in external rotation strength and a trend towards improved functional scores, favoring complete repair.

Francesci et al. compared partial rotator cuff repair to debridement and acromioplasty and found superior functional outcomes and quality-of-life scores for partial repair [8]. Although patients who underwent debridement experienced less pain in the first postoperative month, partial repair of the rotator cuff resulted in significantly increased strength and range of motion.

Longer Term Follow-Up

Shon et al. demonstrated that despite initial improvement in clinical and radiographic parameters, about half of the patients demonstrated worsening of outcomes, including increasing patient dissatisfaction, over a 2-year period of follow-up after partial rotator cuff repair [1]. The authors suggested multiple possibilities to account for this decline, including re-tearing of the cuff and deterioration of the positive effect of subacromial decompression and biceps tenotomy/tenodesis. However, unlike in other studies, the patients in the study by Shon et al. did not receive margin convergence procedures in addition to the partial rotator cuff repair.

Preoperative Factors

Several preoperative factors have been identified as contributing to a poor outcome following rotator cuff repair. These include older age, female sex, smoking, diabetes, longer duration of symptoms, preoperative disability, pseudoparalysis, size and shape of the tear, retraction of the tear, subscapularis tears, and atrophy and fatty infiltration of the muscle [36–40]. One must consider that the factors which portend a poor outcome for complete rotator cuff repairs may also be important determinants of outcomes in partial cuff repairs. Shon et al. identified fatty infiltration of the teres minor muscle, in particular, as a factor associated with worse outcomes following a partial rotator cuff repair [1]. This was confirmed by Godeneche and Barth [41], who found lower functional scores with higher stages of fatty infiltration (greater than Goutallier stage 1). These observations suggest that tears should be treated promptly, and may explain why repair of acute traumatic tears results in better outcomes than chronic degenerative tears [41–43].

Franceschi et al. identified acromiohumeral index (AHI) and patients' daily activity levels as factors predicting a poor outcome for partial repair [8]. They found that for patients with high activity levels or a preoperative AHI grade 2 or worse, that is, acromiohumerus interval of 5 mm or less, partial repair did not have any advantage when compared with debridement and acromioplasty.

Holtby et al. found that although advanced age is correlated with larger tear size, poorer tendon quality, and more U-shaped tears, age was not a predictor of whether a massive tear was amenable to complete or partial repair [44]. In that analysis, men and women were found to have an equal incidence of U-shaped tears, although men had more crescent-shaped tears while women had more L-shaped tears. Crescent-shaped tears had the best outcomes. One factor that did predict reparability was external rotation strength. Patients with stronger external rotation at neutral prior to surgery were significantly more likely to have a complete repair. Interestingly, neither active flexion nor abduction was a significant predictor. High subjective disability, lack of external rotation, poor tendon quality, larger tear size, and U-shaped tears were all associated with inability to achieve a full repair, thus resulting in a partial repair of the cuff. Both patients with partial repairs and full repair achieved significant gains in strength, ROM, and improvement in disability levels. However, those with partial repairs did have slightly higher levels of disability and had less improvement in functional scores at 2 years post-op [44].

There is some disagreement over whether the size of the rotator cuff tear has any bearing on outcome. Some authors argue that tear size does not affect final postoperative functional outcome or patient satisfaction [12, 19, 45, 46]. Others report that larger tears have worse functional outcomes and result in greater levels of disability following repair [47–50]. Godeneche et al. compared two-tendon tears with three tendon tears, and found lower Constant scores for the three-tendon tears. The net improvement in scores was the same, however, for all types of tears. These results are confirmed by Gerber and Bennett [51, 52].

Re-tear Rates

Recurrence of a rotator cuff tear, also known as a re-tear, may be categorized as early (within 6 months postoperatively) or late (at greater than 1 year). In one series, recurrence went from 34% at 3 years to 44% at 10 years postoperatively [43]. The rate at which a rotator cuff re-tears can be evaluated by MRI. Most studies have consistently reported the re-tear rate of partial rotator cuff repairs as ranging from 42 to 56%. This small variation may be due to differences in fatty infiltration and tear size [43]. The finding of a re-tear on MRI, however, does not necessarily correlate with clinical performance. Studies have found only a weak correlation between re-torn rotator cuff tendons and functional shoulder performance [15, 53, 54].

Other Treatment Options

There are several other treatment options that could be effective for the management of a massive irreparable tear. Tuberoplasty is a procedure that involves debriding and reshaping the proximal humerus, thereby establishing a new articulation between the acromion and humeral head. This was proposed by Fenlin et al., who found 95% satisfaction and 68% pain relief [55]. Lee et al. found significant improvements with Constant and UCLA shoulder scores with subacromial decompression and tuberoplasty [56]. Transfer of the latissimus dorsi tendon to the footprint of the rotator cuff has also been studied. Gerber et al. found a significant improvement in subjective shoulder and Constant scores with this procedure [57].

Weaknesses of the Data

There is no consensus as to the proper method for classifying rotator cuff tears. Cofield defined a massive rotator cuff tear as being >5 cm in length [13]. Gerber et al. used the definition of tears involving two or more tendons [27, 51, 58], while others only included tears of more than two tendons [16, 36, 43]. Henry et al. used a definition that includes both the size of the tear and the number of tendons (>3 cm in the coronal plane with complete detachment of both supraspinatus and infraspinatus tendons or >4 cm with complete detachment of one tendon) [51]. Given the varying definition of what constitutes a massive rotator cuff tear, there is low interobserver agreement with any classification system, other than distinguishing partial- from full-thickness tears [59]. This makes comparing results between studies very challenging.

Part of what may explain differences in studies regarding partial rotator cuff tears may also relate to differences in surgeon experience and skill [60]. There are also differences in technique, with some surgeons performing arthroscopic repairs, while others preferring an open exposure and repair. Other associated procedures, such as acromioplasty, distal clavicle excision, and biceps tenotomy/tenodesis, were also variably applied between studies, and could affect the results. Additionally, there are differences in postoperative rehabilitation protocols, with some utilizing relatively long periods of postoperative immobilization, while others advocating earlier active motion. It is not known what effect these differences may have had on the results.

Clinical Pearls/Pitfalls

- Fully inform patients of the difficulty in managing massive retracted rotator cuff tears. Some studies have demonstrated a suboptimal outcome regardless of treatment.
- In elderly low-demand patients or in patients who have significant medical comorbidities, be sure to exhaust all nonoperative measures prior to considering surgical intervention.
- Obtain a high-quality preoperative non-contrast MRI to determine the size of the tear, amount of retraction, and degree of atrophy and fatty infiltration. Be sure to evaluate the subscapularis and biceps tendons.
- Perform a thorough diagnostic shoulder arthroscopy to fully characterize the size and shape of the tear, amount of tendon retraction, amount of scarring, quality of the tendon tissue, and degree to which the torn edge of the cuff can be mobilized.
- Be sure to debride the edges of the tendon as well as the surrounding scar tissue so that the tendon can be mobilized laterally.
- Do not attempt to bring the torn edge of the rotator cuff tendon back to its anatomic footprint if doing so creates a significant amount of tension. A rotator cuff repaired under excessive tension is doomed to failure.
- If a complete repair cannot be performed, perform a margin convergence procedure by bringing together the anterior and posterior edges of the tear in a side-to-side fashion, followed by a partial rotator cuff repair, in which the remaining anterior and posterior edges of the tear are

brought to the articular margin of the greater tuberosity. Parts of the tear that cannot be repaired are left alone. Avoid any repairs that place the tendon under excessive tension.

- Following an initial diagnostic arthroscopy, I prefer to perform massive repairs through a longitudinal incision over the anterolateral acromion. Although some surgeons may prefer an all-arthroscopic approach, I find that an open approach allows better evaluation of the tear and removes any doubt with regard to the integrity of the final repair.
- Postoperatively, protect the patient in a sling for an initial 4–6 weeks followed by a supervised therapy program focused on reestablishing glenohumeral motion and eventual strengthening. Patients should be followed closely to track functional gains and to evaluate for possible re-tear.

References

1. Shon MS, et al. Arthroscopic partial repair of irreparable rotator cuff tears: preoperative factors associated with outcome deterioration over 2 years. Am J Sports Med. 2015;43(8):1965–75.
2. Dines DM, et al. Irreparable rotator cuff tears: what to do and when to do it; the surgeon's dilemma. J Bone Joint Surg Am. 2006;88(10):2294–302.
3. MacDonald PB, Altamimi S. Principles of arthroscopic repair of large and massive rotator cuff tears. Instr Course Lect. 2010;59:269–80.
4. Singh A, et al. Massive rotator cuff tears: arthroscopy to arthroplasty. Instr Course Lect. 2010;59:255–67.
5. Osti L, et al. Comparison of arthroscopic rotator cuff repair in healthy patients over and under 65 years of age. Knee Surg Sports Traumatol Arthrosc. 2010;18(12):1700–6.
6. Ostor AJ, et al. Diagnosis and relation to general health of shoulder disorders presenting to primary care. Rheumatology (Oxford). 2005;44(6):800–5.
7. Papalia R, et al. RC-QOL score for rotator cuff pathology: adaptation to Italian. Knee Surg Sports Traumatol Arthrosc. 2010;18(10):1417–24.

8. Franceschi F, et al. Operative management of partial- and full-thickness rotator cuff tears. Med Sport Sci. 2012;57:100–13.

9. Nakagaki K, et al. Fatty degeneration in the supraspinatus muscle after rotator cuff tear. J Shoulder Elb Surg. 1996;5(3):194–200.

10. Steinbacher P, et al. Effects of rotator cuff ruptures on the cellular and intracellular composition of the human supraspinatus muscle. Tissue Cell. 2010;42(1):37–41.

11. Godeneche A, et al. Should massive rotator cuff tears be reconstructed even when only partially repairable? Knee Surg Sports Traumatol Arthrosc. 2017;25(7):2164–73.

12. Burkhart SS, Danaceau SM, Pearce CE Jr. Arthroscopic rotator cuff repair: analysis of results by tear size and by repair technique-margin convergence versus direct tendon-to-bone repair. Arthroscopy. 2001;17(9):905–12.

13. Cofield RH. Rotator cuff disease of the shoulder. J Bone Joint Surg Am. 1985;67(6):974–9.

14. Galatz LM, et al. The outcome and repair integrity of completely arthroscopically repaired large and massive rotator cuff tears. J Bone Joint Surg Am. 2004;86-A(2):219–24.

15. Zingg PO, et al. Clinical and structural outcomes of nonoperative management of massive rotator cuff tears. J Bone Joint Surg Am. 2007;89(9):1928–34.

16. Zumstein MA, et al. The clinical and structural long-term results of open repair of massive tears of the rotator cuff. J Bone Joint Surg Am. 2008;90(11):2423–31.

17. Goutallier D, et al. Influence of cuff muscle fatty degeneration on anatomic and functional outcomes after simple suture of full-thickness tears. J Shoulder Elb Surg. 2003;12(6):550–4.

18. Bedi A, et al. Massive tears of the rotator cuff. J Bone Joint Surg Am. 2010;92(9):1894–908.

19. Burkhart SS, et al. Partial repair of irreparable rotator cuff tears. Arthroscopy. 1994;10(4):363–70.

20. Burkhart SS. Arthroscopic treatment of massive rotator cuff tears. Clinical results and biomechanical rationale. Clin Orthop Relat Res. 1991;267:45–56.

21. Wellmann M, et al. Results of arthroscopic partial repair of large retracted rotator cuff tears. Arthroscopy. 2013;29(8):1275–82.

22. Gerber C, et al. Effect of selective experimental suprascapular nerve block on abduction and external rotation strength of the shoulder. J Shoulder Elb Surg. 2007;16(6):815–20.

23. Burkhart SS. Partial repair of massive rotator cuff tears: the evolution of a concept. Orthop Clin North Am. 1997;28(1):125–32.

24. van der Zwaal P, et al. Arthroscopic side-to-side repair of massive and contracted rotator cuff tears using a single uninterrupted suture: the shoestring bridge technique. Arthroscopy. 2012;28(6):754–60.
25. Rousseau T, et al. Arthroscopic repair of large and massive rotator cuff tears using the side-to-side suture technique. Mid-term clinical and anatomic evaluation. Orthop Traumatol Surg Res. 2012;98(4 Suppl):S1–8.
26. Kim KC, et al. Repair integrity and functional outcomes for arthroscopic margin convergence of rotator cuff tears. J Bone Joint Surg Am. 2013;95(6):536–41.
27. Iagulli ND, et al. Comparison of partial versus complete arthroscopic repair of massive rotator cuff tears. Am J Sports Med. 2012;40(5):1022–6.
28. Porcellini G, et al. Partial repair of irreparable supraspinatus tendon tears: clinical and radiographic evaluations at long-term follow-up. J Shoulder Elb Surg. 2011;20(7):1170–7.
29. Wolf EM, Pennington WT, Agrawal V. Arthroscopic side-to-side rotator cuff repair. Arthroscopy. 2005;21(7):881–7.
30. Mazzocca AD, et al. Biomechanical evaluation of margin convergence. Arthroscopy. 2011;27(3):330–8.
31. Nove-Josserand L, et al. Open side-to-side repair for non-repairable tendon-to-bone rotator cuff tear. Clinical and anatomic outcome at a mean 5 years' follow-up. Orthop Traumatol Surg Res. 2015;101(7):819–22.
32. Duralde XA, Bair B. Massive rotator cuff tears: the result of partial rotator cuff repair. J Shoulder Elb Surg. 2005;14(2):121–7.
33. Hansen ML, et al. Biomechanics of massive rotator cuff tears: implications for treatment. J Bone Joint Surg Am. 2008;90(2):316–25.
34. Zvijac JE, Levy HJ, Lemak LJ. Arthroscopic subacromial decompression in the treatment of full thickness rotator cuff tears: a 3- to 6-year follow-up. Arthroscopy. 1994;10(5):518–23.
35. Moser M, et al. Functional outcome of surgically treated massive rotator cuff tears: a comparison of complete repair, partial repair, and debridement. Orthopedics. 2007;30(6):479–82.
36. Chung SW, et al. Arthroscopic repair of massive rotator cuff tears: outcome and analysis of factors associated with healing failure or poor postoperative function. Am J Sports Med. 2013;41(7):1674–83.
37. Denard PJ, et al. Pseudoparalysis: the importance of rotator cable integrity. Orthopedics. 2012;35(9):e1353–7.

38. Gerber C, et al. Correlation of atrophy and fatty infiltration on strength and integrity of rotator cuff repairs: a study in thirteen patients. J Shoulder Elb Surg. 2007;16(6):691–6.
39. Le BT, et al. Factors predicting rotator cuff retears: an analysis of 1000 consecutive rotator cuff repairs. Am J Sports Med. 2014;42(5):1134–42.
40. McElvany MD, et al. Rotator cuff repair: published evidence on factors associated with repair integrity and clinical outcome. Am J Sports Med. 2015;43(2):491–500.
41. Barth J, et al. Ultrasonic evaluation of the repair integrity can predict functional outcomes after arthroscopic double-row rotator cuff repair. Knee Surg Sports Traumatol Arthrosc. 2015;23(2):376–85.
42. Thes A, Hardy P, Bak K. Decision-making in massive rotator cuff tear. Knee Surg Sports Traumatol Arthrosc. 2012;23(2):449–59.
43. Heuberer PR, et al. Arthroscopic management of massive rotator cuff tears: an evaluation of debridement, complete, and partial repair with and without force couple restoration. Knee Surg Sports Traumatol Arthrosc. 2016;24(12):3828–37.
44. Holtby R, Razmjou H. Relationship between clinical and surgical findings and reparability of large and massive rotator cuff tears: a longitudinal study. BMC Musculoskelet Disord. 2014;15:180.
45. Baysal D, et al. Functional outcome and health-related quality of life after surgical repair of full-thickness rotator cuff tear using a mini-open technique. Am J Sports Med. 2005;33(9):1346–55.
46. Klepps S, et al. Prospective evaluation of the effect of rotator cuff integrity on the outcome of open rotator cuff repairs. Am J Sports Med. 2004;32(7):1716–22.
47. Kim SH, et al. Arthroscopic versus mini-open salvage repair of the rotator cuff tear: outcome analysis at 2 to 6 years' follow-up. Arthroscopy. 2003;19(7):746–54.
48. Prasad N, et al. Outcome of open rotator cuff repair. An analysis of risk factors. Acta Orthop Belg. 2005;71(6):662–6.
49. Oizumi N, et al. Massive rotator cuff tears repaired on top of humeral head by McLaughlin's procedure. J Shoulder Elb Surg. 2007;16(3):321–6.
50. Sugaya H, et al. Repair integrity and functional outcome after arthroscopic double-row rotator cuff repair. A prospective outcome study. J Bone Joint Surg Am. 2007;89(5):953–60.
51. Gerber C, Fuchs B, Hodler J. The results of repair of massive tears of the rotator cuff. J Bone Joint Surg Am. 2000;82(4):505–15.

52. Bennett WF. Arthroscopic repair of anterosuperior (supraspinatus/subscapularis) rotator cuff tears: a prospective cohort with 2- to 4-year follow-up. Classification of biceps subluxation/instability. Arthroscopy. 2003;19(1):21–33.
53. Ainsworth R. Physiotherapy rehabilitation in patients with massive, irreparable rotator cuff tears. Musculoskeletal Care. 2006;4(3):140–51.
54. Bokor DJ, et al. Results of nonoperative management of full-thickness tears of the rotator cuff. Clin Orthop Relat Res. 1993;294:103–10.
55. Fenlin JM Jr, et al. Tuberoplasty: creation of an acromiohumeral articulation-a treatment option for massive, irreparable rotator cuff tears. J Shoulder Elb Surg. 2002;11(2):136–42.
56. Lee BG, Cho NS, Rhee YG. Results of arthroscopic decompression and tuberoplasty for irreparable massive rotator cuff tears. Arthroscopy. 2011;27(10):1341–50.
57. Gerber C, Maquieira G, Espinosa N. Latissimus dorsi transfer for the treatment of irreparable rotator cuff tears. J Bone Joint Surg Am. 2006;88(1):113–20.
58. Fossati C, et al. How do massive immobile rotator cuff tears behave after arthroscopic interval slides? Comparison with mobile tears. Joints. 2014;2(2):66–70.
59. Kuhn JE, et al. Interobserver agreement in the classification of rotator cuff tears. Am J Sports Med. 2007;35(3):437–41.
60. Anakwenze OA, et al. Arthroscopic repair of large rotator cuff tears using the double-row technique: an analysis of surgeon experience on efficiency and outcomes. J Shoulder Elb Surg. 2013;22(1):26–31.

Chapter 20
Suprascapular Nerve Release with Rotator Cuff Tears

Erik M. Fritz, J. Christoph Katthagen, Robert E. Boykin, and Peter J. Millett

Abbreviations

EMG   Electromyography
NCV   Nerve conduction velocity
RC   Rotator cuff
SSN   Suprascapular neuropathy

E.M. Fritz, M.D.
Steadman Philippon Research Institute,
181 West Meadow Drive Suite 1000, Vail, CO 81657, USA

J.C. Katthagen, M.D.
Steadman Philippon Research Institute,
181 West Meadow Drive Suite 1000, Vail, CO 81657, USA

Department of Trauma, Hand, and Reconstructive Surgery,
Albert-Schweitzer-Campus 1, University Hospital Muenster,
Gebaeude W1, Muenster 48149, Germany

R.E. Boykin, M.D. • P.J. Millett, M.D., M.Sc. (✉)
Steadman Philippon Research Institute,
181 West Meadow Drive Suite 1000, Vail, CO 81657, USA

The Steadman Clinic, 181 West Meadow Drive Suite 400,
Vail, CO 81657, USA
e-mail: drmillett@thesteadmanclinic.com

© Springer International Publishing AG 2018
P.J. McMahon (ed.), *Rotator Cuff Injuries*,
DOI 10.1007/978-3-319-63668-9_20

Case 1

The patient is a 49-year-old right-hand-dominant female former professional tennis player with a history of right rotator cuff (RC) repair and biceps tenodesis 4 years prior to presentation. She did well postoperatively but developed increasing pain over a 1-year timeframe. She began to notice difficulty with serves and high backhands while increasing the amount of tennis she was playing. She was treated with physical therapy and a shoulder injection without significant improvement. Given her continued pain and difficulty with overhead activity she presented to our clinic for further evaluation.

On physical exam of the shoulder, the patient had tenderness of the acromioclavicular (AC) joint and positive impingement signs of Neer and Hawkins. She had full active and passive range of motion, but demonstrated weakness in her supraspinatus and infraspinatus muscles. No muscle atrophy was noted clinically.

Radiographs of the patient's right shoulder demonstrated some cystic changes of the greater tuberosity, AC joint arthritis, and minimal glenohumeral arthritis (Fig. 20.1). An MRI demonstrated a 4–6 mm intrasubstance partial tear of the midportion of the supraspinatus tendon adjacent to the greater tuberosity with an intact infraspinatus and no significant atrophy or fatty infiltration of the rotator cuff musculature (Fig. 20.2).

Diagnosis

The patient's imaging findings were consistent with the diagnosis of a small, partial recurrent supraspinatus tear; however, her weakness on physical exam and continued severe pain with overhead activity appeared out of proportion to her MRI findings. Therefore, the patient was sent for electromyography (EMG)/nerve conduction velocity studies (NCV) which demonstrated suprascapular nerve entrapment at the suprascapular notch along with mild cervical radiculopathy (Fig. 20.3). A cervical spine MRI demonstrated minimal

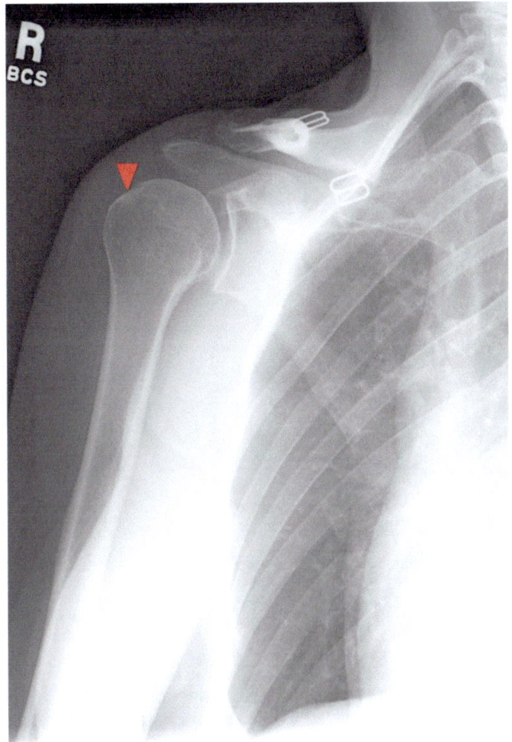

FIGURE 20.1 AP radiograph of the right shoulder showing cystic change of the greater tuberosity (*arrowhead*)

pathology and it was felt that the majority of the changes were due to suprascapular nerve compression.

Given the fact that she had previously undergone nonoperative management and was still experiencing pain and limited function, the patient elected to pursue revision surgery and arthroscopic suprascapular nerve decompression, distal clavicle excision, and intraoperative evaluation of the rotator cuff were recommended. It was felt that the majority of her symptoms were due to traction on the suprascapular nerve in the setting of repetitive overhead activity.

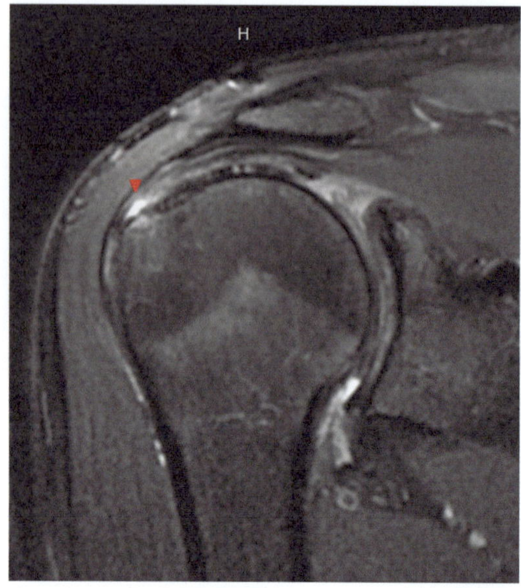

Figure 20.2 MRI of right shoulder showing a supraspinatus tear (*arrowhead*)

ELECTRODIAGNOSTIC RESULTS:

EMG

Side	Muscle	Nerve	Root	Ins Act	Fits	Psw	Amp	Dur	Poly	Recrt	Int Pat	Comment
Right	Pronator Teres	Medium	C6-7	Nml	Nml	Nml	Nml	Nml	0	Nml	Nml	
Right	Brachio Rad	Radial	C5-6	Nml	Nml	Nml	Nml	Nml	0	Nml	Nml	
Right	Biceps	Musculocul	C5-6	Nml	Nml	1+	Decr	>12ms	1+	Reduced	75%	
Right	Triceps	Radial	C6-7-8	Nml	Nml	Nml	Nml	Nml	0	Nml	Nml	
Right	Deltoid	Axillary	C5-6	Nml	Nml	Nml	Nml	Nml	0	Nml	Nml	
Right	Supraspinatus	SupraScap	C5-6	Nml	Nml	Nml	Decr	>12ms	1+	Reduced	75%	
Right	LevatorScap	DorsalScap	C3-5	Nml	1+	Nml	Nml	Nml	0	Reduced	75%	
Right	Infraspinatus	SupraScap	C5-6	Nml	Nml	2+	Decr	>12ms	2+	Reduced	50%	
Right	Rhomboid	DorsalScap	C5	Nml	Nml	Nml	Decr	Nml	2+	Reduced	75%	

Figure 20.3 EMG results. *Red* boxes indicate supraspinatus and infraspinatus muscle testing

Management

A standard posterior portal was used for initial diagnostic arthroscopy with the patient in the beach-chair position. This revealed multiple loose bodies in the glenohumeral joint, synovitis, and a focal full-thickness re-tear of the supraspinatus tendon (Fig. 20.4). Attention was then turned to release of the suprascapular nerve at the suprascapular notch. While viewing

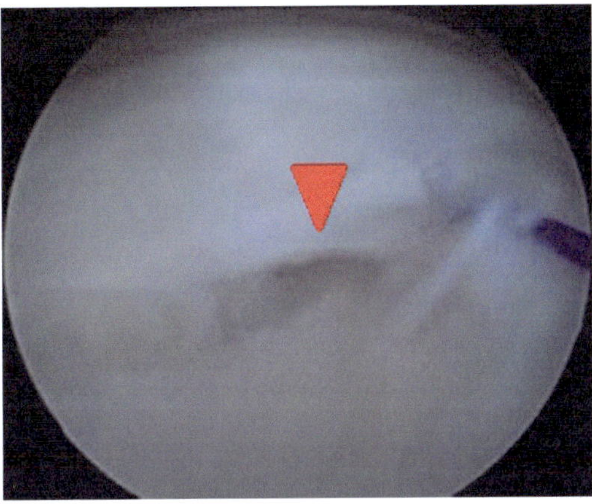

FIGURE 20.4 Arthroscopic posterior-portal view of full-thickness rotator cuff tear (*arrowhead*)

from a posterolateral portal and working from an anterolateral portal, the posterior aspect of the coracoid was identified as was the insertion of the coracoclavicular ligaments. The transverse scapular ligament was carefully identified medial to the conoid ligament and a portal slightly medial to the standard Nevasier accessory superior portal was created to allow an appropriate trajectory for release. The suprascapular artery was identified (running over the ligament) and protected. While the artery is typically not used as a landmark, it can be helpful for orientation. Carefully blunt dissection can prevent injury to the artery and at times branches may need to be cauterized with a radiofrequency device to improve visualization. While protecting the suprascapular nerve (running underneath the ligament), the transverse scapular ligament was resected using a meniscal biter (Fig. 20.5). The nerve was then inspected, which revealed no further compression. The RC repair was then performed arthroscopically using a single-suture anchor and two sutures placed in a simple configuration (Fig. 20.6).

Immediate postoperative rehabilitation included immobilization in a sling and early pendulums and passive range of motion. Active and active-assisted motions were permitted after 5 weeks with return to sport at 4 months.

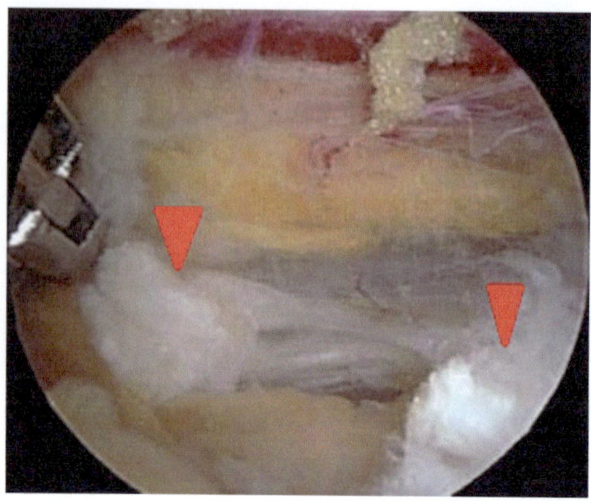

FIGURE 20.5 Arthroscopic view using meniscal biter to resect transverse scapular ligament (*arrowheads*)

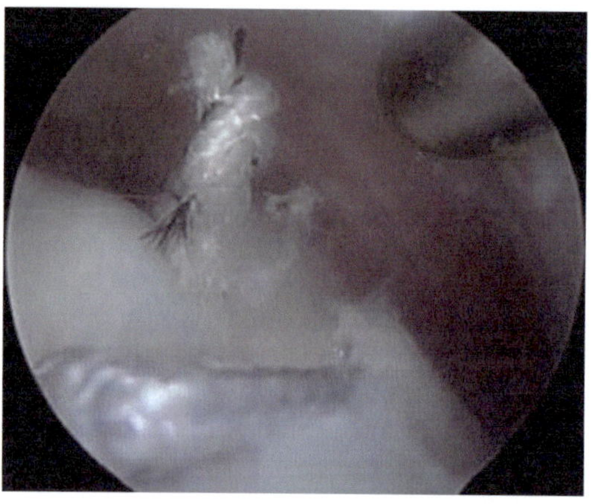

FIGURE 20.6 Arthroscopic view showing repaired rotator cuff

Outcome

The 49-year-old patient with suprascapular neuropathy (SSN) recovered successfully. At 5 weeks postoperatively, her strength had recovered to 4+ out of 5 in all ranges. At 4 months she had minimal further pain with restoration of strength and was allowed to return to tennis. At 10 years postoperatively, her SF-12 PCS score was 48.9, ASES score was 73.3, and DASH score was 27.2 (normative scores for age and gender as mean ± standard deviation 49.7 ± 9.9, 92.2 ± 14.5, and 12 ± 16, respectively) [1–3].

Case 2

The patient is a 60-year-old right-hand-dominant retired male with a history of multiple injuries to his left shoulder including a remote humeral and scapular fractures treated nonoperatively. Prior to presentation he sustained two falls on his left shoulder while skiing and reported that pain and weakness in the left shoulder worsened with external rotation and abduction. Through clinical exam and MRI imaging (Fig. 20.7) he was diagnosed with complete tears of the supraspinatus and infraspinatus without atrophy or fatty infiltration. He underwent arthroscopic repair at an outside facility.

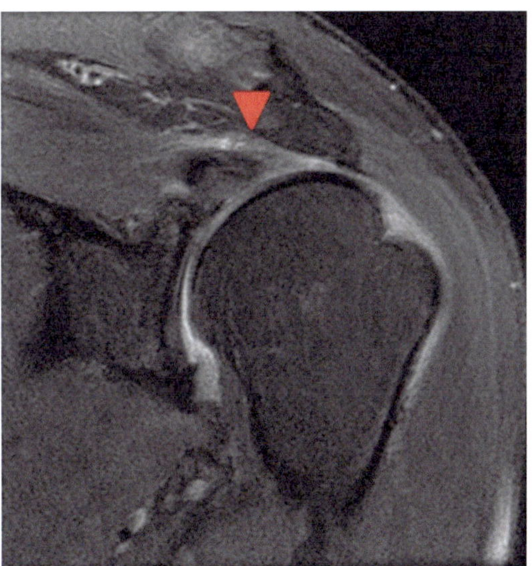

FIGURE 20.7 MRI of left shoulder demonstrating tear of the infraspinatus and supraspinatus (*arrowhead*) tendons with retraction

The patient's rehabilitation went well until approximately 3 months postoperatively when he again fell and hurt his shoulder. At that point, he presented to clinic with increasing shoulder pain. Physical exam of the left shoulder demonstrated a preserved range of motion; strength examination revealed −5/5 strength on external rotation and forward flexion. Radiographs were unchanged from the previous images. A repeat MRI demonstrated a 25% partial bursal tear of the infraspinatus with an intact repair otherwise. There was mild atrophy of the supraspinatus and mild-to-moderate atrophy of the infraspinatus muscles noted on the new imaging (Fig. 20.8). Due to his increasing pain in the setting of a predominately intact RC and some early findings of atrophy, the patient underwent EMG/NCV which demonstrated SSN at the suprascapular notch (Fig. 20.9).

Diagnosis

The patient's clinical course, examination, imaging studies, and EMG findings were consistent with the diagnosis of supra-

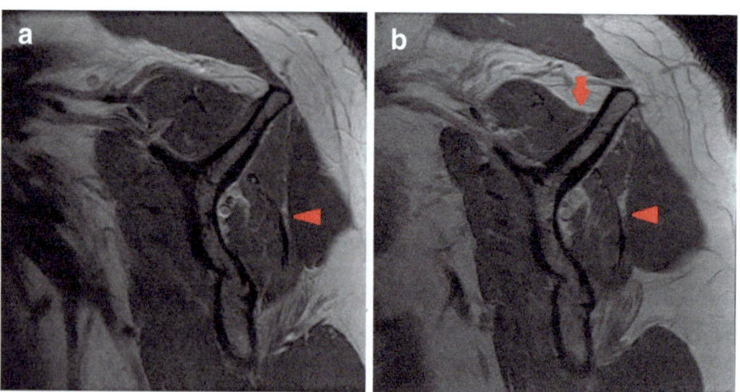

FIGURE 20.8 (**a**) Left-shoulder sagittal-view T1 MRI performed prior to first surgery demonstrating infraspinatus (*arrowhead*) without atrophy. (**b**) Left-shoulder sagittal-view T1 MRI performed following first surgery demonstrating infraspinatus (*arrowhead*) and supraspinatus (*arrow*) with atrophy

EMG

Side	Muscle	Nerve	Root	Ins Act	Fibs	Fascle	Psw	Amp	Dur	Poly	Recrt	Int Pat	Comment
Left	Biceps	Musculocul	C5-6	Nml	Nml	Nml	Nml	Nml	Nml	0	Nml	Nml	
Left	Triceps	Radial	C6-7-8	Nml	Nml	Nml	Nml	Nml	Nml	0	Nml	Nml	
Left	Pronator Teres	Medium	C6-7	Nml	Nml	Nml	Nml	Nml	Nml	0	Nml	Nml	
Left	IslDorini	Ulnar	C8-T1	Nml	Nml	Nml	Nml	Nml	Nml	0	Nml	Nml	
Left	Brachio Rad	Radial	C5-6	Nml	Nml	Nml	Nml	Nml	Nml	0	Nml	Nml	
Left	Deltoid	Axillary	C5-6	Nml	Nml	Nml	Nml	Nml	Nml	0	Nml	Nml	
Left	Supraspinatus	SupraScap	C5-6	Nml	Nml	Nml	Nml	Nml	>12ms	1+	Reduced	75%	
Left	Infraspinatus	SupraScap	C5-6	Nml	Nml	Nml	Nml	Incr	>12ms	1+	Reduced	75%	
Left	Teres Major	SubScap	C5-6	Nml	Nml	Nml	Nml	Nml	Nml	0	Nml	Nml	

FIGURE 20.9 EMG results. *Red* box indicates supraspinatus and infraspinatus muscle testing

scapular neuropathy in the setting of only mild recurrent RC pathology. The diagnosis and treatment options were discussed with the patient; he elected to pursue surgical management.

Management

A standard posterior portal was used for initial diagnostic arthroscopy with the patient in the beach-chair position. This revealed a healed RC, chronic biceps tendon rupture, and mild early glenohumeral arthritic changes. Following glenohumeral debridement and revision subacromial decompression, the suprascapular nerve release was performed at the suprascapular notch. Posterolateral (viewing) and anterolateral (working) portals were established. Dissection was carefully carried medially using a combination of a full-radius shaver and a radiofrequency ablation wand. The leading edge of the intact supraspinatus was followed medially to identify the posterior aspect of the coracoid. The posterior aspect of the conoid ligament was then identified and dissected to its insertion on the coracoid. At this level the transverse scapular ligament originates and runs medially across the notch forming an L-shape (or reverse L-shape depending on laterality) with the conoid ligament (Fig. 20.10). The suprascapular artery was identified (Fig. 20.11) followed by nerve running under the ligament.

Inspection of the suprascapular nerve revealed obvious entrapment; the nerve appeared flat within a stenotic suprascapular notch. For this case two additional suprascapular portals were created medially through the trape-

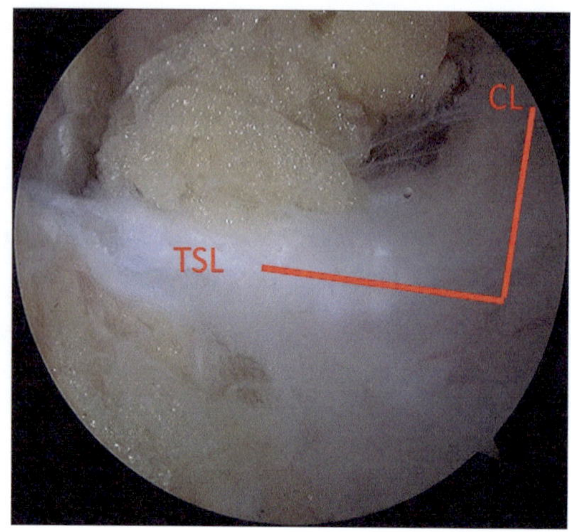

FIGURE 20.10 Arthroscopic image demonstrating the reverse L-shape created by the posterior aspect of the conoid ligament (CL) and transverse scapular ligament (TSL)

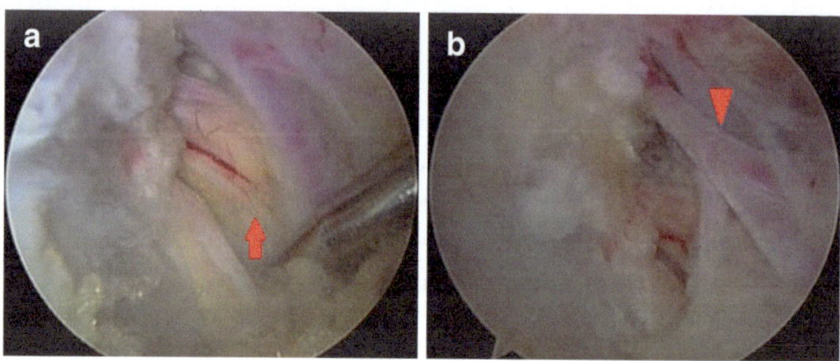

FIGURE 20.11 (**a** and **b**) Two views of the suprascapular artery (*arrowhead*), transverse scapular ligament, and suprascapular nerve (*arrow*)

zius. A switching stick was placed to protect the nerve while the ligament was released from the second medial portal. A neurolysis was then performed proximally and distally to the suprascapular notch so as to carefully free the nerve and prevent any additional tethering to the stenotic notch.

A subpectoral biceps tenodesis was performed for his chronic rupture.

For postoperative rehabilitation, the patient was allowed immediate pendulums and passive range of motion. Within a few days he was permitted to begin active and active-assisted motion and weaned out of the sling.

Outcome

The 60-year-old patient with a history of a rotator cuff repair and increasing pain, mild weakness, and atrophy after a fall recovered quite well. At 3 months postoperatively, he had regained full range of motion and strength in his shoulder. As of 3 years postoperatively, his SF-12 PCS score was 47, ASES score was 94.9, and DASH score was 11.3 (normative scores for age and gender as mean ± standard deviation 51.4 ± 7.3, 92.2 ± 14.5, and 11 ± 16, respectively) [1–3].

Literature Review

In cases of isolated suprascapular neuropathy (SSN) not due to space-occupying lesions, it is generally accepted that the best initial treatment is nonoperative management [4]. However, in cases of SSN secondary to a RC tear, the role of surgical intervention is far less clear. This is partly due to lack of consensus with diagnosis. The prevalence of SSN among massive RC tears has been reported to range between 2 and 60.5% [5, 6]. Collin et al. note that this range is due to inaccuracy and variability in EMG results, lack of EMG validation, and absence of definitive EMG diagnostic criteria. Given the unclear diagnostic criteria and prevalence, it is not surprising that studies in optimal management of SSN with RC tears are lacking.

Some authors have demonstrated resolution of SSN with isolated RC repair without concomitant suprascapular nerve release [7, 8]. Because of these findings, along with the widely varying prevalence, some authors recommend avoiding routine release of the transverse scapular ligament along with rotator cuff repair if the cuff can be adequately repaired [6–8]. The thought process is that the nerve injury is created by traction on the nerve as the RC retracts medially where the nerve can be tethered. This is then resolved with reduction of the tendon.

There is a considerable scarcity of data in the orthopedic literature regarding the outcomes for treatment of SSN secondary to traction from RC tears; only a few case series are available. Costouros et al. [7] reported on seven patients with SSN in the setting of massive RC tear with associated retraction and fatty infiltration of the supraspinatus and infraspinatus. SSN was confirmed with EMG/NCV. Of these seven RC tears, six were repairable arthroscopically, either with complete or partial repair. In all six of these patients, 6-month follow-up demonstrated pain relief, functional improvement, and EMG/NCV-confirmed partial recovery in two patients and full recovery in four patients of the SSN.

Mallon et al. [8] reported on eight patients with EMG-confirmed SSN associated with massive RC tear. Of these eight patients, four underwent partial surgical repair. All four patients demonstrated significant improvement in function at mean follow-up of 24 months; two consented to follow-up EMG studies which revealed significant SSN recovery.

In patients who present with pain after a prior rotator cuff repair, SSN should be considered on the differential. Symptoms can include pain which is typically posterosuperior and weakness in forward flexion and/or external rotation. Atrophy and/or fatty infiltration of the muscle belly can be seen on CT or MRI (most easily visualized on sagittal T1 images). In both of the cases presented above, the severity of the recurrent RC injury did not seem to warrant the amount of pain and weakness seen clinically. EMG/NCV studies were used to confirm the diagnosis of SSN. When these are ordered the surgeon should specifically ask for evaluation of the suprascapular nerve and these must carefully be interpreted to identity the location of injury either at the suprascapular notch or at the spinoglenoid notch. Release should be considered in refractory cases and can be accomplished safely with an arthroscopic approach at either location. Care must be taken to thoroughly evaluate the morphology of the suprascapular or spinoglenoid notch on preoperative imaging to assess for ossification, which is more commonly seen in the transverse scapular ligament. Instruments for resection (typically Kerrison type rongeurs or small osteotomes) should be readily available.

Clinical Pearls/Pitfalls

- Though the prevalence is low, suprascapular nerve injury is an important condition to recognize since surgical correction can result in marked functional improvement for patients.
- If suprascapular neuropathy is present with a retracted RC tear, RC repair alone will resolve the SSN in a majority of patients by correcting the traction on the nerve.
- If SSN is present following RC repair with an intact repair, surgical decompression of the nerve may be warranted.
- The location of the suprascapular nerve lesion should be elucidated preoperatively through electrodiagnostic studies to determine whether the nerve is entrapped at the suprascapular notch or at the spinoglenoid notch.
- When performing a release at the suprascapular notch it is important to identify the posterior aspect of the conoid ligament and carefully proceed medially with blunt dissection to identify the transverse scapular ligament.
- At the level of the suprascapular notch the artery typically runs over the transverse ligament and the nerve below.
- When performing a release at the spinoglenoid notch there may be a variable presence and thickness of the spinoglenoid ligament, which is less consistent than the transverse scapular ligament. The nerve can be carefully identified as it proceeds around the base of the scapular spine.
- Postoperative management includes immobilization in a sling for comfort; early motion is encouraged. Strengthening,

throwing, and overhead activities are typically based on concomitant pathology treated at the time of surgery [9].

References

1. Aasheim T, Finsen V. The DASH and QuickDASH instruments. Normative values in the general population in Norway. J Hand Surg Eur Vol. 2014;39(2):140–144.
2. Mols F, Pelle AJ, Kupper N. Normative data of the SF-12 health survey with validation using postmyocardial infarction patients in the Dutch population. Qual Life Res. 2009;18(4):403–14.
3. Sallay PI, Reed L. The measurement of normative American Shoulder and Elbow Surgeon scores. J Shoulder Elb Surg. 2003;12(6):622–7.
4. Martin SD, Warren RF, Martin TL, Kennedy K, O'Brien SJ, Wickiewicz TL. Suprascapular neuropathy. Results of non-operative treatment. J Bone Joint Surg Am. 1997;79(8):1159–65.
5. Boykin RE, Friedman DJ, Zimmer ZR, Oaklander AL, Higgins LD, Warner JJ. Suprascapular neuropathy in a shoulder referral practice. J Shoulder Elb Surg. 2011;20(6):983–8.
6. Collin P, Treseder T, Lädermann A, Benkalfate T, Mourtada R, Courage O, Favard L. Neuropathy of the suprscapular nerve and massive rotator cuff tears: a prospective electromyographic study. J Shoulder Elb Surg. 2014;23(1):28–34.
7. Costouros JG, Porramatikul M, Lie DT, Warner JJ. Reversal of suprascapular neuropathy following arthroscopic repair of massive supraspinatus and infraspinatus rotator cuff tears. Arthroscopy. 2007;23(11):1152–61.
8. Mallon WJ, Wilson RJ, Basamania CJ. The association of suprascapular neuropathy with massive rotator cuff tears: a preliminary report. J Shoulder Elb Surg. 2006;15(4):395–8.
9. Millett PJ, Barton RS, Pacheco IH, Gobezie R. Suprascapular nerve entrapment: technique for arthroscopic release. Tech Should Elb Surg. 2006;7(2):89–94.

Chapter 21
Redo Rotator Cuff Repair

Edward G. McFarland, Seyedali R. Ghasemi, and Alexander Bitzer

Case Presentation

A 56-year-old woman presented to the office with a 10-year history of right, dominant shoulder pain, loss of motion, and loss of function after treatment for injuries sustained 10 years prior to the evaluation. Her first injury was at the age of 46 years, when she fell at work, sustaining a, full-thickness tear of her supraspinatus tendon. Through imaging and subsequent arthroscopic rotator cuff repair the tear was discovered to be full-thickness involvement of the supraspinatus, which was 3 by 1 cm. After repair, she continued to have pain and loss of motion so, at the urging of her physical therapist, she underwent a repeat MRI, which demonstrated a full-thickness retracted tear of the supraspinatus tendon. She underwent immediate repeat arthroscopic partial rotator cuff repair

E.G. McFarland, M.D. (✉) • S.R. Ghasemi, M.D. • A. Bitzer, M.D.
Division of Surgery, Department of Orthopaedic Surgery,
The Johns Hopkins University, Baltimore, MD, USA
e-mail: emcfarl1@jhmi.edu; samirghasemi@yahoo.com;
abitzer1@jhmi.edu

© Springer International Publishing AG 2018
P.J. McMahon (ed.), *Rotator Cuff Injuries*,
DOI 10.1007/978-3-319-63668-9_21

of the supraspinatus tendon because complete repair was not possible. She also had a biceps tenodesis and a distal clavicle excision. Postoperatively she had some mild drainage from one portal successfully treated with oral antibiotics and local wound care. She continued to have pain and loss of motion and was unable to return to work. Another MRI demonstrated a retracted tear of the supraspinatus tendon and the upper infraspinatus tendons (Fig. 21.1). She subsequently underwent an arthroscopic repair with dermal grafting material. She failed to regain her motion and continued to have pain and loss of function. Radiographs demonstrated a high-riding humeral head with moderate arthritic changes (Fig. 21.2). Repeat MRI showed what appeared to be an intact grafting material of a couple millimeters thick, a slight effusion, significant atrophy of her supraspinatus and infraspinatus muscles, and thickening of the inferior capsule consistent

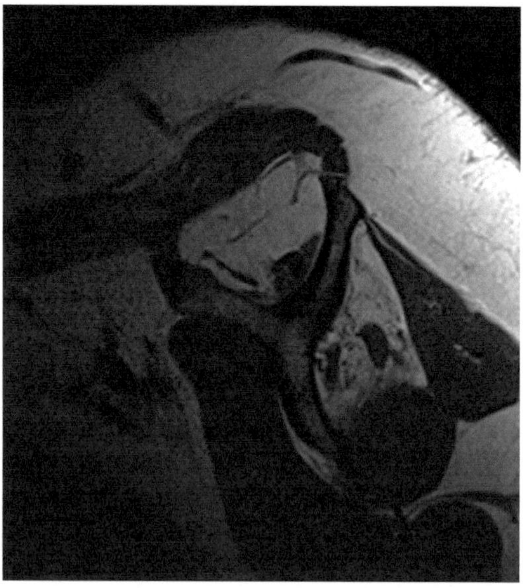

FIGURE 21.1 Sagittal view of an MRI of the shoulder showing muscle atrophy and fatty replacement of the supraspinatus and infraspinatus

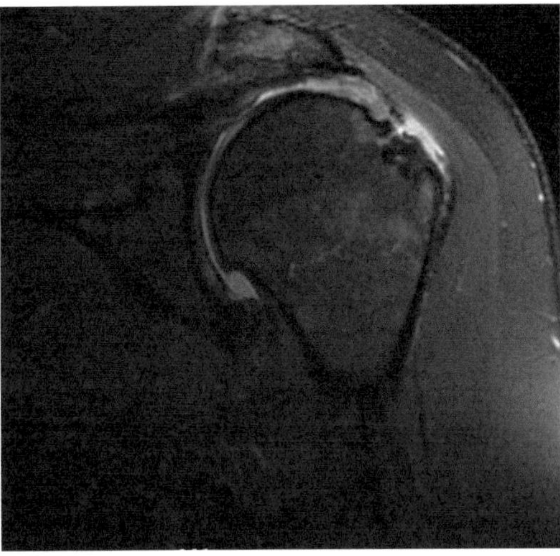

FIGURE 21.2 Oblique coronal view of the left-shoulder MRI showing torn and retracted rotator cuff tendon

with adhesive capsulitis. Upon presentation she was clearly unhappy with her shoulder pain, weakness, loss of motion, and loss of function. She had pain at night and a constant ache in the shoulder. She was on permanent disability but wanted a functioning shoulder. Upon examination, she had global stiffness with loss of 30° compared with the other side for elevation and all other rotations. She had "endpoint pain" in that, when she reached the extremes of motion, most of her pain was reproduced. She was weak, with 3/5 strength in elevation, 4/5 strength in internal rotation, and 2/5 strength in external rotation and a positive external rotation lag sign. She was neurologically intact.

Diagnosis/Assessment

For patients who have had multiple surgeries, it is particularly important to obtain a good history, paying special attention to complications and to why the pain has not been alleviated.

Similarly, the physical examination of this patient needs to be meticulous to understand what is contributing the most to her pain. The most concerning aspect of this patient's history was the presence of wound drainage, so it is critical to evaluate for erythema, warmth, swelling, and drainage. Laboratory studies such as white blood cell count (WBC), sedimentation rate, and C-reactive protein should be obtained. MRI scanning can also be helpful in the assessment because, in addition to characteristics of the rotator cuff tear, findings of effusion, bone edema, soft-tissue edema, or debris in the joint are indicative of infection. Typically, patients who have a previous infection after rotator cuff repair will have little tendon tissue remaining to repair [1]. If there are concerns about infection, the patient should undergo repeat arthroscopic debridement, removal of anchor and suture material if possible, and intravenous antibiotics. Re-repair should not be attempted at the time of debridement, and decisions about re-repair can be made after the infection is cleared. However, in our experience, typically in patients with infections after rotator cuff surgery, the rotator cuff tendons cannot be repaired. Instead, it is imperative to diminish the patient's stiffness.

The other confounding issue in this patient is the role of stiffness in her pain. It is important to establish whether the loss of motion is due to neural causes or not, so questioning the patient about paresthesias and neck pain is important. Similarly, the physical examination should include a complete neurological examination. The most commonly injured nerves with rotator cuff repair surgery are the axillary nerve and the musculocutaneous nerve. However, there can rarely be a brachial plexopathy caused by traction from arm suspension used in surgery or from regional anesthesia, specifically an interscalene block.

Evaluating the range of motion in a patient whose previous surgery has failed can be challenging if there is pain. If the patient has a large shrug sign [2] or a positive drop-arm sign [3], it is important to determine whether these are due to stiffness, pain, or mechanical problems with the shoulder.

When testing range of motion, typically the patient is asked to perform the motions actively, such as elevation in flexion or abduction in the plane of the scapula. Often, patients will attempt to elevate their arms, which they proceed to do in the plane of their body with their thumbs down. This maneuver will undoubtedly produce less-than-normal motion, especially if the patient has secondary gain. In some patients, range of motion can be tested better with the patients supine because gravity is eliminated. If the patient's active and passive motions are similarly diminished, then frozen shoulder, osteoarthritis, fixed glenohumeral dislocation, or avascular necrosis should be considered.

If the patient has not had a distal clavicle excision, the acromioclavicular (AC) joint should also be tested for signs of inflammation. Local tenderness of the AC joint is the most important test but the active-compression test, cross-arm adduction stress test, and the arm-extension test have all been shown to be helpful in localizing pain to the AC joint [4, 5].

Lastly, the patient should be examined to determine the extent of rotator cuff injury. The supraspinatus can be tested with resisted abduction and the infraspinatus with resisted external rotation at the side. The patient should be tested for an external rotation lag sign, which is performed with the arm at the side and the elbow bent 90°. The arm is externally rotated to the maximum and then internally rotated a few degrees. The patient is asked to hold the arm in that position, and if they cannot, the arm falls into internal rotation, then the patient has involvement of the supraspinatus and infraspinatus tendons.

The integrity of the subscapularis tendon should also be evaluated in several ways. The first is increased external rotation of the shoulder on the side with the subscapularis tear. The second is the liftoff test, in which the patient is asked to lift the arm off the back; inability to do this is a positive test [6]. A liftoff lag sign is also very helpful for determining integrity of the subscapularis tendon [7]. In this test, the patient places the arm in internal rotation up the back, and the examiner then lifts the hand off the back and asks the patient to hold it there. A positive test is when the arm falls to the back or the elbow falls into extension, and this means that the subscapularis tendon also is irreparable.

This series of examinations should give the examiner a good sense of what can be achieved with an individual patient. Imaging should be performed, beginning with plain radiographs, including a true anterior-posterior radiograph (i.e., Grashey view) [8] of the shoulder, an anterior-posterior view in internal rotation, and an axillary view. A scapular Y view does not add much to the evaluation because it is neither reliable nor reproducible and has been shown to have no effect on the clinical result [9]. A plain radiograph with superior humeral head subluxation or with erosion of the acromion and greater tuberosity suggests that the rotator cuff tear is long-standing and irreparable [10]. It is important to look for spurs consistent with osteoarthritis and for joint space narrowing, because cartilage loss may be contributing to the patient's pain and limited motion.

MRI can be helpful to confirm the integrity of the tendons and, in the case of rotator cuff tears, the size of the tear. Multiple studies have confirmed that the best predictor of rotator cuff surgery is the size of the rotator cuff tear [11–13]. Muscle atrophy has also been shown to be a negative prognostic sign for success of rotator cuff surgery [11] (Fig. 21.3). MRI also can demonstrate edema in the bone or soft tissues, which might suggest infection; however, edema in the muscles can be seen after acute injury or with Parsonage-Turner syndrome [14].

In this patient, blood work would be helpful to rule out infection. Although the WBC is usually normal, if the sedimentation rate and C-reactive protein level are elevated, then aspiration of the shoulder could be considered. Long-standing infections of the glenohumeral joint are often accompanied by glenohumeral arthritis due to destruction of the cartilage by the infection. In a chronically infected shoulder, MRI can also show edema in the humeral head, debris in

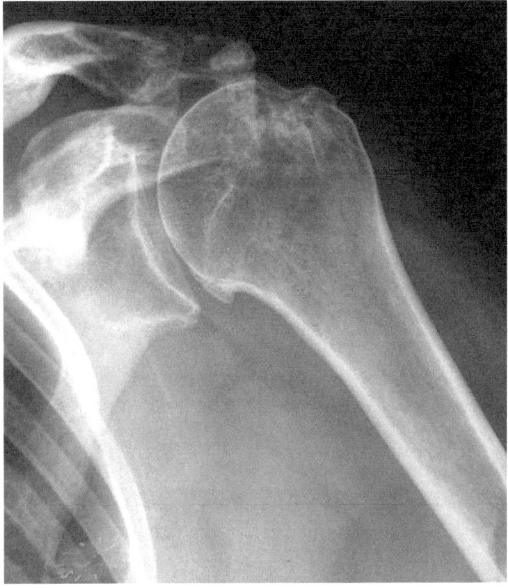

FIGURE 21.3 Plain radiograph showing anterior-posterior view of the shoulder with a high-riding humeral head, wear of the greater tuberosity, and moderate glenohumeral joint arthritis

the joint, lymph node enlargement, joint effusion, and diffuse muscle edema [15].

Plain radiographs of our patient revealed a small spur on the humeral head but no glenohumeral joint-space narrowing. There was narrowing of the humeral head to acromial distance of 3 mm. Her WBC count, C-reactive protein level, and sedimentation rate were normal, and an aspiration of her shoulder was negative for cultures over 15 days. Her MRI showed tendon retraction of the supraspinatus and infraspinatus to the glenoid with atrophy and grade III–IV fatty infiltration of the muscles (grade III begins equal fat and muscle and grade IV begins more fat than muscle) using the system of Goutallier [16, 17]. The MRI showed no signs of chronic infection and only mild osteoarthritis of the glenohumeral joint.

Management

The patient was treated without surgery using a program that included changing her expectations, avoiding things that aggravated her shoulder, cryotherapy, daily range-of-motion exercises, judicious use of NSAIDs, and occasional intra-articular cortisone injections.

Outcome

She regained function of the shoulder for activities of daily living but was weak when using the arm overhead and away from her body. She retired and settled with her employer for work-related injuries. Ten years later, at last follow-up, she had nearly full range of motion and little pain. She was anticipating shoulder replacement in the future but her shoulder was not painful enough to warrant surgery.

Literature Review

Decision making for any patient with a rotator cuff tear, whether recurrent or not, involves many factors. The major variables shown to determine the success or failure of rotator cuff surgery are the size of the rotator cuff tear and the patient's age [18–20]. Another factor that should be considered is whether the patient has pain; it is difficult to rationalize an operation with limited success when the patient has no pain. Whether it is the dominant side can be a consideration, with less compelling need for operating on a nondominant shoulder. The degree to which the patient has limitation of function, including activities of daily living, also is a factor. The goals of the patient in terms of returning to work or sport should be considered but the patient should have realistic expectations of what can be accomplished with further surgery. The health of the patient is an important consideration; in patients for whom an operation is risky such as patients with American Society of Anesthesiologists (ASA) classification of 3 or 4, the risk of death for better shoulder function requires special counseling and considerations.

The last consideration for repeat surgery in patients with failed rotator cuff repair is the natural history of rotator cuff disease, especially in the face of failed previous surgeries. The success rate of surgery for failed rotator cuff repair has been found to be acceptable for pain relief but not function [21]. The re-tear rate (or perhaps the lack of healing rate) after surgery for large-to-massive rotator cuff tears has been reported to be 30% to 95% [22, 23]; a patient should be informed of these rates before any surgical treatment of the rotator cuff, especially if they have had multiple failed operations.

The patient should be counseled that the natural history of rotator cuff surgery is not entirely known. Although many patients believe that their shoulders are doomed with torn rotator cuff tendons, the reality is that many can be functional with some limitations. Gerber et al. evaluated 19 patients with massive rotator cuff tears for 4 years and found little progression of their degenerative changes [24]. Another study found that rotator cuff repair does not prevent the progression of rotator cuff pathology over time [25]. When considering surgery, patients should know that degeneration of the shoulder is not certain, and surgery is the last resort.

The main goal for the patient with multiple failed rotator cuff surgeries is to manage the existing pathologies, which can include stiffness, arthritis, biceps tendon pathologies, and wear of the tuberosity against the acromion and AC joint. In our experience, the most common symptom in patients with multiple failed surgeries is stiffness. A program to improve their range of motion should include cryotherapy, medication for pain relief, physical therapy, a home-stretching program, and injections of corticosteroids. The patient should ice the shoulder as often as needed for pain control, after any stretching session, after physical therapy, prior to before bedtime, and whenever the pain is severe. Cryotherapy is an inexpensive treatment and can be applied easily by most patients. Medication should include acetaminophen, nonsteroidal anti-inflammatory drugs, glucosamine with or without chondroitin sulfate, and pain medication. Physical therapy should emphasize range of motion until full motion is attained. A twice-a-week program of physical therapy appears to create less stress and inflammation than three or more times a week. A home pulley program of stretching is recommended on the days when the patient is not seeing the physical therapist.

Oral corticosteroids can be very effective in these patients. There is no known limit to the number of oral steroid tapers that can be prescribed over time but judicious use is recommended. Often, oral corticosteroids will allow the patient to make major gains in motion. Intra-articular injections have also been shown to be effective in the treatment of stiffness [26]. Although damage to the cartilage with repeated injections is a hypothetical concern, the risk is usually less than the risk of continued pain and loss of motion.

Lastly, examination of the shoulder under anesthesia with closed manipulation can be attempted. Diagnostic arthroscopy can also be performed to evaluate the status of the articular cartilage and the biceps tendon if it is present. Then, if needed, debridement of the articular cartilage lesions and extensive bursectomy along with release of adhesions may be effective. After surgery, the patient should undergo a program similar to the one described previously.

For patients who have undergone multiple failed surgeries, there are no good options regarding re-repair of the tendons. Although some surgeons contend that all rotator cuff tears can be repaired, that has not been our experience [27]. To our knowledge, there is no surgical option currently available that will alleviate the pain and restore normal function to the shoulder. In patients seeking disability benefits or those involved in worker's compensation claims, the goals of surgery should be weighed carefully against the final disposition of the patient; some will not return to work with or without surgery. Other surgical options include tendon transfers and reverse total shoulder arthroplasty.

Clinical Pearls/Pitfalls

- Patients with multiple failed rotator cuff surgeries should be evaluated very carefully for other pathologies contributing to their pain, including biceps tendon pathologies, stiffness, arthritis, and infection.
- Stiffness is a common cause of continued pain and disability in patients with multiple failed rotator cuff surgeries.
- A multi-modality approach can often provide these patients with improved motion and function without surgery.
- Most surgical options in this population will not result in a completely pain-free and normally functioning shoulder. Surgery, including repair, tendon transfers, and hemiarthroplasty, should be performed with complete understanding of the goals and possible outcomes.
- Currently, the final surgical solution for patients after multiple failed rotator cuff surgeries is reverse total shoulder arthroplasty but the limitations, complications, and uncertain long-term results warrant caution.

References

1. Mirzayan R, Itamura JM, Vangsness CT Jr, Holtom PD, Sherman R, Patzakis MJ. Management of chronic deep infection following rotator cuff repair. J Bone Joint Surg Am. 2000;82-A(8):1115–21.
2. Jia X, Ji JH, Petersen SA, Keefer J, McFarland EG. Clinical evaluation of the shoulder shrug sign. Clin Orthop Relat Res. 2008;466(11):2813–9. doi:10.1007/s11999-008-0331-3. Epub 2008 Jun 10
3. van Kampen DA, van den Berg T, van der Woude HJ, Castelein RM, Scholtes VA, Terwee CB, Willems WJ. The diagnostic value of the combination of patient characteristics, history, and clinical shoulder tests for the diagnosis of rotator cuff tear. J Orthop Surg Res. 2014;9:70. doi:10.1186/s13018-014-0070-y.
4. O'Brien SJ, Pagnani MJ, Fealy S, McGlynn SR, Wilson JB. The active compression test: a new and effective test for diagnosing labral tears and acromioclavicular joint abnormality. Am J Sports Med. 1998;26(5):610–3.

5. Chronopoulos E, Kim TK, Park HB, Ashenbrenner D, McFarland EG. Diagnostic value of physical tests for isolated chronic acromioclavicular lesions. Am J Sports Med. 2004;32(3):655–61.

6. Bartsch M, Greiner S, Haas NP, Scheibel M. Diagnostic values of clinical tests for subscapularis lesions. Knee Surg Sports Traumatol Arthrosc. 2010;18(12):1712–7. doi:10.1007/s00167-010-1109-1. Epub 2010 Apr 8

7. Yoon JP, Chung SW, Kim SH, Oh JH. Diagnostic value of four clinical tests for the evaluation of subscapularis integrity. J Shoulder Elb Surg. 2013;22(9):1186–92. doi:10.1016/j.jse.2012.12.002. Epub 2013 Feb 20

8. Koh KH, Han KY, Yoon YC, Lee SW, Yoo JC. True anteroposterior (Grashey) view as a screening radiograph for further imaging study in rotator cuff tear. J Shoulder Elb Surg. 2013;22(7):901–7. doi:10.1016/j.jse.2012.09.015. Epub 2013 Jan 10

9. Liotard JP, Cochard P, Walch G. Critical analysis of the supraspinatus outlet view: rationale for a standard scapular Y-view. J Shoulder Elb Surg. 1998;7(2):134–9.

10. Hamada K, Fukuda H, Mikasa M, Kobayashi Y. Roentgenographic findings in massive rotator cuff tears. A long-term observation. Clin Orthop Relat Res. 1990;254:92–6.

11. Harryman DT 2nd, Mack LA, Wang KY, Jackins SE, Richardson ML, Matsen FA 3rd. Repairs of the rotator cuff. Correlation of functional results with integrity of the cuff. J Bone Joint Surg Am. 1991;73(7):982–9.

12. Lädermann A, Denard PJ, Burkhart SS. Management of failed rotator cuff repair: a systematic review. J ISAKOS. 2016;1(1):32–7. Epub 2016 Jan 21

13. Collin P, Abdullah A, Kherad O, Gain S, Denard PJ, Lädermann A. Prospective evaluation of clinical and radiologic factors predicting return to activity within 6 months after arthroscopic rotator cuff repair. J Shoulder Elb Surg. 2015;24(3):439–45. doi:10.1016/j.jse.2014.08.014. Epub 2014 Oct 16

14. Monteiro Dos Santos RB, Dos Santos SM, Carneiro Leal FJ, Lins OG, Magalhães C, Mertens Fittipaldi RB. Parsonage-turner syndrome. Rev Bras Ortop. 2015;50(3):336–41. doi:10.1016/j.rboe.2015.04.002. eCollection 2015 May–Jun

15. Sperling JW, Potter HG, Craig EV, Flatow E, Warren RF. Magnetic resonance imaging of painful shoulder arthroplasty. J Shoulder Elb Surg. 2002;11(4):315–21.

16. Fuchs B, Weishaupt D, Zanetti M, Hodler J, Gerber C. Fatty degeneration of the muscles of the rotator cuff: assessment by computed tomography versus magnetic resonance imaging. J Shoulder Elbow Surg. 1999;8(6):599–605.
17. Goutallier D, Postel JM, Bernageau J, Lavau L, Voisin MC. Fatty muscle degeneration in cuff ruptures. Pre- and postoperative evaluation by CT scan. Clin Orthop Relat Res. 1994;304:78–83.
18. Keener JD. Revision rotator cuff repair. Clin Sports Med. 2012;31(4):713–25. doi:10.1016/j.csm.2012.07.007. Epub 2012 Sep 1. Review
19. Liem D, Lichtenberg S, Magosch P, Habermeyer P. Magnetic resonance imaging of arthroscopic supraspinatus tendon repair. J Bone Joint Surg Am. 2007;89(8):1770–6. doi:10.2106/JBJS.F.00749.
20. Liem D, Buschmann VE, Schmidt C, Gosheger G, Vogler T, Schulte TL, Balke M. The prevalence of rotator cuff tears: is the contralateral shoulder at risk? Am J Sports Med. 2014;42(4):826–30. doi:10.1177/0363546513519324. Epub 2014 Feb 5. PMID: 24500916
21. DeOrio JK, Cofield RH. Results of a second attempt at surgical repair of a failed initial rotator-cuff repair. J Bone Joint Surg Am. 1984;66(4):563–7.
22. Galatz LM, Ball CM, Teefey SA, Middleton WD, Yamaguchi K. The outcome and repair integrity of completely arthroscopically repaired large and massive rotator cuff tears. J Bone Joint Surg Am. 2004;86-A(2):219–24.
23. Paxton ES, Teefey SA, Dahiya N, Keener JD, Yamaguchi K, Galatz LM. Clinical and radiographic outcomes of failed repairs of large or massive rotator cuff tears: minimum ten-year follow-up. J Bone Joint Surg Am. 2013;95(7):627–32. doi:10.2106/JBJS.L.00255.
24. Zingg PO, Jost B, Sukthankar A, Buhler M, Pfirrmann CW, Gerber C. Clinical and structural outcomes of nonoperative management of massive rotator cuff tears. J Bone Joint Surg Am. 2007;89(9):1928–34. doi:10.2106/JBJS.F.01073.
25. Gladstone JN, Bishop JY, Lo IK, Flatow EL. Fatty infiltration and atrophy of the rotator cuff do not improve after rotator cuff repair and correlate with poor functional outcome. Am J Sports Med. 2007;35(5):719–28. Epub 2007 Mar 2
26. Jacobs LG, Smith MG, Khan SA, Smith K, Joshi M. Manipulation or intra-articular steroids in the management of adhesive capsulitis

of the shoulder? A prospective randomized trial. J Shoulder Elb Surg. 2009;18(3):348–53. doi:10.1016/j.jse.2009.02.002.
27. Lädermann A, Denard PJ, Burkhart SS. Midterm outcome of arthroscopic revision repair of massive and nonmassive rotator cuff tears. Arthroscopy. 2011;27(12):1620–7. doi:10.1016/j.arthro.2011.08.290. Epub 2011 Oct 29

Chapter 22
Nonoperative Treatment of Rotator Cuff Tears

John E. Kuhn and Richard Blalock

Case Presentation

A 63-year-old male presented with right-shoulder pain ongoing for 4 months without a history of an injury. He noted pain laterally over his shoulder, and had pain at night, as well as pain during activity. He denied having any pain at rest. On physical examination he had very limited function with active forward elevation to 80° (Fig. 22.1), abduction to 20 (Fig. 22.2), internal rotation to his back pocket, and external rotation to 50. He was also noted to have weakness in shoulder abduction, forward flexion, and external rotation. He had positive drop-arm, Neer, and Hawkins impingement signs. He was able to elevate his arm over head while lying supine. He was also able to perform the "hand-over-fist" sign (Fig. 22.3) and the "hallelujah" sign (Fig. 22.4). His

J.E. Kuhn, M.D., M.S. (✉) • R. Blalock, M.D.
Vanderbilt University Medical Center, 3200 MCE South Tower, 1215 21st Avenue South, Nashville, TN 37205, USA
e-mail: j.kuhn@vanderbilt.edu; blalock2@gmail.com

© Springer International Publishing AG 2018

P.J. McMahon (ed.), *Rotator Cuff Injuries,*
DOI 10.1007/978-3-319-63668-9_22

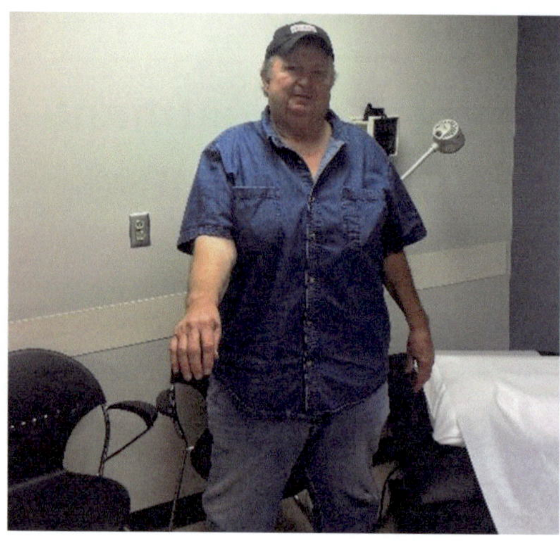

FIGURE 22.1 Clinical photograph showing the patient's forward flexion on his injured shoulder prior to physical therapy

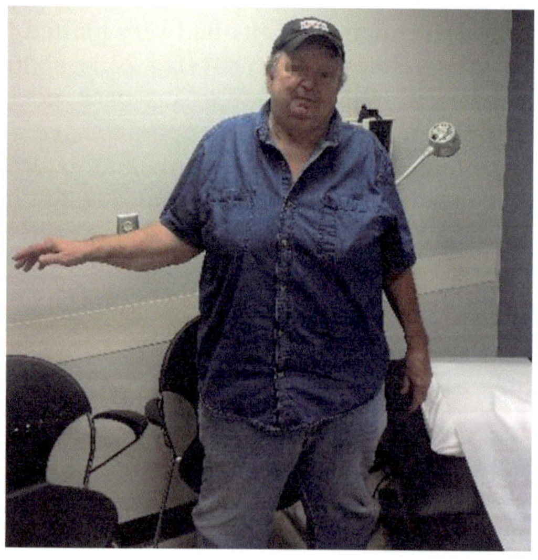

FIGURE 22.2 Clinical photograph showing the patient's shoulder abduction on his injured shoulder prior to physical therapy

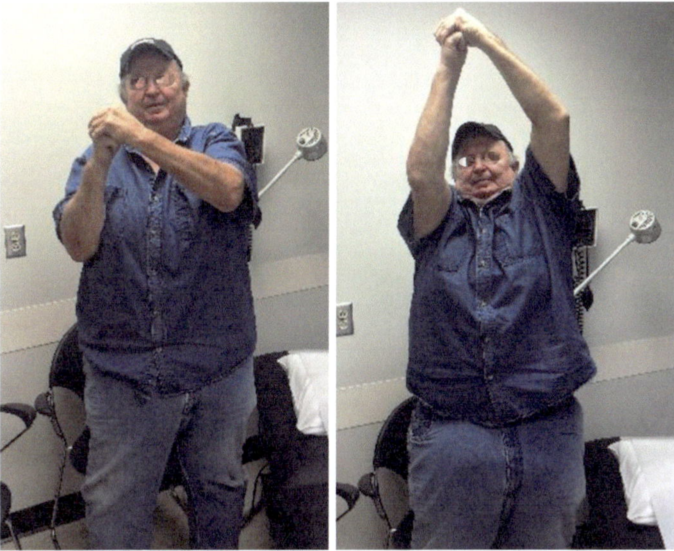

FIGURE 22.3 Clinic photographs showing the "hand-over-fist" sign

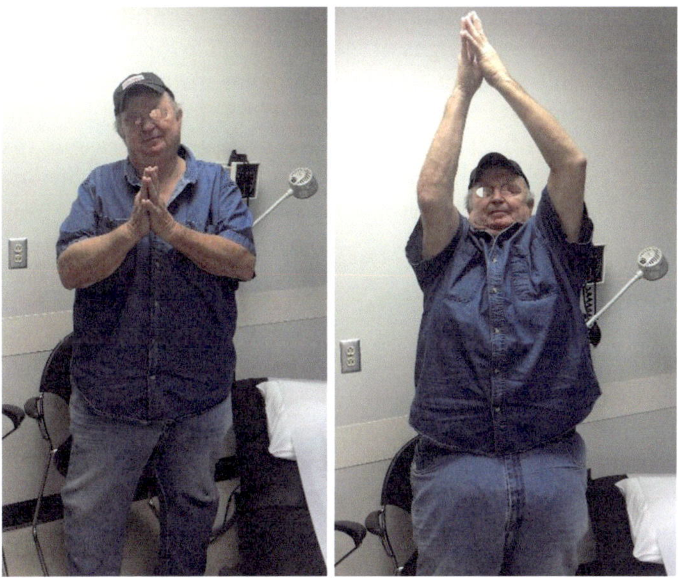

FIGURE 22.4 Clinical photographs showing the "hallelujah" sign

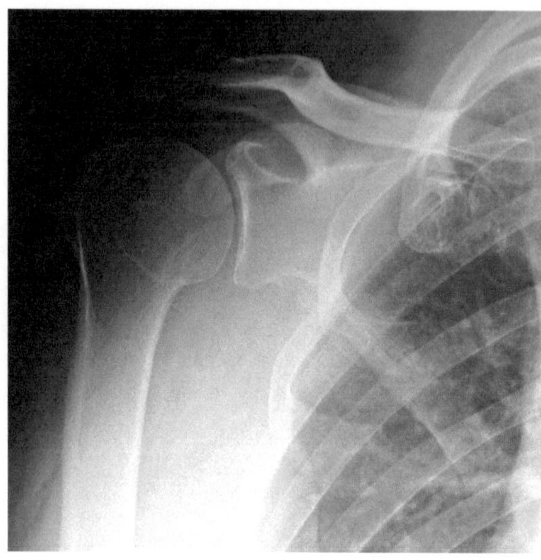

FIGURE 22.5 AP radiograph of symptomatic shoulder without signs of advanced osteoarthritis

passive range of motion was normal, but painful. His plain films showed early signs of glenohumeral arthritis; however there were no signs of a significant rotator cuff tear (Fig. 22.5). MRI showed a massive rotator cuff tear with atrophy of infraspinatus, subscapularis, and supraspinatus muscles (Fig. 22.6). He was also noted to have a chronic draining wound on his lower leg.

Diagnosis/Assessment

The patient's history, physical exam, and radiographic findings were consistent with a chronic massive rotator cuff tear. Rotator cuff tears are common and become more prevalent as patients age [1]. A systematic review of the many studies assessing prevalence of rotator cuff tears demonstrates that the prevalence of full-thickness tears in the population over 40 years is between 11.8 and 40.8% [2].

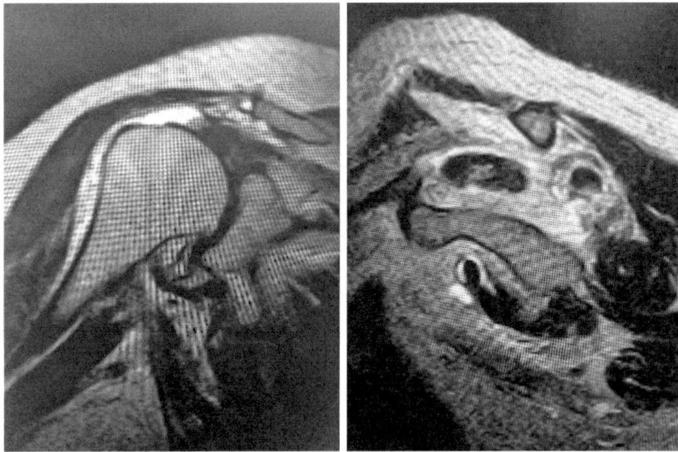

Figure 22.6 MRI of patients' symptomatic shoulder. (a) Coronal image showing full-thickness supraspinatus tear. (b) Sagittal image showing significant rotator cuff muscle atrophy

It is important to understand that not all rotator cuff tears are the same and there are marked differences among acute traumatic tears, acute-on-chronic tears, and chronic atraumatic tears. Patients with *traumatic tears* will typically present with an event that caused acute and severe pain in the shoulder with immediate loss of function. Patients with *acute-on-chronic tears* typically had a history of some mild symptoms prior to a relatively low-energy injury which exacerbated their symptoms. Their pain is significant, but seems to improve over the course of a few days. They may have lost some function, but return of function occurs over a few days. *Chronic atraumatic tears* are degenerative and are often seen in patients over 60 years old [1–3]. These classically present with insidious onset of shoulder pain with pain at night and loss of function, but typically are related to pain. These tears usually have some degree of muscle atrophy, poor tissue quality, and tendon retraction, making a rotator cuff repair less likely to heal.

Physical examination that employs lag signs can be very helpful to identify large rotator cuff tears [4]. These lag signs can be performed with the arm at the side and externally rotated, the arm held in 90 of abduction and externally rotated, and with the arm behind the back and held away from the spine. When the patient fails to hold this position when the arm is let go, it could be considered a positive test. Lag signs, a drop-arm test, or the inability to raise the arm are the ultimate expression of the weakness associated with massive rotator cuff tears. Interestingly, patients who present with chronic rotator cuff tears and are able to perform either the "hallelujah" sign or the "hand-over-fist" sign will have a high likelihood of successful treatment with physical therapy [5].

Physical examination signs are not particularly useful when patients have small rotator cuff tears [6], and combinations of physical examination tests may be more useful. Murrell et al. found that patients who demonstrated supraspinatus weakness, weakness in external rotation, and positive impingement signs had a 98% chance of having a rotator cuff tear [7]. It must be noted that patients with a rotator cuff tear can present atypically with a full range of motion and good muscle strength due to functional compensation [8]. These patients may require imaging to accurately diagnose the rotator cuff tear.

To evaluate for a suspected rotator cuff tear, multiple imaging modalities can be utilized. Plain radiographs are typically the first imaging modality obtained for shoulder pain. In reviewing plain films, if superior migration of the humeral head is noted on the AP film, a rotator cuff tear is highly suspect. This finding indicates a loss of function of the rotator cuff and appears with long-standing tears. The normal acromiohumeral distance measures from 9 to 10 mm with a range of 7 to 14 mm [9]. An acromiohumeral distance less than 7 mm is consistent with a rotator cuff tear, and a space less than 5 mm indicates a massive rotator cuff tear [10, 11]. Chronic rotator cuff arthropathies can show joint space narrowing, rounding of the greater tuberosity, acetabularization of the undersurface of the acromion, superomedial glenoid wear, and humeral head collapse [12].

Additional imaging modalities include ultrasound and magnetic resonance imaging [MRI]. Ultrasound allows quick and reliable diagnostic imaging for rotator cuff tears; however its accuracy is highly operator dependent [13]. A meta-analysis showed that the sensitivity for ultrasound can range from 66 to 92% and specificity can range from 86 to 94% depending on the size of the tear and the operator [14]. MRI allows for visualization of the tear, as well as muscle atrophy, fatty infiltration, and tendon retraction [15–17]. The sensitivity for MRI ranges from 64 to 92% and specificity ranges from 81 to 93%. MRI arthrography improves the sensitivity range to 91–95% and specificity range to 95–99% [14].

Management

The patient in the case study presented with a chronic rotator cuff tear. At his initial clinic visit he was given an intra-articular steroid injection and a physical therapy prescription specifying the MOON (Multi-center Orthopaedic Outcomes Network) massive rotator cuff tear protocol. This protocol was based on a systematic review of Level 1 studies that demonstrate effectiveness of exercise for treating rotator cuff disease [18]. This protocol was also used in a large prospective cohort study of patients with symptomatic atraumatic full-thickness rotator cuff tears, with over 75% success [19]. This protocol is available on www.moonshoulder.com.

The protocol begins with supervised physical therapy, two to three times a week with the addition of joint and soft-tissue mobilization. Patients who no longer need joint and soft-tissue mobilization and have developed proficiency with the protocol can be moved to a home-exercise program. Scapular range-of-motion exercises should include shrugs, shoulder retraction, and protraction exercises. Glenohumeral motion should start with pendulum exercises and progress to active-assisted motion and then to active motion as comfort dictates. Active assist exercises can be performed with a cane, suspended with pulleys, or simply with just the uninvolved arm. Stretching should emphasize anterior and posterior shoulder capsule stretching. Strengthening exercises should focus on the rotator cuff and scapular stabilizing muscles. Exercises should focus on internal and external rotation with the arm adducted, as well as scaption provided that the patient does not experience pain with these motions. Scapular exercises should include chair presses, push-ups with a plus, and upright rows [18].

Patients with massive rotator cuff tears and poor function are better served by the protocol described by Levy et al. [5]. This protocol starts with pendulum exercises and active-assist warm-up for the affected shoulder. Once the patient is able to elevate the affected arm in forward flexion with the assistance of the uninjured arm while supine, the patient may then start to try active arm-elevation exercises. After the patient is comfortable with lifting the affected arm alone, resistance training may be initiated using an 8 ounce can progressing to a 1 pound weight. When the patient has become comfortable doing all these exercises while laying supine the bed is then elevated 20 and the steps are repeated until the patient is able to perform all exercises upright.

Importantly, this protocol also calls for strengthening the muscles surrounding the glenohumeral joint, including the deltoid and periscapular muscles. The deltoid muscle is strengthened using resisted exercises involving three motions: shoulder extension, abduction, and forward punches. Lastly, strengthening the periscapular muscles is important so as to control the glenoid during shoulder motion to maximize shoulder function. The two primary exercises the protocol utilizes for periscapular strengthening include serratus punch exercises and upright rows. The serratus punch is performed with the patient lying supine, holding the affected arm at 90 with elbow extended, and then bringing the scapula around the side of the chest wall to "punch" the ceiling, emphasizing scapular protraction. The other exercise is upright rows emphasizing shoulder retraction. The patient is seated in an upright position and then squeezes his shoulder blades together holding for 2 s. Both of these exercises are started with no resistance and then progressed using Theraband resistance bands [5].

Outcome

This 63-year-old male underwent a total of 12 weeks of physical therapy. On the patients' 6-week follow-up he was able to forward elevate his arm to 140 and his pain had improved by 50%; however, external rotation was still limited to 50 and he still had shoulder weakness with abduction and external rotation. With a positive response in symptoms and motion, therapy was continued for another 6 weeks.

After 12 weeks of physical therapy he subjectively felt 80% better in regard to his pain and function. His shoulder forward elevation as well as abduction had improved to 180 (Fig. 22.7). His external rotation was improved to

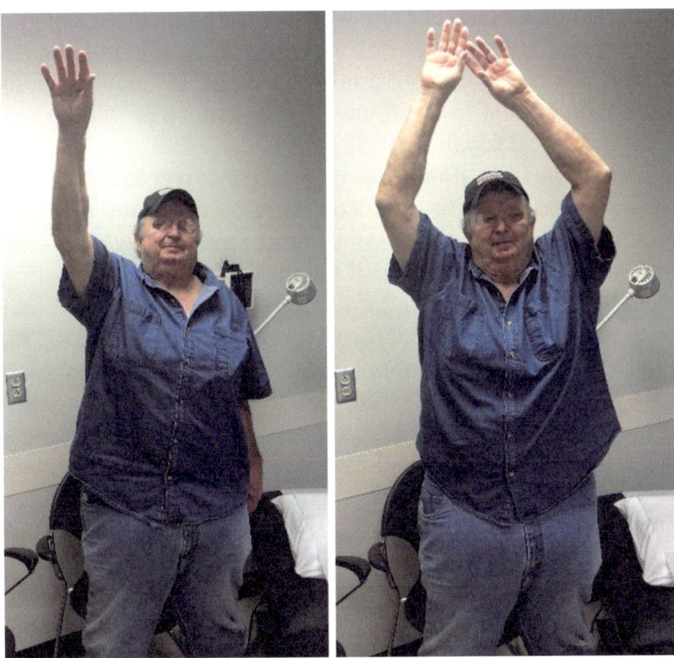

FIGURE 22.7 Clinical photograph showing the patients' range of motion 12 weeks after the physical therapy program. (**a**) Right-shoulder forward flexion active motion. (**b**) Right-shoulder abduction active motion

70 and internal rotation to L3. He still had weakness in external rotation and abduction; however he was very satisfied with his results.

Literature Review

The indications for surgery for rotator cuff tears are not well defined and there is no consensus on who should have surgery. This is demonstrated by the large geographic variation in rotator cuff repair rates [20], and by the great variation in approaches to the same patient as demonstrated by surveys of surgeons [21]. Systematic reviews of the literature demonstrate a paucity of high-level studies, but using the best evidence available (Level 3 and 4), it seems that acute traumatic rotator cuff tears do better if repaired early, age and gender should not affect the decision to have surgery, and strength and/or functional loss will have better outcomes with a successful surgical repair [22, 23].

Pain as an indication for surgery is controversial. The rotator cuff tear severity does not seem to correlate with the patient's pain, duration of symptoms, or activity level [24–26]. Patient-reported outcomes of failed rotator cuff repair using validated patient-reported outcomes are typically good and cannot be distinguished from successful repairs [27, 28]. Physical therapy for atraumatic tears is successful in over 75% of patients [19, 29, 30]. Finally, while natural history studies of rotator cuff tears demonstrate that some patients will have progression and these patients will statistically have more pain, patients can have progression without pain, or may develop pain without progression making pain a relatively poor predictor of rotator cuff tear progression [31].

Weakness and functional loss may be better indications for surgery than pain. The literature supports this concept, particularly with regard to weakness, where exercise therapy may improve function, but not necessarily strength [32, 33], and in patients in whom rotator cuff repairs have failed, they generally report good pain relief, but are found to be weaker than those whose repairs heal [27, 28]. In summary, indications for surgery should include acute tears, acute on chronic tears with loss of function, and chronic tears with weakness or loss of function. Pain in a patient with a chronic, atraumatic tear may not be a strong indication for surgery and nonoperative treatment should be employed.

Multiple small case series have demonstrated that nonoperative treatment can be helpful in patients. These case series are promising although limited, as they are retrospective in design, subject to selection bias, including only patients with massive rotator cuff tears, or systemic illness in which surgery cannot be performed [34–37].

Several prospective studies looking at success rates of nonoperative treatment of rotator cuff tears have also been performed. One prospective cohort included 103 shoulders with rotator cuff tears treated without surgery. This study showed lasting pain relief up to 13 years after diagnosis, and 72% of patients had no disturbance in activities of daily living [38]. A second prospective study enrolled all patients with atraumatic rotator cuff tears into a physical therapy program [19]. The study enrolled 422 patients and followed them for more than 2 years. After 12 weeks of physical therapy, 15% of patients had opted to undergo surgery. After 2 years only an additional 11% of patients in the cohort had undergone surgery for their rotator cuff tears. This study suggests that 74% of patients with atraumatic rotator cuff tears can be successfully treated with physical therapy. All of the patient-reported outcomes showed improvement at 6 and 12 weeks in those patients who were treated nonoperatively, and most patients who elected to undergo surgery did so in the first 12 weeks of treatment [19]. Of interest, failure or success of nonoperative treatment was predicted strongly by the patient's expectations of treatment [39]. If the patient *believed* that the therapy program would work it would; patients who did not have confidence in the effect of exercise would fail. The failure had no relationship to the anatomy of the rotator cuff [18].

It is reasonable to consider prevention of tear progression as an indication for surgical repair of rotator cuff tears. It is known that some rotator cuff tears progress in size, and these patients are statistically more likely going to develop symptoms [31, 40, 41]. However, one cannot effectively use pain as a predictor of rotator cuff tear enlargement as some tears progress without pain, and some patients develop pain without progression [31]. We do know that older patients with larger tears are less likely to heal their degenerative rotator cuff tears, and therefore one might surmise that surgical repair for younger patients with smaller tears might prevent rotator cuff tear progression. There is some data to suggest that repair might delay the muscle changes associated with tear progression [42]. Alternatively, one could argue that younger patients with degenerative rotator cuff disease may have a genetic predisposition toward rotator cuff tears, and that surgical repair may only delay the inevitable rotator cuff failure [43]. Clearly we need better natural history studies to identify who would benefit best from surgical repair of their rotator cuff tear.

Clinical Pearls/Pitfalls

- Weakness or functional loss is an indication for surgery. Pain is not as clear and may not relate to the presence of the rotator cuff tear.
- Exercise therapy is an effective treatment for chronic rotator cuff tears.
- Patients who do not respond to physical therapy will typically withdraw themselves in the first 12 weeks of therapy.
- Physical therapy is effective in improving pain and dysfunction, but not necessarily strength.
- Physical therapy should emphasize glenohumeral and scapular range of motion, along with rotator cuff and periscapular muscle strengthening.
- Patient expectations drive the outcome. If a patient does not believe that exercise will be effective, he or she will likely fail nonoperative treatment.

References

1. Teunis T, Lubberts B, Reilly BT, Ring D. A systematic review and pooled analysis of the prevalence of rotator cuff disease with increasing age. J Bone Joint Surg Am. 2014;23(12):1913–21. doi:10.1016/j.jse.2014.08.001.
2. Reilly P, McLeod I, MacFarlane R, Windley J, Emery RJH. Dead men and radiologists don't lie: a review of cadaveric and radiological studies of rotator cuff tear prevalence. Ann R Coll Surg Engl. 2006;88:116–21.
3. Norwood LA, Barrack R, Jacobson KE. Clinical presentation of complete tears of the rotator cuff. J Bone Joint Surg. 1989;71(4):499–505.
4. Hertel R, Ballmer FT, Lombert SM, et al. Lag signs in the diagnosis of rotator cuff rupture. J Shoulder Elb Surg. 1996;5:307–13.
5. Levy O, Mullett H, Roberts S, Copeland S. The role of anterior deltoid reeducation in patients with massive irreparable degenerative rotator cuff tears. J Shoulder Elb Surg. 2008;17(6):863–70.
6. Hegedus EJ, Goode A, Campbell S, Morin A, Tamaddoni M, Moorman CT III, Cook C. Physical examination tests of the shoulder: a systematic review with meta-analysis of individual tests. Br J Sports Med. 2008;42:80–92.
7. Murrell GA, Walton JR. Diagnosis of rotator cuff tears. Lancet. 2001;357(9258):769–70.
8. Neviaser JS. Ruptures of the rotator cuff of the shoulder. Arch Surg. 1971;102(5):483–5.
9. Petersson CJ, Redlund-Johnell I. The subacromial space in normal shoulder radiographs. Acta Orthop Scand. 1984;55(1):57–8.
10. Cotton RE, Rideout DF. Tears of the humeral rotator cuff; a radiological and pathological necropsy survey. J Bone Joint Surg Br. 1964;46:314–28.
11. Neer CS. Impingement lesions. Clin Orthop Relat Res. 1983;173:70–7.
12. Hamada K, Fukuda H, Mikasa M, Kobayashi Y. Roentgenographic findings in massive rotator cuff tears. A long-term observation. Clin Orthop Relat Res. 1990;254:92–6.
13. Teefey SA, Hasan SA, Middleton WD, Patel M, Wright RW, Yamaguchi K. Ultrasonography of the rotator cuff. A comparison of ultrasonographic and arthroscopic findings in one hundred consecutive cases. J Bone Joint Surg. 2000;82(4):498–504.
14. De Jesus JO, Parker L, Frangos AJ, Nazarian LN. Accuracy of MRI, MR arthrography, and ultrasound in the diagnosis

of rotator cuff tears: a meta-analysis. Am J Roentgenol. 2009;192(6):1701–7.

15. Thomazeau H, Rolland Y, Lucas C, Duval J-M, Langlais F. Atrophy of the supraspinatus belly Assessment by MRI in 55 patients with rotator cuff pathology. Acta Orthop Scand. 1996;67(3):264–8.

16. Patte D. Classification of rotator cuff lesions. Clin Orthop Relat Res. 1990;254:81–6.

17. Fuchs B, Weishaupt D, Zanetti M, Hodler J, Gerber C. Fatty degeneration of the muscles of the rotator cuff: assessment by computed tomography versus magnetic resonance imaging. J Shoulder Elb Surg. 1999;8(6):599–605.

18. Kuhn JE. Exercise in the treatment of rotator cuff impingement: a systematic review and a synthesized evidence-based rehabilitation protocol. J Shoulder Elb Surg. 2009;18(1):138–60.

19. Kuhn JE, Dunn WR, Sanders R, An Q, Baumgarten KM, Bishop JY, et al. Effectiveness of physical therapy in treating atraumatic full-thickness rotator cuff tears: a multicenter prospective cohort study. J Shoulder Elb Surg. 2013;22(10):1371–9.

20. Vitale MG, Krant JJ, Gelijns AC, Heitjan DF, Arons RR, Bigliani LU, et al. Geographic variations in the rates of operative procedures involving the shoulder, including total shoulder replacement, humeral head replacement, and rotator cuff repair. J Bone Joint Surg Am. 1999;81:763–72.

21. Dunn WR, Schackman BR, Walsh C, Lyman S, Jones EC, Warren RF, et al. Variation in orthopaedic surgeons' perceptions about the indications for rotator cuff surgery. J Bone Joint Surg Am. 2005;87:1978–84. doi:10.2106/jbjs.d.02944.

22. Wolf BR, Dunn WR, Wright RW. Indications for repair of full thickness rotator cuff tears. Am J Sports Med. 2007;35:1007–16. doi:10.1177/0363546506295079.

23. Oh LS, Wolf BR, Hall MP, Levy BA, Marx RG. Indications for rotator cuff repair: a systematic review. Clin Orthop Relat Res. 2007;455:52–63. doi:10.1097/BLO.0b013e31802fc175.

24. Dunn WR, Kuhn JE, Sanders R, Baumgarten KM, Bishop JY, Brophy RH, Carey JL, Holloway BG, Jones GL, Ma CB, Marx RG, McCarty EC, Poddar SK, Smith MV, Spencer EE, Vidal AF, Wolf BR, Wright RW. Symptoms of pain do not correlate with rotator cuff tear severity. A cross sectional study of 393 patients with symptomatic atraumatic full thickness rotator cuff tears. J Bone Joint Surg. 2014;96(10):793–800.

25. Unruh KP, Kuhn JE, Sanders R, An Q, Baumgarten KM, Bishop JY, Brophy RH, Carey JL, Holloway BG, Jones GL, Ma BC, Marx RG, McCarty E, Poddar SK, Smith MV, Spencer EE, Vidal AF, Wolf BR, Wright RW, Dunn WR. The duration of symptoms does not correlate with rotator cuff tear severity or other patient related features. A cross sectional study of patients with atraumatic, full thickness rotator cuff tears. J Shoulder Elb Surg. 2014;23(13):1052–8.
26. Brophy RH, Dunn WR, Kuhn JE, Sanders R, Baumgarten KM, Bishop JY, Carey JL, Holloway BG, Jones GL, Ma CB, Marx RG, McCarty EC, Poddar SK, Smith MV, Spencer EE, Vidal AF, Wolf BR, Wright RW. Shoulder activity is not associated with the severity of symptomatic, atraumatic rotator cuff tears on MRI. Am J Sports Med. 2014;42(5):1150–4.
27. Slabaugh MA, Nho SJ, Grumet RC, Wilson JB, Seroyer ST, Frank RM, et al. Does the literature confirm superior clinical results in radiographically healed rotator cuffs after rotator cuff repair? Arthroscopy. 2010;26(3):393–403.
28. Russell RD, Knight JR, Mulligan E, Khazzam MS. Structural integrity after rotator cuff repair does not correlate with patient function and pain: a meta-analysis. J Bone Joint Surg. 2014;96-A(4):265–71.
29. Moosmayer S, Lund G, Seljom US, Haldorsen B, Svege IC, Hennig T, Pripp AH, Smith HJ. Tendon repair compared with physiotherapy in the treatment of rotator cuff tears: a randomized controlled study in 103 cases with a five-year follow-up. J Bone Joint Surg Am. 2014;96(18):1504–14.
30. Kukkonen J, Joukainen A, Lehtinen J, Mattila KT, Tuominen EKJ, Kauko T, et al. Treatment of non-traumatic rotator cuff tears. A randomized controlled trial with one-year clinical results. Bone Joint J. 2014;96-B(1):75–81.
31. Keener JD, Galatz LM, Teefey SA, Middleton WD, Steger-May K, Stobbs-Cucchi G, Patton R, Yamaguchi K. A prospective evaluation of survivorship of asymptomatic degenerative rotator cuff tears. J Bone Joint Surg Am. 2015;97(2):89–98. doi:10.2106/JBJS.N.00099. PMID: 25609434
32. Bang MD, Deyle GD. Comparison of supervised exercise with and without manual physical therapy for patients with shoulder impingement syndrome. J Orthop Sports Phys Ther. 2000;30(3):126–37.
33. Haahr JP. Exercises versus arthroscopic decompression in patients with subacromial impingement: a randomized,

controlled study in 90 cases with a one year follow up. Ann Rheum Dis. 2005;64(5):760–4.

34. Ainsworth R, Lewis JS. Exercise therapy for the conservative management of full thickness tears of the rotator cuff: a systematic review. Br J Sports Med. 2007;41(4):200–10.

35. Goldberg BA, Nowinski RJ, Matsen FA. Outcome of nonoperative management of full-thickness rotator cuff tears. Clin Orthop Relat Res. 2001;382:99–107.

36. Koubaa S, Ben Salah FZ, Lebib S, et al. Conservative management of full thickness rotator cuff tears. A prospective study of 24 patients. Ann Readapt Med Phys. 2006;49(2):62–7.

37. Yamada N, Hamada K, Nakajima T, Kobayashi K, Fukuda H. Comparison of conservative and operative treatments of massive rotator cuff tears. Tokai J Exp Clin Med. 2000;25(4):151–63.

38. Kijima H, Minagawa H, Nishi T, Kikuchi K, Shimada Y. Long-term follow-up of cases of rotator cuff tear treated conservatively. J Shoulder Elb Surg. 2012;21(4):491–4.

39. Dunn WR, Kuhn JE, Sanders R, An Q, Baumgarten KM, Bishop JY, Brophy RH, Carey JL, Holloway BG, Jones GL, Ma CB, Marx RG, McCarty EC, Poddar SK, Smith MV, Spencer EE, Vidal AF, Wolf BR, Wright RW. 2013 Neer Award: predictors of failure of nonoperative treatment of chronic, symptomatic, full-thickness rotator cuff tears. J Shoulder Elb Surg. 2016;25(8):1303–11. doi:10.1016/j.jse.2016.04.030. PMID: 27422460

40. Moosmayer S, Tariq R, Stiris M, Smith HJ. The natural history of asymptomatic rotator cuff tears: a three-year follow-up of fifty cases. J Bone Joint Surg Am. 2013;95(14):1249–55.

41. Mall NA, Kim HM, Keener JD, et al. Symptomatic progression of asymptomatic rotator cuff tears: a prospective study of clinical and sonographic variables. J Bone Joint Surg Am. 2010;92(16):2623–33.

42. Fabbri M, Ciompi A, Lanzetti RM, Vadalà A, Lupariello D, Iorio C, Serlorenzi P, Argento G, Ferretti A, De Carli A. Muscle atrophy and fatty infiltration in rotator cuff tears: can surgery stop muscular degenerative changes? J Orthop Sci. 2016;21(5):614–8.

43. Kuhn JE. Are atraumatic rotator cuff tears painful? A model to describe the relationship between pain and rotator cuff tears. Minerva Orthop Traumatol. 2015;66(Suppl 1):51–61.

Index

© Springer International Publishing AG 2018   357
P.J. McMahon (ed.), *Rotator Cuff Injuries*,
DOI 10.1007/978-3-319-63668-9

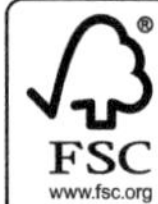